Stress and the Heart

Psychosocial pathways to coronary heart disease

Stress and the Heart
Psychosocial pathways to coronary heart disease

Edited by

Stephen Stansfeld

Department of Psychiatry, Queen Mary, University of London, London

and

Michael Marmot

Department of Epidemiology and Public Health, Royal Free and University College London, London

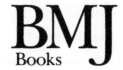

BMJ Books is an imprint of the BMJ publishing Group

First published in 2002
by BMJ Books, BMA House, Tavistock Square,
London WC1H 9JR

www.bmjbooks.com

British Library Cataloguing in Publication Data
A catalogue record for this book is available from the British Library

ISBN 0-7279-1277-1

Typeset by Newgen Imaging Systems Pvt. Ltd., Chennai, India

Printed and bound in Spain by GraphyCems, Navarra

Contents

Contributors

Mel Bartley
International Centre for Health and Society, University College London,
London, UK

Yoav Ben-Shlomo
Department of Social Medicine, Bristol, UK

Lisa Berkman
Harvard School of Public Health, Boston, USA

Eric Brunner
International Centre for Health and Society, Department of
Epidemiology and Public Health, University College London,
London, UK

Kamaldeep Bhui
Barts and the London, Queen Mary's School of Medicine and Dentistry,
Queen Mary, University of London, London, UK

Matthew Burg
Harvard School of Public Health, Boston, USA

George Davey Smith
Department of Social Medicine, University of Bristol, UK

Rebecca Fuhrer
Department of Epidemiology and Public Health,
University College London, London, UK

E Leigh Gibson
ICRF Health Behaviour Unit, Department of Epidemiology and Public
Health, University College London, London, UK

Harry Hemingway
International Centre for Health and Society, Department of
Epidemiology and Public Health, University College London, London
and Director of Research and Development, Department of Research and
Development, Kensington & Chelsea and Westminster Health Authority,
London, UK

Steve Humphries
Centre for Cardiovascular Genetics, British Heart Foundation
Laboratories, The Rayne Building, Royal Free and University College
London Medical School, London, UK

Martin Jarvis
ICRF Health Behaviour Unit, Department of Epidemiology and Public
Health, University College London, London, UK

John Lynch
Department of Epidemiology,
University of Michigan, Ann Arbor, MI, USA

Michael Marmot
International Centre for Health and Society,
University College London, London, UK

Hugh Montgomery
Senior Lecturer, Centre for Cardiovascular Genetics, British Heart
Foundation Laboratories, The Rayne Building, Royal Free and University
College London Medical School, London, UK

Johannes Siegrist
Institute of Medical Sociology, Medical Faculty,
University of Düsseldorf, Düsseldorf, Germany

Stephen Stansfeld
Barts and the London, Queen Mary's School of Medicine and Dentistry,
Queen Mary, University of London, London, UK

Andrew Steptoe
Department of Epidemiology and Public Health, University College
London, London, UK

Tores Theorell
National Institute for Psychosocial Factors and Health,
Stockholm, Sweden

Jane Wardle
ICRF Health Behaviour Unit, Department of Epidemiology and Public
Health, University College London, London, UK

Gonneke Willemsen
Department of Psychology, Free University,
Amsterdam, The Netherlands

Redford Williams
Professor of Psychiatry and Behavioral Sciences, Professor of Psychology,
Professor of Medicine, Co-Director, Center for Integrative Medicine, and
Director, Behavioral Medicine Research Center, Duke University Medical
Center, Durham, USA

Foreword

There was a time early in the last century when almost all of the research then being done on psychosocial factors and disease centred around the concept of "stress". This work was dealt a deadly blow in 1976 when the most prominent researcher in the field at that time, Professor John Cassel, gave a devastating critique of the concept in the last paper he wrote before he died.[1] In that paper, he suggested that as soon as one discusses the role of psychosocial factors in disease aetiology, one inevitably thinks about stress and disease. He said, "I think the simple-minded invocation of the word stress in such thinking has done as much to retard research in this area as did the concept of the miasmas at the time of the discovery of microorganisms." Cassel was concerned that the concept of stress was being uncritically used by researchers as if it were capable of having a direct pathogenic effect, analogous to that of a physicochemical or microbiological disease agent, while all the evidence available at that time suggested that this was not the case. As a consequence, most of us working in this area of research studiously avoided using the term. And now, 25 years later, we have a book entitled *Stress and the Heart: Psychosocial Pathways to Coronary Heart Disease*.

I was at first shocked to see so boldly and recklessly flaunted this forbidden word. After examining the contents of the chapters in this book, however, I began to see that the idea of stress is being used here in the most useful way: as a sensitising concept. It alerts us to a range of psychosocial factors that influence health and disease either indirectly, by influencing risk behaviour, or directly, by affecting neuroendocrine or immune functioning. This is an approach that John Cassel would have appreciated and endorsed.

As a person who has struggled in this field for over forty years, I am truly impressed by the progress that has been made during this time. Perhaps the clearest way to convey this message is to contrast the contents of this book with one published in 1967, *Social Stress and Cardiovascular Disease*.[2] That book was a report of a conference to which were invited all the US researchers working at that time in the new field of psychosocial factors and heart disease. Among the 27 attenders were Sol Levine, David Jenkins, Bruce Dohrenwend, Saxon Graham, Adrian Ostfeld, Norman Scotch and, of course, John Cassel, who perhaps after listening to the proceedings for three days, first developed his criticism of the concept of stress.

The state of the art in 1967 consisted of three categories of findings. The first category focused on the study of rapid changes among groups of people and on the challenges people faced adapting to such changes. The second category of finding dealt with research on social and demographic factors with particular emphasis on income, and occupational and educational status. The third was concerned with psychological and interpersonal factors (including type A behaviour, the most prominent psychosocial risk factor at that time). Very few of the findings and conclusions from that conference have survived to the present day (except, of course, the fact that people lower in social class still have higher rates of disease—an observation that has been with us since the beginning of recorded history). However, that conference did serve several important purposes: it provided for the first time recognition that this field of research did in fact exist; it stimulated subsequent longterm research collaborations among the attendees; it emphasised the serious gaps and inconsistencies in the findings then available; and finally, it encouraged the attenders to think hard about needed new research.

It is stunning to review the progress that has been made in this field some thirty years later. Today, the major issues include a far more specific and broad set of topics including inequalities, social class, work, social support, hostility, and, most importantly, considerations of biological mechanisms that link these psychosocial factors to disease. And while gaps in knowledge and inconsistencies in findings continue to exist, they now, instead of leading to despair and frustration, lead to new hypotheses and concepts.

The work in this field is not merely interesting. We are all aware of the burden that is imposed on society by attempting to provide high quality and timely medical care to all those in need. As populations all over the world continue to live longer, this burden will increase enormously. Clearly, we must do a better job of preventing disease. Some progress in this will be achieved as we continue to understand the genetic basis of health; but the impressive advances in genome research will not help in reducing massive income inequalities in the world, or relieve discrimination, or help in providing social support to those who are isolated. To address these issues, we will need to better understand the importance of specified social and psychological factors and how they affect bodily functioning. This knowledge may help in the development of intervention efforts to prevent disease, not only among individuals, but in society as well. This is a huge task, but the disease challenges we face are also huge. This book represents an important and impressive contribution to the effort.

S LEONARD SYME
Professor of Epidemiology
University of California, Berkeley

References

1 Cassel J. The contribution of the social environment to host resistance. *Am J Epidemiol* 1976;**104**:107–23.
2 Syme SL, Reeder LG, eds. Social Stress and Cardiovascular Disease. *Milbank Mem Fund Q* 1967;**45**:175–80.

1: Introduction

STEPHEN STANSFELD AND MICHAEL MARMOT

There has been discordance between the hard science and the lay views of heart disease causation. The hard science view, to the degree that it embraced epidemiology and prevention, acknowledged the vital importance of smoking and other risk factors for heart disease. The role of cholesterol had to wait for the advent of lipid lowering drugs before it was accepted by cardiologists. The lay view, endorsed by many clinicians, acknowledged stress as a dominant cause of coronary heart disease.

For many years, small groups of scientists have been working hard to produce the evidence base needed for the acceptance or rejection of the importance of stress. Their intellectual forebears were Osler, Selye, and others: Osler, as an astute clinician, recognised the type of personality and behaviour he saw in his coronary patients;[1] Selye made the biological study of stress both respectable and plausible.[2]

There have been significant advances in this field of endeavour, the discussion of which has been largely confined to those with a specialised interest in this research. It is our view, and indeed that of the *British Medical Journal*, who commissioned this volume, that the research has now accumulated an evidence base that means it should be part of wider discussion of causation, prevention and treatment of coronary heart disease. The aim of this book, therefore, is to provide an overview of the topic for a wider audience.

We are not so bold as to pretend that this is the first time an attempt has been made to present psychosocial factors in a serious way to the wider scientific community. There have been many, with varying degrees of success. Yet there appears to be resistance to its acceptance. If that resistance relates to mind–body dualism, to a scepticism that mental processes could have an effect on physiology sufficiently profound to cause myocardial infarction, then this book will have little success in changing minds. Our hope is that if the resistance comes from a view that the evidence on stress is at best patchy, then this book might indeed have some success by presenting a view of the substantial evidence that has accumulated on this subject.

Stress and psychosocial factors

In the early days of research, the issue of what constituted stress threatened to create an intellectual tower of Babel. To the outside critic, what was stress for one person was stimulus and challenge to another. The concept of stress was close to indefinable, in which case it could not be measured—and without measurement, scientific progress was impossible. Researchers were split into those who defined stress, as an engineer might, as an external force applied to the organism; and those following Selye, who conceived of it as the reaction of the organism to the external load. In passing, it is worth mentioning that the concept of allostatic load might be far more useful for this latter view of stress.[3]

Recognising that this split adds further to difficulties of definition and measurement, it is no surprise that many of us working in this field do not find it necessary to use the word "stress". To put it more strongly, we avoid it. We have come to use the umbrella term "psychosocial" to denote psychological processes linked to the social environment, but use more specific concepts and measurements. These are represented in the chapters in this book. "Stress" is retained in the title of the book for its value in orienting the potential reader. It makes little appearance subsequently. In fact, we gave no specific instruction to the authors as to their use of the word "stress".

One model of how psychosocial factors might be causally involved in coronary heart disease

Len Syme used always to pose the challenge that we needed to understand how psychosocial factors got "under the skin". An important part of the research endeavour is to go further, and trace causation from social and psychosocial processes through behaviour and biology to disease. One simple model that we have been using to guide our research is presented in Figure 1.1. It is important to note that psychosocial factors may act by influencing behaviours such as smoking, eating, and drinking. Three chapters of this book deal explicitly with the determinants of eating, smoking, and physical activity. The other type of pathway is that more usually thought of under the rubric "stress". Psychosocial factors may influence psychological processes that may have direct effects on the neuroendocrine and immune systems. Four of the chapters deal with the types of biological pathways that are represented as something of a "black box" in Figure 1.1. The figure also acknowledges that these processes will act on a genetic substrate, and this theme is dealt with in Chapter 15.

One factor or many?

Much of the book reviews the evidence on specific psychosocial factors. There are separate strands of the scientific literature devoted to each of these. Redford Williams, a few years ago, wrote a thoughtful piece entitled, "What if we rounded up the usual suspects and they all belonged to the same gang?" His question was whether, in the end, each of these psychosocial factors was a different way of addressing the balance between

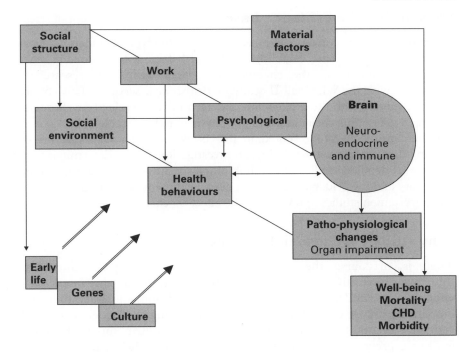

Figure 1.1 Potential psychological pathways to coronary heart disease.

the individual's resources and the challenges faced.[4] Whether there turns out to be one final common pathway or several more specific pathways is not altogether clear. It has been proposed that one type of psychosocial factor is related to the sympathoadrenomedullary axis, and a different type is related to the hypothalamic–pituitary–adrenocortical axis.

At this stage of our knowledge we can say that some of the factors represented in this book have independent effects on coronary heart disease risk. Social support, for example, seems to be independent of work characteristics in predicting coronary heart disease. This area has, however, been insufficiently explored and will clearly be the next stage of research. These factors may interact and there may be a limited number of biological pathways by which they act.

One important specific type of interaction is that between factors acting at various points in the life course. Two streams of work have pointed to the origins of coronary heart disease early in life. In the atherosclerosis literature, the findings of evidence of atherosclerosis in young soldiers killed in war alerted people to the early origins of coronary disease. A second stream comes from the work of Barker and others showing that characteristics of newborn infants, related to influences acting in utero, affect subsequent development of risk of coronary heart disease and diabetes.[5] The third chapter in this book draws on a further developing theme: that social factors may act through the life course to affect coronary heart disease risk.

3

Developing the evidence base

Much of the advance in this field has come from the type of epidemiological cohort studies that have established other risk factors for coronary heart disease. A number of the chapters have been written by researchers connected with the Whitehall II study of British civil servants. This cohort study was set up with the explicit aim of determining the role of psychosocial factors in generating social gradients in physical and mental health.

Other approaches represented in this book are secondary analyses of existing data sets, social psychological investigations of the determinants of behaviour, detailed studies of psychobiological pathways in the psychology laboratory and the field, biochemical studies of gene–environment interactions, and intervention studies to investigate the effect on changing disease risk.

Why study psychosocial factors?

There is, of course, the bigger question—why bother? Our answer is threefold. First, this research has been important in the intellectual endeavour to understand how the psyche and soma interact to cause human disease. It offers the prospect of improving the understanding of aetiology. Second, the overall aim of most of the contributors to this book is disease prevention and health promotion. Knowledge of both types of pathway is important here, i.e. the psychosocial determinants of health behaviours such as smoking and diet, and the psychosocial processes that affect disease more directly. Knowledge that social supports or aspects of the psychosocial work environment increase disease risk may well be the basis for programmes to reduce this risk.

The third reason is treatment. Understanding people's social and psychological state has always been important to the good clinician. The scientific information reviewed here bolsters this approach.

The signs are now encouraging that plans to reduce the burden of coronary heart disease in society are leading to serious consideration of the social determinants of health. Psychosocial factors have an important part to play.

References

1   Osler W. The Lumleian Lectures on angina pectoris. *Lancet* 1892;**i**:829–44.
2   Selye H. *The stress of life*. New York: McGraw-Hill, 1956.
3   McEwen BS. Protective and damaging effects of stress mediators. *N Engl J Med* 1998;**338**:171–9.
4   Williams RB, Barefoot JC, Blumenthal JA et al. Psychosocial correlates of job strain in a sample of working women. Arch Gen Psychiatry 1997;**54**:543–8.
5   Barker DJP. *Fetal and infant origins of adult disease*. London: BMJ Books, 1992.

2: Social class and coronary heart disease

MICHAEL MARMOT AND MEL BARTLEY

One of the most common ways in which studies present the relationship between psychosocial factors such as stress and coronary heart disease is by means of its social distribution. This often takes the form of showing different rates of coronary heart disease in different social classes. Social class is a contested concept: there are longstanding debates as to how best to define and measure it.[1-3] The practice of referring to "higher" and "lower" social classes implies that class is a measure of social rank or status, and that it is the stress of low levels of general standing in the community that may constitute a coronary risk. Other studies using only income or education as a marker of socioeconomic position have, however, found equally powerful relationships of these variables to disease.[4-6] This makes it all the more striking that studies from different times and places have consistently shown similar gradients in coronary heart disease risk: lowest in the social groups with greatest advantage, and highest in the most disadvantaged groups.

Changes in the distribution of coronary heart disease

It is worth reviewing the changing distribution of coronary heart disease internationally to put into context the possible contribution of work stress to the development of ill health and disease. There have been two major changes in the epidemiology of coronary heart disease over recent years: shifts in the social class distribution of the disease,[7] and its rise and fall in different countries.[8] In many European countries, as in the USA, as coronary heart disease became a mass disease, it rose first in higher socioeconomic groups and subsequently in lower socioeconomic groups, to the extent that the social distribution changed to the now familiar pattern of an inverse social gradient: higher rates as the social hierarchy is descended. More recently, the decline in coronary heart disease mortality both in the United Kingdom and the USA has been enjoyed to a greater extent by higher socioeconomic groups, leading to a widening of the social gap.[9] Concerns that the predominance of coronary heart disease in higher socioeconomic groups may relate to the stress of their occupations go back at least to Osler,[10] who wrote that work and worry were major causes of the disease (see Chapter 4). The fact that coronary heart disease is now more common in lower socioeconomic groups does not, by itself, refute the potential importance of work "stress". Research has moved on from the simplistic notion that high responsibility or dealing with multiple tasks represents work stress.

At a time when cardiovascular mortality has been declining in North America, Australia, and many countries of western Europe, it has been on the rise in the countries of central and eastern Europe and in the newly independent states of the former Soviet Union. Of the 6 year life expectancy gap between eastern and western Europe, more than half is due to cardiovascular disease, especially to coronary heart disease. This gap in life expectancy grew from around the late 1960s to the present,[11] corresponding to the time when cardiovascular disease was on the rise in the east and declining in the west. The concepts and data reviewed in this chapter may provide some reasons for the inverse social gradient in cardiovascular disease in the west and rising mortality in the east.

Explanations of the social distribution of coronary heart disease

There is now a widely validated body of knowledge on risk factors for coronary heart disease relating to development of atherosclerosis, and a somewhat less secure body of knowledge relating to predisposition to thrombosis. The major risk factors are high levels of blood pressure, plasma total cholesterol concentration, and smoking. Although smoking, in particular, shows a strong social gradient,[12] these risk factors account for no more than a third of the social gradient in cardiovascular disease.[13] Similarly, smoking is high in many countries of central and eastern Europe and may relate to the high rates of cardiovascular disease,[11] but data from the international MONICA studies (the World Health Organization project to MONITOR trends in Cardiovascular diseases) show that international variations in smoking, high blood pressure, and raised plasma cholesterol levels account for less than half of the international variation in coronary heart disease mortality rates.[14]

We are left then with two types of question. First, what accounts for the social and international variation in unhealthy behaviours such as atherogenic diet, smoking, and sedentary lifestyle? Second, given that these factors appear to be inadequate explanations of social and international variations in cardiovascular mortality, what else could account for the observed differences? We have argued elsewhere that one must look for explanations in the nature of social and economic organisation of societies.[15] One way in which the relationships between health and social organisation are often studied is by investigating differences in health and health related behaviours in groups with different levels of prestige, material advantage and disadvantage, and different relationships to the structure of employment. In the UK, these forms of social variation in health are often referred to as "class differences". In the next sections of this chapter we look more closely at the concept of "social class" and try to clarify the concept in a way which makes it more useful for aetiological research.

The concept of social class

It is increasingly acknowledged that in order to move beyond description towards explanation of social patterns of cardiovascular disease, the concept of socioeconomic status needs to be unpacked. It is true that research has revealed similar social patterns regardless of the measure used.[16] However, the strength of the relationships between social position and cardiovascular risk factors varies according to which definition of social position is used.[17–23] There is little discussion of the degree of consistency between the size of the social effects in studies that use different measures of social position, or of variation between studies in the effect of adjustment for confounders and possible mediating variables. As a result it is difficult to be clear about the nature of the evidence about either the degree or the causes of health inequality for purposes of policy discussion. Simple questions such as "how great is the effect of social inequality on heart disease?" and "what are the best policies for reducing this?" therefore receive vague answers.

Inconsistencies between studies are not surprising in view of the differences between the (explicit or implicit) conceptual bases of the measures of social position they use. If the conceptual basis of the measure of social position used in each study is not clear, inconsistencies will be difficult to interpret, and may be mistakenly regarded as confirming or disconfirming specific causal models of health inequality. Causal processes cannot be understood without clear definitions of the independent as well as the dependent variables.

Epidemiological information on the social distribution of cardiovascular disease in the UK and other European countries, in contrast to the practice in the USA, is often presented in terms of rates in different social classes. However, "social class" is only one of a number of ways in which socioeconomic position has been defined and measured. Sociologists in the USA use a variety of measures of socioeconomic position in studies of health inequality. Krieger and colleagues define socioeconomic position as "an aggregate concept that includes both resource-based income, wealth, education and prestige-based rank in the social hierarchy measures".[2] The practice of mixing these elements together in the same measure, and the use of the term "socioeconomic status" which confuses social class, economic resources, and prestige (status) has been criticised.[2,24,25] Here we will try to draw clear distinctions between different dimensions of socioeconomic position: class, status, and indicators of material living standards.

The measures most often used in US research are what Krieger et al. refer to as "socioeconomic indices",[2] which combine information on the income and/or prestige of an occupation with that on the education and income of the individual. These include the Nam–Powers[26] occupational status score based on median income and education of persons employed in a given occupation; the Nam–Powers socioeconomic status score combines the Nam–Powers occupational status score for an individual's job with that individual's education and household income; the Duncan[27] socioeconomic index, which combines information on occupational prestige with income and education; and the Hollingshead index of social position, which combines the education of the individual combined with the rank of the occupation (as judged by Hollingshead himself in the 1960s)[28].

The concept of social class has been most intensively developed in the USA by Erik Olin Wright.[29] His defining criteria of social class membership are ownership of capital (land, factories), control of other's work (managers and supervisors), and the degree of autonomy individuals exercise over the work process in which they are involved. These are all important to Wright because they affect the power relations between people. The owner of a farm or factory controls what happens there; managers control what happens in their departments; more autonomous workers have greater control over the course of their own work life. In each case, those with less control can be exploited by those with more. The term "exploitation" is used to describe any situation where the efforts of one person benefit another more than the person who has made the effort. The classical form is the control that owners of businesses exert over the proceeds of selling the products. Only a part of these proceeds are used to pay the wages of those who actually made the products and the costs of machinery: the rest is profit. However, in a modern economy there are many other forms of exploitation. Managerial or supervisory control also enables individuals to benefit from the work of others.

Social class in the UK

There are several different ways to measure socioeconomic position in the UK. The Registrar-General's social classification, used in all official health statistics in the UK, is a good example of the type of hybrid measure criticised by Krieger. At the time of the 1981 census, the classification was described as one that operationalised "general standing in the community".[30] At the time of the 1991 census, the conceptual basis was described as "occupational skill". However, there has been no systematic study measuring the changing skill content of the Registrar-General's classes over time, or of possible changes in the "standing" of different occupations in the eyes of the general public.[31] There has never been any attempt to measure the degrees of skill involved in the occupations in the different Registrar-General classes, nor to measure the degree of prestige allocated by citizens to different skills: does the skill of a nurse rank higher or lower than that of a business manager?[32] Table 2.1 shows the distribution of men of working age into the Registrar-General's classes, and the relative risk of mortality in each class, compared with all men (set to the value of 1).

Outside the sphere of official statistics, sociological and political research has used three main classifications, only one of which may be regarded as a

Table 2.1 Numbers of men aged 15–64 years in Registrar-General's classes and hazard ratio for mortality in the Office of National Statistics Longitudinal Study 1986–1995.

Social class		Number of men	Hazard ratio (95% CI)
I	Professional	32 643	0·69 (0·63–0·76)
II	Managerial	17 231	0·81 (0·77–0·84)
IIIN	Skilled non-manual	52 905	0·92 (0·88–0·99)
IIIM	Skilled manual	25 162	1·05 (1·02–1·09)
IV	Semiskilled manual	9 092	1·17 (1·12–1·22)
V	Unskilled manual	2 505	1·32 (1·24–1·41)

Source: Fitzpatrick et al.[78]
CI, confidence interval.

measure of "social class". The Hope–Goldthorpe scale is a true prestige measure, which is based on rankings of occupations by surveys in which people are asked to order a large number of job titles.[33] The Cambridge scale is unique in that it is derived not from preset rules for placing occupations into categories, nor from rankings of occupations, but from observed social behaviour. The Cambridge scale was originally derived from surveys asking the occupations of the best friends and marriage partners of respondents, on the grounds that marriage and friendship choices are the most important expression of perceived equality.[34,35] Pairs of occupations whose members seldom cited each other as friends were regarded as separated by a greater social distance than those frequently cited. Having ascertained the relative distances between all pairs of occupations, multidimensional scaling was used to extract the principal dimensions of the space so defined. This exercise yielded a single major dimension, supporting the concept of a single hierarchy of social interaction and social advantage:[36,37] the score on this factor is the Cambridge score. The Cambridge scale, therefore, makes no reference to employment relations or conditions as a source of social inequality.

The Erikson–Goldthorpe schema has a more similar conceptual basis to that of Erik Olin Wright, in that it is based on economic relations rather than hierarchies of skill or status. Social classes within this schema are characterised by different relationships within the structure of employment. Owners of businesses are distinguished from employees. However, the second organising principle of the Erikson–Goldthorpe schema is the concept of the "form of employment regulation". This can take the form of a "service contract" or a "labour contract". The former is characterised by a relatively high degree of autonomy over one's own work, job security, and a career ladder. The motivation for work is, therefore, a matter of positive incentives. The "labour contract" mode of regulation involves a simpler exchange of money for work, relatively closely supervised, with less job security and no career opportunities. Thus managers and supervisors are distinguished from those without supervisory responsibility, and those with more from those with less discretion over their own work. There is a degree of order in this classification, but it is not a hierarchy and its associations with skills, income and prestige (status) are only contingent. For example, a self employed baker would be located differently to a baker in a large organisation, but there is no implicit or explicit hierarchical relationship between them. For Erikson and Goldthorpe, as for Olin Wright, social class is about the economic relationships between the individual and the structure of employment, and relationships of power and control between individuals within this structure (employer to employee, manager to subordinate).[38,39] However, the Erikson–Goldthorpe schema also makes a distinction between manual and non-manual work, which Wright does not. Table 2.2 shows the distribution of working age men into Erikson–Goldthorpe classes in the mid-1980s, and shows the relative risk of mortality for each class.

As a result of widespread dissatisfaction with the ad hoc nature of the Registrar-General's classes and the socioeconomic groupings, a review of social classifications was commissioned by the Office of National Statistics (ONS) for England and Wales. This was a largescale exercise, intended first to decide what type of classification was needed, and then to design and validate one. The ONS socioeconomic classification (ONS-SEC), like

Table 2.2 Numbers of men aged 15–64 years in Erikson–Goldthorpe classes and relative risk of mortality in the Office of National Statistics Longitudinal Study 1986–1989.

Erikson–Goldthorpe class	Number of men	Relative risk of mortality (95% CI)
1 Higher professionals, senior managers, owners of large firms	14 317	0·71 (0·63–0·79)
2 Lower professionals, managers in small firms, higher technicians or manual supervisors	20 912	0·84 (0·77–0·92)
3a Higher routine non-manual	9 641	1·00 (0·89–1·13)
3b Lower routine non-manual	1 450	1·47 (1·03–2·10)
4a Self employed, small proprietors with employees	3 044	1·02 (0·83–1·25)
4b Self employed without employees	7 189	0·84 (0·72–0·98)
4c Farmers	1 687	0·97 (0·75–1·26)
5 Lower technicians, manual supervisors	8 287	1·02 (0·91–1·15)
6 Skilled manual	28 164	1·10 (1·02–1·18)
7a Semiskilled and unskilled manual	34 251	1·18 (1·11–1·25)
7b Agricultural and primary production workers	1 527	0·60 (0·40–0·90)

Source: Bartley et al.[32]
CI, confidence interval.

10

the Erikson–Goldthorpe schema, is based on employment relations and conditions. It has been adopted for use in the 2001 UK census and in other official and vital statistics.

The primary distinction made by this schema is between employers and employees. Within the category of employees, distinctions are made between those whose work involves higher or lower amounts of planning, supervision of their own work and that of others, degrees of job security, and the existence or not of a career structure.[40] The classification does not distinguish between "manual" and "non-manual" work because "changes in the nature and structure of both industry and occupations have rendered this distinction both outmoded and misleading".[40] The concept of "routine" work has replaced that of "skill". In the modern context, and most importantly in relation to women's occupations, it is far more relevant to know the degree to which employees determine the content of their own work or have this laid down as a routine set by others, rather than the degree to which it involves manual skills.

The development of the classification has involved extensive validation studies.[41] The new measure, the ONS-SEC, is furthermore intended to be consistent with existing classifications such as that of the Registrar-General.[41] This feature of the ONS-SEC is particularly important for health studies, because of the contested and policy-relevant nature of research on health inequality. Throughout the first forty years of the British welfare state, public health experts (most prominently successive Registrars-General) reported that differences in health between the social classes had not reduced, and may even have widened.[42–44] If a new classification were not comparable to the Registrar-General's, it would be impossible to continue this monitoring of population trends. Table 2.3 shows the full version of the ONS-SEC and the simplified one which is most commonly adopted for health studies. Table 2.4 shows the distribution of working age men into the seven category version of the schema, with the relative risk of mortality in each group for the period 1985–1996 (numbers differ from Table 2.1 owing to missing data on the component variables from which the two measures are derived).[45] Taken together, Tables 2.1–2.3 show that the ONS-SEC, although it shares a theoretical basis with the Erikson–Goldthorpe schema, displays a mortality gradient almost the same as the Registrar-General's classification.

Social class and coronary heart disease

The association of measures of socioeconomic position with coronary heart disease has been demonstrated in a large number of studies, and appears to hold in all Western industrialised nations, regardless of the measure of socioeconomic position used. These studies have established the fact of social variation and for this purpose the variety of measures has been an advantage. By no means all studies use any measure of class strictly speaking, either the Registrar-General's measure or any of the theoretically derived measures discussed above. One of the best known of these is the

11

Table 2.3 The Office of National Statistics socioeconomic classification (ONS-SEC).

Full 13-category ONS-SEC classes	Description of 13-category class	Seven-category ONS-SEC classes	Description of seven-category class
L1	Employers in large firms (over 25 staff)	1	Higher managerial and professional
L2	Managers in large firms		
L3	Professionals		
L4	Associate professionals	2	Lower managerial and professionals
L5	Managers in small firms		
L6	Higher supervisors (supervisors of intermediate workers)		
L7.1	Clerical and secretarial	3	Intermediate occupations
L7.2	Intermediate public service occupations		
L7.3	Intermediate technical occupations		
L8.1, 8.2	Employers in small firms	4	Small employers and own account occupations
L9.1, 9.2	Non-professional self employed occupations		
L10	Supervisors of craft and routine occupations	5	Lower supervisors, craft and related occupations
L11	Craft and related occupations		
L12	Semiroutine occupations	6	Semiroutine occupations
L13	Routine occupations	7	Routine occupations

Table 2.4 Numbers of men aged 15–64 years and relative risk of mortality for each ONS-SEC class in the ONS Longitudinal Study 1985–1996.

ONS-SEC class	n	Relative risk (95% CI)
1 Higher managerial and professional	20 179	0·74 (0·70–0·77)
2 Lower managerial and professional	23 497	0·86 (0·82–0·90)
3 Intermediate employees	11 029	0·96 (0·91–1·02)
4 Small employers/own account	11 992	0·94 (0·89–0·99)
5 Lower supervisors, craft and related	26 242	1·09 (1·05–1·13)
6 Employees in semiroutine occupations	41 342	1·18 (1·14–1·21)
7 Employees in routine occupations	10475	1·38 (1·31–1·45)

Source: Office of National Statistics Longitudinal Study.
ONS-SEC, Office of National Statistics socioeconomic classification.

Whitehall study of health in civil servants in London. Table 2.5 shows the extent to which civil service employment grade, a measure that includes employment relations, income, and prestige, distinguishes groups with widely different levels of morbidity and cardiovascular risk factors.

The Registrar-General's social classification is, for obvious reasons, another of the most widely used measures in the UK.[46–49] Mainland European and Nordic studies have used their own national definitions,[50,51] or the Erikson–Goldthorpe classification, which is suitable for use in international comparisons.[52–55] One German study derived a measure of social position from a combination of qualifications, skills, and how heavy the work of an occupation was.[56] Education is widely used as a measure in all countries, either on its own,[57–59] or in combination with other measures.[4,44,60] Some US studies have used an official measure derived from a combination of education and income.[61,62]

Although this diversity of measures has been a strength of previous research, one implication is that studies attempting to investigate pathways between social position and health might easily obtain contradictory findings owing to their choice of indicators of social position. For example, Bartley et al. compared the relationship of cardiovascular risk factors with three different measures of socioeconomic position: social class according to the Erikson–Goldthorpe classification, general social advantage (the Cambridge scale), and ownership of home and cars.[63] Social class (Erikson–Goldthorpe) was strongly related to work control and variety,

Table 2.5 Social variation in morbidity and cardiovascular risk factors by civil service grade in the Whitehall II study.

Condition or risk factor	Sex	Civil service grade						Significance
		1	2	3	4	5	6	
Probable/possible ischaemia on ECG/angina (%)	M	7·6	7·0	7·3	9·3	8·4	12·3	0·001
	F	4·5	5·0	5·5	9·8	13·3	11·1	0·001
Average or worse self-rated health (%)	M	15·3	19·5	21·5	22·8	27·5	33·7	0·001
	F	26·2	25·5	28·7	28·9	34·4	42·1	0·001
Regular cough with phlegm in winter (%)	M	6·7	7·3	6·9	9·2	11·0	10·9	0·001
	F	4·2	6·1	10·3	6·4	6·5	8·6	0·05<0·01
Obesity (%)	M	4·1	3·7	4·6	5·1	6·0	10·7	0·001
	F	7·4	4·6	7·9	7·8	10·3	13·2	0·001
Regular smokers (%)	M	8·3	10·2	13·0	18·4	21·9	33·6	0·001
	F	18·3	11·6	15·2	20·3	22·7	27·5	0·001
Longstanding illness (%)	M	29·9	30·4	30·1	31·6	31·8	36·4	0·01–0·001
	F	30·2	35·8	26·7	33·7	31·6	30·5	

Source: Marmot et al.[12]
ECG, electrocardiogram.

even when adjusting for the other socioeconomic measures; however, the relationships to behavioural risk factors and blood pressure were explained by adjustment for general social advantage (Cambridge scale). Much, but not all, of the apparent relationship of Erikson–Goldthorpe social class to risk factors therefore appeared to be due to material and cultural influences. However, we need to do more than adopt better defined measures of the dimensions of social inequality. The interpretation of results will depend on identifying the aetiological pathways between aspects of social position and circumstances, and health.[20] Neither "class" nor "status" can be literally causes of illness, nor indeed of risky behaviour.

Before attempting to construct and test more precise models of the causal processes linking class to coronary heart disease, it is useful to return to the rich existing literature with clearer definitions in mind. The adoption of such definitions of different dimensions of social inequality, together with a more explicit model of aetiological pathways, has implications for the ways in which these may be interpreted. In different studies, adjustment for risk factors results in various degrees of attenuation of relationships between social position and cardiovascular disease outcomes.[47,52,64] One variable may attenuate the effect of another for two reasons: because it is a confounder, or because it lies on the aetiological pathway between the other two.[65] Much research on health inequality, while referring to risk behaviours as "confounders", in fact implicitly treats risk behaviour as part of the aetiological process linking social position to disease.[66] Although we may not know enough about why those in less (materially or culturally) privileged circumstances behave more riskily than others,[60] explicitly regarding risk behaviours as part of an aetiological pathway is helpful, at least in framing the next questions.[16] We need to ask: what is it about being in social position x that increases or decreases the likelihood of behaviour y? This is easier to do once a specific dimension of social position has been chosen.

The evidence to date from studies that have used theoretically based measures such as Erikson–Goldthorpe class or the Cambridge scale indicate, for example, that relationships between social position and cardiovascular disease outcomes may be more substantially attenuated by behavioural variables when social position is defined in terms of shared lifestyle or culture, and less so when it is defined in terms of employment relations, income, or other indicators of living standards. This would be expected if the pathway between social position and cardiovascular disease is one that mainly involves culturally determined health-related behaviour. However, if socioeconomic position is defined and measured in terms of employment relations and conditions, attenuation by behavioural risk factors would be expected to be somewhat less, and attenuation by variables measuring work stress greater. Confusion is likely when measures of socioeconomic position derived from one conceptual basis are used in combination with mediating factors more appropriate to another pathway.

Examples of this problem can indeed be found in the literature. Woodward *et al.* reported on coronary heart disease incidence according to occupational social class (Registrar-General's definition), level of educational attainment, and housing tenure.[47] All of these were significantly related to mortality before adjustment for behavioural risk factors. Differences according to educational level (a "cultural" measure) were by far the most attenuated by adjustment for risk factors in multivariate analysis. Brunner *et al.* reported similar findings in respect of fibrinogen: the relationships with civil service grade and housing tenure survived adjustment for behavioural risk factors, whereas that with education did not.[67] Differences between income groups in the incidence of acute myocardial infarction in Finnish men,[65] and all cause mortality in the Americans' Changing Lives survey,[68] were not explained away by behavioural risk factors, while differences between educational groups were. In contrast, studies that define social position using an employment based measure ("true social class" according to Kreiger's definition discussed above) and examine relationships with disease, show less attenuation of the effect of social position by adjustment for behaviours than those using education or prestige based measures.[13,47,52,59] What we can expect from any variable in this sort of model depends upon its theoretical basis, and the interpretations of statistical adjustments depend on the nature of the aetiological hypothesis being tested.

Adopting this kind of explanatory strategy helps us to interpret the different effects of adjustment for behavioural risk factors found in the Whitehall I study (which reports that only a small amount of the social variance in cardiovascular disease status is explained by behaviour) and the British regional heart study (in which class differences in cardiovascular events were accounted for to a far greater extent by adjustment for health behaviours).[13,46] If we accept the 1981 definition of the conceptual basis of the Registrar-General's social classes as "general standing in the community" (prestige), and civil service grade as a better indicator of conditions and relationships in the workplace, it becomes clearer how these differences may occur. If it is prestige and shared culture that most strongly affect health behaviours, the inclusion of health behaviour in a statistical model including a measure of "general standing in the community" (a prestige measure with a strong cultural component) will result in considerable attenuation of the univariate relationship between class and health. On the other hand, in models where the measure of social position is a better indicator of employment relations and conditions, the inclusion of work control and variety will have a greater effect whereas the introduction of behavioural variables may have a weaker effect. By using measures of social position with different theoretical bases, studies are in fact testing different hypotheses. Rather than passing over the contradictory results which accumulate in the literature without comment, these can be used to improve understanding.

Linking social structure, work, and stress

Although this would not be the sole reason to adopt social class (as opposed to other measures of socioeconomic position) as an indicator of inequality for health studies, there is a growing body of recent research pointing to the

15

possible importance in the aetiology of cardiovascular disease, of employment conditions and relationships themselves.[69-75] These studies can be roughly divided into two types: those that focus on work strain, and those that emphasise a process known as "effort–reward imbalance" (see Chapter 4). The concept of job strain as developed by Karasek is based on the idea that work combining high levels of demand with low levels of personal control over the pace and scheduling of work may produce an increased risk of cardiovascular risk factors such as high blood pressure,[76] and eventually of heart disease itself.[69,77] Siegrist has developed an alternative but closely related concept of effort–reward imbalance.[71] His research has shown that men in jobs involving high degrees of effort but providing lower levels of reward—in terms of remuneration, job security and prospects for promotion—are at higher risk of developing several of the biological precursors of heart attack such as raised cholesterol level and blood pressure.[72] Job strain and effort–reward imbalance have also been found to be associated with high risk health behaviours[78] and psychological illness.[79]

The pathways leading from social class based on employment relations via work control, job strain, and effort–reward imbalance will therefore combine with others relating, for example, income to respiratory disease (through an effect of income on housing quality) and culturally based measures of social position such as the Cambridge scale on health related behaviours. We would expect individuals in less favoured positions on all of these dimensions to be at greater risk than those disadvantaged on only one. Building up models of the dimensions of inequality and their likely pathways of influence, it is possible to take careful steps, each one accompanied by clear conceptualisation and measurement, from the social to the biological. Greater clarity with respect to the definition and measurement of social class is only the first of such steps.

Acknowledgements

The authors thank the Office of National Statistics for allowing use of the ONS Longitudinal Study, and Kevin Lynch of the LS Support Programme at the Centre for Longitudinal Studies, Institute of Education, London University for technical advice and assistance with analysis of the LS data. The views expressed in this publication are not necessarily those of the Office of National Statistics or Centre for Longitudinal Studies.

References

1 Davey Smith G, Hart C, Hole D *et al*. Education and occupational social class: which is the more important indicator of mortality risk? *J Epidemiol Community Health* 1998;52:153–60.

2 Krieger N, Williams DR, Moss NE. Measuring social class in US public health research: Concepts, methodologies, and guidelines. *Annu Rev Public Health* 1997;18:341–78.

3 O'Reilly K, Rose D. Criterion validation of the interim revised social classification. In: Rose D, O'Reilly K, eds. *Constructing classes: toward a new social classification for the UK*. Swindon: ESRC/ONS, 1997.

4 Bucher HC, Ragland DR. Socioeconomic indicators and mortality from coronary heart-disease and cancer—a 22-year follow-up of middle-aged men. *Am J Public Health* 1995;**85**:1231–6.

5 Elo IT, Preston SH. Educational differentials in mortality—United States, 1979–85. *Soc Sci Med* 1996;**42**:47–57.

6 Smith GD, Neaton JD, Wentworth D, Stamler R, Stamler J. Socio-economic differentials in mortality risk among men screened for the Multiple Risk Factor Intervention Trial: I. White men. *Am J Public Health* 1996;**86**:486–96.

7 Marmot MG. Coronary heart disease: rise and fall of a modern epidemic. In: Marmot MG, Elliott P, eds. *Coronary heart disease epidemiology.* Oxford: Oxford University Press, 1992.

8 Uemura K, Pisa Z. Trends in cardiovascular disease mortality in industrialized countries since 1950. *World Health Stat Q* 1988;**41**:155–78.

9 Wing S, Barnett E, Casper M, Tyroler HA. Geographic and socioeconomic variation in the onset of decline of coronary heart disease mortality in white women. *Am J Public Health* 1992;**82**:204–9.

10 Osler W. The Lumleian Lectures on angina pectoris. *Lancet* 1910;**i**:839–44.

11 Bobak M, Marmot M. East-West mortality divide and its potential explanations: proposed research agenda. *BMJ* 1996;**312**:421–5.

12 Marmot MG, Smith GD, Stansfeld S *et al.* Health inequalities among British civil servants—the Whitehall II study. *Lancet* 1991;**337**:1387–93.

13 Marmot MG, Rose G, Shipley M, Hamilton PJS. Employment grade and coronary heart disease in British civil servants. *J Epidemiol Community Health* 1978;**32**:244–9.

14 MONICA. The World Health Organization MONICA Project. Ecological analyses of the assocation between mortality and major risk factors of cardiovascular disease. *Int J Epidemiol* 1994;**23**:505–16.

15 Marmot M. Social differentials in health within and between populations. *Daedalus* 1994;**123**:197–216.

16 Marmot M, Ryff CD, Bumpass LL, Shipley M, Marks NF. Social inequalities in health: next questions and converging evidence. *Soc Sci Med* 1997;**44**:901–10.

17 Winkleby MA, Jatulis DE, Frank E, Fortmann SP. Socioeconomic status and health: how education, income, and occupation contribute to risk factors for cardiovascular disease. *Am J Public Health* 1992;**82**:816–20.

18 Adler NE, Boyce T, Chesney MA *et al.* Socioeconomic status and health. The challenge of the gradient. *Am Psychol* 1994;**49**:15–24.

19 Wannamethee SG, Shaper AG. Socioeconomic status within social class and mortality: a prospective study in middle-aged British men. *Int J Epidemiol* 1997;**26**:532–41.

20 Wohlfarth T. Socioeconomic inequality and psychopathology: are socioeconomic status and social class interchangeable? *Soc Sci Med* 1997;**45**:399–410.

21 Lewis G, Bebbington P, Brugha T, Farrell M, Gill B, Jenkins R. Socioeconomic status, standard of living, and neurotic disorder. *Lancet* 1998;**352**:605–9.

22 Wohlfarth T, van den Brink W. Social class and substance use disorders: the value of social class as distinct from socioeconomic status. *Soc Sci Med* 1998;**47**:51–8.

23 Krieger N, Chen JT, Selby JV. Comparing individual and household based measures of social class to assess class inequalities in women's health. *J Epidemiol Community Health* 1999;**53**:612–23.

24 Joung IM, van de Mheen H, Stronks K, van Poppel FW, Mackenbach JP. Differences in self-reported morbidity by marital status and by living arrangement. *Int J Epidemiol* 1994;**23**:91–7.

25 Mackenbach JP, van den Bos J, Joung IM, van de Mheen H, Stronks K. The determinants of excellent health: different from the determinants of ill-health? *Int J Epidemiol* 1994;**23**:1273–81.

26 Nam, CB, Terrie WE. Measurement of socioeconomic status from United States census data. In: Rosse PH, Nock SL, eds. *Measuring Social Judgments.* Beverly Hills: Sage Publications, 1982.

27 Duncan OB. A socioeconomic index for all occupations. In: Reiss Jr AJ, ed. *Occupations and Social Status.* New York: Free Press, 1961.

28 Coxon APM, Davies PM, Jones CL. *Images of Social Stratification.* London: Sage Publications, 1986.

29 Wright EO. *Classes.* London: Verso, 1985.

30 Office of Population Censuses and Surveys. *Classification of Occupations.* London: HMSO, 1980.

31 Heath A. The sociology of social class. In: Mascie-Taylor CGN, ed. *Biosocial Aspects of Social Class.* Oxford: Oxford University Press, 1989.

17

32 Bartley M, Carpenter L, Dunnell K, Fitzpatrick R. Measuring inequalities in health—an analysis of mortality patterns using 2 social classifications. *Sociol Health Illness* 1996;**18**:455–74.

33 Goldthorpe JH, Llewellyn C, Payne C. *Social mobility and class structure in modern Britain.* Oxford: Clarendon, 1980.

34 Stewart A, Prandy K, Blackburn RM. *Social Stratification and Occupations.* London: Macmillan, 1980.

35 Marsh C, Blackburn RM. Class differences in access to higher education in Britain. In: Burrows R, Marsh C, eds. *Consumption and Class: Divisions and Change.* London: Macmillan, 1992.

36 Prandy K. The revised Cambridge scale of occupations. *Sociology* 1990;**24**:629–55.

37 Prandy K. *Social and Political Sciences,* Sociological Research Group Working Paper 18. Cambridge: Cambridge University Press, 1990.

38 Erikson R, Goldthorpe JH. *The Constant Flux.* Oxford: Clarendon, 1992.

39 Goldthorpe JH. The 'Goldthorpe' class schema: some observations on conceptual and operational issues in relation to the ESRC review of government social classification. In: Rose D, O'Reilly K, eds. *Constructing Classes: towards a new social classification for the UK.* Swindon: ONS/ESRC, 1997.

40 Rose D, O'Reilly K. Final report of the ESRC review of government social classifications. Swindon: ESRC/ONS, 1998.

41 Rose D, O'Reilly K. *Constructing Classes: towards a new social classification for the UK.* Swindon: ESRC/Office for National Statistics, 1997.

42 Davey Smith G, Blane D, Bartley M. Explanations for socio-economic differentials in mortality: evidence from Britain and elsewhere. *Eur J Public Health* 1994;**4**:131–44.

43 Blane D, Bartley M, Smith GD. Disease aetiology and materialist explanations of socioeconomic mortality differentials. *Eur J Public Health* 1997;**7**:385–91.

44 Drever F, Whitehead M. *Health Inequalities.* London: HMSO, 1997.

45 Sacker A, Firth D, Fitzpatrick R, Lynch K, Bartley M. Comparing health inequality in men and women: prospective study of mortality 1986–96. *BMJ* 2000;**320**:1303–7.

46 Pocock SJ, Shaper AG, Cook DG, Phillips AN, Walker M. Social class differences in ischaemic heart disease in British men. *Lancet* 1987;**ii**:197–201.

47 Woodward M, Shewry MC, Smith WCS, Tunstall-Pedoe H. Social status and coronary heart disease: results from the Scottish Heart Health Study. *Prev Med* 1992;**21**:136–48.

48 Shewry MC, Smith WCS, Woodward M, Tunstall-Pedoe H. Variation in coronary risk-factors by social-status—results from the Scottish Heart Health Study. *Br J Gen Pract* 1992;**42**:406–10.

49 Harding S, Bethune A, Maxwell R, Brown J. Mortality trends using the Longitudinal Study. In: Drever F, Whitehead M, eds. *Health Inequality.* London: HMSO, 1998.

50 Luoto R, Pekkanen J, Uutela A, Tuomilehto J. Cardiovascular risks and socioeconomic-status—differences between men and women in Finland. *J Epidemiol Community Health* 1994;**48**:348–54.

51 Kaprio J, Sarna S, Fogelholm M, Koskenvuo M. Total and occupationally active life expectancies in relation to social class and marital status in men classified as healthy at 20 in Finland. *J Epidemiol Community Health* 1996;**50**:653–60.

52 Lundberg O. Causal explanations for class inequality in health—an empirical analysis. *Soc Sci Med* 1991;**32**:385–93.

53 Stronks K, van de Mheen H, van den Bos J, Mackenbach JP. The interrelationship between income, health and employment status. *Int J Epidemiol* 1997;**26**:592–600.

54 Mackenbach JP, Kunst AE, Cavelaars AEJM, Groenhof F, Geurts JJM. Socioeconomic inequalities in morbidity and mortality in western Europe. *Lancet* 1997;**349**:1655–9.

55 Cavelaars AEJM, Kunst AE, Geurts JJM *et al.* Morbidity differences by occupational class among men in seven European countries: an application of the Erikson–Goldthorpe social class scheme. *Int J Epidemiol* 1998;**27**:222–30.

56 Helmert U, Mielck A, Classen E. Social inequities in cardiovascular-disease risk-factors in East and West Germany. *Soc Sci Med* 1992;**35**:1283–92.

57 Gran B. Major differences in cardiovascular risk indicators by educational status. *Scand J Soc Med* 1995;**23**:9–16.

58 Hoeymans N, Smit HA, Verkleij H, Kromhout D. Cardiovascular risk-factors in relation to educational level in 36000 men and women in the Netherlands. *Eur Heart J* 1996;**17**:518–25.

59 Cavelaars AE, Kunst AE, Geurts JJ et al. Differences in self reported morbidity by educational level: a comparison of 11 western European countries. *J Epidemiol Community Health* 1998;**52**:219–27.

60 Lynch JW, Kaplan GA, Salonen JT. Why do poor people behave poorly? Variation in adult health behaviours and psychosocial characteristics by stages of the socioeconomic lifecourse. *Soc Sci Med* 1997;**44**:809–19.

61 Diezroux AV, Nieto FJ, Tyroler HA, Crum LD, Szklo M. Social inequalities and atherosclerosis—the atherosclerosis risk in communities study. *Am J Epidemiol* 1995;**141**:960–72.

62 Winkleby MA. Accelerating cardiovascular risk factor change in ethnic minority and low socioeconomic groups. *Ann Epidemiol* 1997;**7**:S96–S103.

63 Bartley M, Sacker A, Firth D, Fitzpatrick R. Social position, social roles and women's health in England: changing relationships 1984–1993. *Soc Sci Med* 1999;**48**:99–115.

64 Suadicani P, Hein HO, Gyntelberg F. Strong mediators of social inequalities in risk of ischaemic heart disease: a six-year follow-up in the Copenhagen male study. *Int J Epidemiol* 1997;**26**:516–22.

65 Lynch JW, Kaplan GA, Cohen RD, Tuomilehto J, Salonen JT. Do cardiovascular risk-factors explain the relation between socioeconomic-status, risk of all-cause mortality, cardiovascular mortality, and acute myocardial-infarction. *Am J Epidemiol* 1996;**144**:934–42.

66 MacIntyre S. The Black Report and beyond: What are the issues? *Soc Sci Med* 1997;**44**:723–45.

67 Brunner E, Davey Smith G, Marmot M, Canner R, Beksinska M, O'Brien J. Childhood social circumstances and psychosocial and behavioural factors as determinants of plasma fibrinogen. *Lancet* 1996;**347**:1008–13.

68 Lantz PM, House JS, Lepowski JM, Williams DR, Mero RP, Chen J. Socioeconomic factors, health behaviours and mortality. *JAMA* 1998;**279**:1703–8.

69 Karasek R. Job strain and the prevalence and outcome of coronary-artery disease. *Circulation* 1996;**94**:1140–1.

70 Theorell T, Karasek RA. Current issues relating to psychosocial job strain and cardiovascular disease research. *J Occup Health Psychol* 1996;**1**:9–26.

71 Siegrist J, Klein D, Voigt KH. Linking sociological with physiological data: the model of effort-reward imbalance at work. *Acta Physiol Scand* 1997;**161**:112–16.

72 Peter R, Alfredsson L, Hammar N, Siegrist J, Theorell T, Westerholm S. High effort, low reward, and cardiovascular risk factors in employed Swedish men and women: baseline results from the WOLF Study. *J Epidemiol Community Health* 1998;**52**:540–7.

73 Peter R, Geissler H, Siegrist J. Associations of effort-reward imbalance at work and reported symptoms in different groups of male and female public transport workers. *Stress Med* 1998;**14**:175–82.

74 Schnall PL, Schwartz JE, Landsbergis PA, Warren K, Pickering TG. A longitudinal study of job strain and ambulatory blood pressure: Results from a three-year follow-up. *Psychosom Med* 1998;**60**:697–706.

75 Bosma H, Peter R, Siegrist J, Marmot M. Two alternative job stress models and the risk of coronary heart disease. *Am J Public Health* 1998;**88**:68–74.

76 Landsbergis PA, Schnall PL, Warren K, Pickering TG, Schwartz JE. Association between ambulatory blood-pressure and alternative formulations of job strain. *Scand J Work Environ Health* 1994;**20**:349–63.

77 Karasek RA, Theorell T, Schwartz JE, Schnall PL, Pieper CF, Michela JL. Job characteristics in relation to the prevalence of myocardial infarction in the United States Health Examination Survey (HES) and the Health and Nutrition Examination Survey (HANES). *Am J Public Health* 1988;**78**:910–8.

78 Landsbergis PA, Schnall PL, Deitz DK, Warren K, Pickering TG. Job strain and health behaviors: Results of a prospective study. *Am J Health Prom* 1998;**12**:237–45.

79 Stansfeld SA, Fuhrer R, Shipley MJ, Marmot MG. Work characteristics predict psychiatric disorder: prospective results from the Whitehall II Study. *Occup Environ Med* 1999;**56**:302–7.

80 Fitzpatrick R, Bartley M, Dodgeon B, Firth D, Lynch K. Social variations in health: relationship of mortality to the interim revised social classification. In: Rose D, O'Reilly K, eds. *Constructing Classes—towards a new social classification for the UK*. Swindon: ONS/ESRC, 1997.

3: Life course approaches to inequalities in coronary heart disease risk

GEORGE DAVEY SMITH, YOAV BEN-SHLOMO, AND JOHN LYNCH

There are large social class inequalities in mortality from coronary heart disease among men and women of working ages in the UK (these inequalities are described in greater detail in Chapter 2). This socioeconomic distribution is also seen with respect to morbidity rates.[1,2] For example, in a survey of over 20 000 people aged 35 and over in Somerset and Avon, histories of angina, myocardial infarction (heart attack), and stroke, were all more common among individuals living in deprived areas compared with those in affluent areas (Table 3.1). Socioeconomic position is also related to the early stages of developing cardiovascular disease. In a Finnish study, low income, manual occupation, and little education were all related to a higher severity and greater 4 year progression of carotid atherosclerosis.[3,4] Coronary artery calcification—an index of coronary plaque volume—was greater among young adults in manual rather than non-manual jobs and

Table 3.1 Age standardised prevalence per 100 of self reported illness by deprivation category, in the Somerset and Avon Study of Health.

Condition	1st fifth (least deprived)	2nd fifth	3rd fifth	4th fifth	5th fifth (most deprived)	p value (test for trend)
Men						
Angina	4·4	5·5	5·5	5·5	6·9	<0·001
Myocardial infarction	3·2	3·7	4·0	4·5	4·8	<0·001
Stroke	2·0	1·8	1·3	2·3	2·6	0·03
Women						
Angina	3·8	4·4	4·6	4·4	5·8	<0·002
Myocardial infarction	1·5	1·9	1·7	1·8	2·5	0·03
Stroke	1·6	2·0	2·1	2·2	2·4	0·04

Source: Eachus *et al.*[2]

20

among those who left fulltime education at an early age, in a cross-sectional London study.[5]

Until recently the debate regarding inequalities in health generally concerned the association of illness with socioeconomic circumstances in adulthood. There has now been a revival of interest in the effects of poor social circumstances in early life on health in adulthood. The UK Department of Health report, *Variations in Health,* recognised the importance of a life course perspective on inequalities in health. It concluded that it "is likely that accumulative differential lifetime exposure to health-damaging or health-promoting physical and social environments is the main explanation for observed variations in health and life expectancy". This is not a new idea. In 1941 Antonio Ciocco and colleagues concluded that the findings of their follow up study of Maryland schoolchildren "reinforce the views held by many that disease in adulthood is often brought about by the cumulative effects over a long period of time of many pathological conditions, many incidents, some of which take place and are even perceived in infancy."[6] This life course approach to chronic disease lost favour over the subsequent half century, but has subsequently been revived.[7] It recognises that factors acting in early life accumulate and interact with factors acting in later life in the production of adulthood disease. Coronary heart disease (CHD) is in many ways the paradigmatic adulthood health problem, illustrating the importance of a life course perspective. Genomic and non-genomic intergenerational factors,[8,9] intrauterine environment,[10] growth, nutrition, health, and social circumstances in childhood,[11-13] and a variety of behavioural and socioeconomic factors in adulthood may all contribute to the development of CHD. The high prevalence of atherosclerosis and coronary artery narrowing among young American men killed in war in the early 1950s and late 1960s demonstrates that the risk of coronary heart disease is already established in young adulthood (Table 3.2). The declining trends in coronary heart disease incidence and mortality in the USA since the 1970s appear to have been heralded by a declining prevalence of atherosclerosis in young men. This suggests that the degree to which the disease process is initiated in early life might have some influence on population trends in coronary heart disease. Furthermore, conventional CHD risk factors—blood

Table 3.2   Coronary artery disease in young US soldiers killed in the Korean war in the early 1950s and in the Vietnam war in the late 1960s.

	Korean war	Vietnam war
Number of autopsied combatants	200	105
Mean age (yr)	22	22
Evidence of atherosclerosis (%)	77	45
Clinically significant narrowing of vessel(s) (%)	15	5

Source: Korean war data from Enos *et al.*;[104] Vietnam war data from McNamara *et al.*[105]

pressure, obesity, and blood cholesterol—measured in adolescents and young adults predict CHD risk many decades later.[14] These findings, coupled with substantial evidence that modifying risk factors such as smoking, blood pressure, and blood cholesterol level in adulthood modifies CHD risk, indicates that processes both in early life and in adulthood are of importance. Approaches to coronary heart disease epidemiology that focus exclusively on early life or later life will miss an important part of the picture.

Understanding the influence of life course on health and health inequalities

When considering specific factors underlying socioeconomic inequalities in CHD risk, issues pertinent to inequalities in health in general also need to be addressed. Indeed, considering coronary heart disease in isolation can hinder understanding of the basis for health inequalities, by obscuring issues of common concern. There are three important issues related to the level at which causes of health inequalities should be sought:

- the distinction between fundamental and proximal causes of health inequalities
- the problems of separating proximal causes from mere markers of socioeconomic position
- the question whether general processes underlie inequalities in a wide variety of health outcomes, or whether particular health problems have particular reasons for their socioeconomic distribution.

Fundamental and proximal causes of health inequalities

If studies show that cigarette smoking or low micronutrient intake statistically account for the socioeconomic distribution of CHD, does this mean that these behavioural patterns "explain" the inequalities? If so, should interventions aimed at reducing inequalities be targeted at improving these health related behaviours at the individual level? When considering these questions the Black report committee made a distinction between fundamental and proximal causes of inequalities in health, concluding, for example, that "smoking behaviour cannot be taken as a fundamental cause of ill-health, it is rather an epiphenomenon, a secondary symptom of deeper underlying features of economic society" and therefore policy makers needed to ask "about the social and economic factors which explain ... the prevalence of smoking in the first place, and whether these, independent of individual education and counselling, have to be given priority in reducing the differentials".[15]

Recognition of the distinction between fundamental and proximal causes of health inequalities should broaden the explanatory framework and emphasise the need to account for the distribution of proximal causes, as well as demonstrate the role of these proximal causes in mediating between social factors and the distribution of disease. If, for example, it is shown that differences in dietary patterns between socioeconomic groups account for at least some of the differentials in CHD mortality, then the elements of social organisation of dietary practices should be considered as the antecedent causes. These antecedents include inequitable income and wealth distribution, the profit driven organisation of food retailing, unequal educational opportunities and the failure of collective resistance to such inequities. The concentration of interventions upon proximal rather than fundamental causes of disease may underlie the disappointing outcomes of many health promotion programmes. Thus risk factor modification approaches to reducing CHD risk among the general population have had unimpressive effects,[16,17] at the same time as secular changes in the social circumstances of population groups have been associated with dramatic decreases or increases in CHD mortality. These secular mortality trends indicate that social change can result in sizeable changes in disease risk within populations, while interventions targeted at individuals have little specific impact on risk.

Separating proximal causes from markers of socioeconomic position

As with all approaches to understanding factors influencing the distribution of ill health, it is important that factors postulated to underlie socioeconomic differentials in mortality are actual causes of the diseases in question, rather than merely being markers of socioeconomic position whose association with disease outcome is due to confounding by socially patterned determinants of disease. The importance of such confounding has long been recognised. George Bernard Shaw wrote in 1906 that "it is easy to prove that the wearing of tall hats and the carrying of umbrellas enlarges the chest, prolongs life, and confers comparative immunity from disease; for the statistics show that the classes which use these articles are bigger, healthier, and live longer than the class which never dreams of possessing such things."[18]

In a similar vein, he noted that "had the jewellers thought of claiming that the possession of a gold watch and chain is an infallible prophylactic against smallpox, their statistics would have been quite as convincing as those of the vaccinists."[19]

In both these cases, if studies had been set up, naive statistical analyses of the observational data would suggest that not wearing tall hats and not owning jewellery were causes of ill health. However, if people had been randomised to wearing or not wearing tall hats, there would have been no finding of a causal effect on health status.

The possibility that factors thought to explain socioeconomic differentials in health are in fact associated with health outcomes because of confounding by concomitants of socioeconomic position is of particular concern in this area of work. The importance of considering these issues of residual confounding in making causal interpretations of the exposure–disease links revealed in observational studies can be highlighted by considering the example of the effects of antioxidant vitamin intake on cardiovascular disease. A large number of observational studies suggested that higher levels of β-carotene, vitamin E and vitamin C intake were associated with substantially lower rates of cardiovascular disease incidence and mortality. However, when largescale, longterm, randomised controlled trials of vitamin supplementation were carried out, they produced no evidence of benefit; indeed, in the case of β-carotene there was a suggestion of increased cardiovascular disease incidence and mortality in those randomised to supplementation (Figure 3.1). The explanation for this discrepancy is probably that antioxidant intake is strongly related to a wide range of socially patterned environmental and behavioural risk factors for cardiovascular disease. For example, Nyyssönen et al. demonstrated an association between plasma vitamin C levels and risk of myocardial infarction (Table 3.3).[20] Risk was increased mainly among those with very low plasma vitamin C levels. However, as Table 3.4 makes clear, the study participants with low plasma vitamin C levels were markedly different in a variety of ways from the participants with higher levels. They were of poorer socioeconomic background, they were much more likely to be smokers, they engaged in considerably less leisure time physical activity, they were less physically fit, their blood white cell count was raised (perhaps indicating higher rates of minor illnesses), and they drank more alcohol. These two groups are so

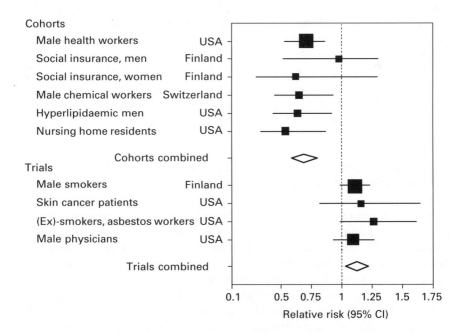

Figure 3.1 Findings from observational cohort studies and randomised controlled trials of β-carotene and cardiovascular disease mortality. Source: Egger et al.[102]

Table 3.3 Relative risks (95% confidence intervals) of myocardial infarction in 1605 men according to plasma vitamin C concentration at baseline.

Plasma vitamin C (μmol/L)	Relative risk adjusted for age, season, and examination year
< 11·4	4·03 (1·74 to 9·36)
11·4–32·9	1·46 (0·71 to 3·01)
33·0–49·9	0·95 (0·42 to 2·12)
50·0–64·8	1·08 (0·49 to 2·38)
> 64·8	1·00

Source: Nyyssönen et al.[20]

Table 3.4 Major coronary risk factors in men with and without vitamin C deficiency.

Characteristic	Plasma vitamin C level $\leq 11\cdot4$ μmol/L ($n = 91$)	> 11·4 μmol/L ($n = 1514$)	p value
Age (yr)	54·7 (0·42)	52·1 (0·14)	< 0·001
Smoking (no. of pack yr)	18·9 (2·2)	7·0 (0·4)	< 0·001
No. (%) of smokers	57 (63)	424 (28)	< 0·001
Adulthood socioeconomic group (0–26)*	9·92 (0·37)	7·76 (0·11)	< 0·001
Dietary carotene (μg/d)	1226 (110)	2723 (86)	< 0·001
Maximal oxygen uptake (mL/min/kg)	29·5 (0·6)	32·6 (0·2)	< 0·001
Moderate to vigorous physical activity during leisure time (kJ/d)	144 (24)	214 (7)	0·005
Blood leucocyte count ($\times 10^9$/L)	6·2 (0·2)	5·6 (0·0)	0·001
Coffee intake (g/d)	645 (34)	562 (7)	0·019
Alcohol intake (g/wk)	116 (18)	72 (3)	0·019

Values are mean (standard error) unless stated otherwise.
*High value denotes low socioeconomic position.
Source: Nyyssönen et al.[20]

different they would probably be distinguishable simply by looking at them (for example, although height was not reported, they would probably be considerably shorter). Given these differences, it is not surprising that the risk of myocardial infarction was higher among the men with low plasma vitamin C levels. The authors attempted to take this into account by statistically adjusting for these risk factors, which considerably attenuated the elevated risk among the men with low plasma vitamin C levels, but left a residual doubling (rather than a fourfold elevation) of risk (Table 3.5). Given the limitations of multivariable adjustment in the presence of measurement imprecision (which would certainly be considerable for several of the risk factors in this study), it is likely that this residual effect represents confounding by other factors.[21,22]

Table 3.5 Relative risks (95% confidence intervals) of myocardial infarction in 1605 men according to plasma vitamin C concentration at baseline.

Plasma vitamin C (μmol/L)	Adjusted for age, season, and examination year	Adjusted for risk factors
< 11·4	4·03 (1·74 to 9·36)	2·08 (0·82 to 5·30)
11·4–32·9	1·46 (0·71 to 3·01)	0·87 (0·40 to 1·87)
33·0–49·9	0·95 (0·42 to 2·12)	0·62 (0·26 to 1·45)
50·0–64·8	1·08 (0·49 to 2·38)	0·92 (0·41 to 2·07)
> 64·8	1·00	1·00

Source: Nyyssönen et al.[20]

This general issue of residual confounding relates to many of the factors that are potential mediators between indicators of social position and CHD risk. For example, a prominent contemporary perspective on understanding social inequalities in CHD has involved the idea that a particular form of job stress—that associated with a low degree of control over activity at work—is a major contributor to socioeconomic differentials in cardiovascular mortality. Indeed, statistical adjustment for self reported job control essentially abolished the socioeconomic gradient in CHD incidence in the Whitehall II study of London civil servants.[23] These results are impressive, but they also raise questions regarding collinearity—is job control just another sensitive marker of socioeconomic position, like the wearing of tall hats? This issue was addressed in the Whitehall II study and it was concluded that, in these data, there was a contribution of job control that was independent of socioeconomic position.

As this is only one—albeit important—study, it is worth while to consider how job control and socioeconomic position might be linked within the broader context. In some circumstances, low control over work can be virtually synonymous with other indicators of low socioeconomic position. In the Whitehall II study,[23] the links between job control and employment grade may have been especially close. In other populations comprising more than one employer and more diverse occupational classifications, the links between the degree of job control and other markers of socioeconomic position (such as occupation or income) may not be as tight. For instance, it is unlikely that levels of job control reveal as much about the socioeconomic conditions of farmers or those working in the home, or the unemployed, as they do about particular job hierarchies within one workplace.[23] This is not to deny that there might be a role of job control as a mediator between socioeconomic position and CHD—this possibility has been raised by analyses of the Whitehall II study.[23] Rather, we are using it as an example to pose the larger questions of the potential for a high degree of collinearity between socioeconomic indicators within particular occupational contexts, and in regard to the potential for residual confounding. Both collinearity and residual confounding should be considered before judging potential mediators to be causal. For all the factors we posit as potential mediators of the link between socioeconomic position and health, we need to ask what evidence can be brought to bear to support a belief that randomising individuals to such factors as cigarette smoking, high and low job control conditions, or high and low social support, would causally affect their CHD risk, given that every other aspect of their lives was identical.

The ability to "control work" should be considered a structural characteristic of particular jobs rather than a characteristic of the individuals reporting low control over those jobs.[24] Low control jobs cluster at the bottom of the occupational hierarchy and are much more likely to be occupied by those from poorer childhood circumstances, who have had less education. Poor socioeconomic conditions early in life and low education restrict the range of occupations, and therefore the range of job control that is available in adulthood. Thus, it is possible that in some circumstances, job control could be a good marker of lifetime social circumstances, although adjustment for childhood social class had little effect on job control associations in the Whitehall II study.[23] While it is possible that a sense of job control *per se* may causally affect health via psycho-neuroendocrine and immune pathways, the causal effect of job control is less well understood than is the case for some other variables on the causal pathway between socioeconomic indicators and health, such as smoking. Ongoing research—such as that linking job control to fibrinogen—may contribute in this regard.[59]

Data from other sources are also important when considering the role of low job control in the social distribution of CHD. Earlier in the twentieth century, when most women were not in formal employment—and thus job control was not the key issue—the socioeconomic gradient in CHD was much steeper for women than for men.[25] This issue can be further explored by analysing the association between socioeconomic position and mortality among people in or out of work. Table 3.6 presents all cause and CHD mortality over a 13 year follow up according to household car access (0, 1, or more) for people in England and Wales who were in fulltime or part-time employment, and those who were seeking work or waiting to take up a job in 1981. The mortality differentials according to car access are similar for those in work and for those not working,[26] whereas if socioeconomic differentials in CHD were largely caused by job stress, as has been suggested,[23] then they should be considerably more marked among those in work. Control over other areas of life could, of course, also be of importance, but generalising the hypothesis in this way may make it both less testable and less useful for planning interventions.

A demonstration of how factors related to socioeconomic position can apparently be "independent" risk factors for disease is given by an examination of the association between car ownership and mortality in the first Whitehall study.[27] Not owning a car was associated with a 49% higher risk of all cause mortality than owning a car. Adjustment for employment grade left a significant excess mortality of 28%, just as adjustment for socioeconomic position left a residual association between vitamin C intake

27

Table 3.6 Hazard ratios and 95% confidence intervals for all causes and coronary heart disease (CHD), 1981–1994, by access to cars: women and men, working ages at the 1981 census, in the Office of National Statistics Longitudinal Study.

	Employed 1981	Not employed 1981
Women		
All cause		
No car	1·00	1·00
Car	0·69 (0·64–0·75)	0·81 (0·61–1·07)
CHD		
No car	1·00	1·00
Car	0·61 (0·50–0·74)	0·72 (0·37–1·40)
Men		
All cause		
No car	1·00	1·00
Car	0·70 (0·67–0·73)	0·70 (0·63–0·77)
CHD		
No car	1·00	1·00
Car	0·78 (0·73–0·85)	0·70 (0·59–0·83)

Adapted from: Davey Smith and Harding.[26]

and myocardial infarction in the Nyyssönen study,[20] and adjustment for employment grade in the Whitehall II study left a residual significant influence of job control on CHD risk.[23] Until we have strong evidence that not owning a car is an actual cause of increased mortality, it would be more conservative to treat it as a sensitive indicator of lifetime socioeconomic position (ownership of a car indexes wealth as well as income); the same may be true for vitamin C levels and job control.

As with all areas of epidemiology, the full range of considerations regarding the robustness of evidence that factors are causally related to disease outcomes need to be applied. In addition, it is also important to consider the plausibility of potential mediators against the broader picture of the changes in the distribution of disease over time and across the population as a whole. This approach is highlighted when a life course perspective on CHD is adopted, as it is explicitly recognised that life courses are lived in particular contexts.

Life course approaches to CHD inequalities

Coronary heart disease is the major single cause of death among men in most of the industrialised world, an important cause of death in women, and an increasingly important cause of death in urban areas of industrialising countries. It is a cause of death that illustrates the life course perspective well, since risk is associated with parental health, with intrauterine development, with growth and health in childhood, and with several socioeconomic and behavioural factors in adulthood. While the social patterning of CHD according to adulthood social position has been investigated extensively—and in most industrialised countries marked gradients of increasing risk with worsening social circumstances are seen—there has been relatively little investigation of life course socioeconomic influences on CHD risk.

Early life social circumstances and CHD risk

Some of the early epidemiological studies of CHD were interested in a potential role of socioeconomic position in early life, but this mostly related to the investigation of hypothetical influences of social incongruity—for example, the possible stress of moving from a disadvantaged background into the (perceived) stressful environment of the professional and managerial world.[28] Interest in the possible specific effects of socioeconomic deprivation in early life on later health was stimulated by the work of Forsdahl,[29,30] and subsequently developed by Barker and Osmond,[31] who demonstrated that areas with high infant mortality rates earlier in the twentieth century had high coronary heart disease rates at the time of study. Forsdahl interpreted this as demonstrating that deprivation in early life, followed by later affluence, worked together to increase coronary risk, in part mediated by elevation of blood cholesterol concentrations.[32]

These ideas can be empirically tested with data on childhood and adulthood social circumstances from the West of Scotland Collaborative Study (Table 3.7). Father's social class—as a measure of childhood social circumstances—was predictive of CHD mortality, with a 50% higher risk for men whose fathers were in manual occupations compared with those whose fathers were in non-manual jobs.[33] There were three measures of adulthood social position available: own occupation in middle age; deprivation level of the area of residence; and car driving (as an indicator of car access—a useful marker for available income in UK studies). Adjustment for these markers of adulthood social circumstances attenuated the association between father's social class and CHD mortality by about half. This analysis may lead to underestimation of the importance of early life social circumstances, since early and later life social circumstances are linked and the measures of

Table 3.7 Mortality from coronary heart disease according to social class at screening and fathers' social class in the West of Scotland Collaborative Study. Values are relative rates (95% confidence intervals) adjusted for socioeconomic factors and risk factors profiles.

	Subject non-manual at screening		Subject manual at screening	
	Non-manual father	Manual father	Non-manual father	Manual father
Age	1	1·51 (1·16 to 1·96)	1·68 (1·09 to 2·58)	1·82 (1·43 to 2·32)
Risk factors[*]	1	1·43 (1·10 to 1·86)	1·59 (1·02 to 2·48)	1·67 (1·27 to 2·13)

[*]Age, smoking, diastolic blood pressure, cholesterol, body mass index, forced expiratory volume (FEV_1) score, deprivation category, and car.
Source: Davey Smith et al.[33]

adulthood circumstances are clearly superior, both in being multidimensional and in being likely to contain less measurement error than father's occupation reported by middleaged men. The data therefore provide evidence that both early life and later life social circumstances contribute to CHD risk. There was no suggestion that upward mobility increased the risk of CHD.[33] The influence of childhood and adulthood socioeconomic position was cumulative rather demonstrating any particular influence of intergenerational social mobility, whether upwards or downwards.

Other studies that have looked for an interaction between childhood and adulthood social circumstances have also failed to find evidence to support this component of the Forsdahl hypothesis.[34-36] The suggestion that the effects of early life deprivation are mediated through high blood cholesterol concentrations in adulthood has also received little support, with studies finding no evidence of higher cholesterol levels among those who had been in worse socioeconomic circumstances in early life.[35-37]

Most,[34-36,38-41] but not all,[42-44] studies that have examined the association between childhood social circumstances and CHD risk have found a link which is apparently not purely due to adverse socioeconomic destinations of those born into poor circumstances. A recent study showed effects of both early and later life socioeconomic disadvantage on coronary heart disease risk in women.[45] Figure 3.2 shows how these cumulative lifetime effects of socioeconomic disadvantage increase CHD risk, especially among shorter women. If adult height is the result of both genetic potential and factors such as childhood nutrition, this figure shows how greater

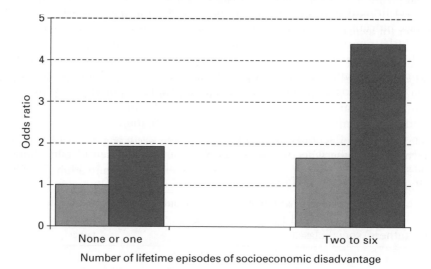

Figure 3.2   Episodes of socioeconomic disadvantage across the life course, adult height, and risk of CHD among 584 women in Stockholm, Sweden, 1991–1994. Left hand column of each pair represents women taller than 160 cm, right hand column represents women shorter than 160 cm. Adapted from Wamala et al.[45]

cumulative disadvantage over the life course increases risk even among taller women; but by far the highest CHD risk is among women who were both shorter and had the most cumulative disadvantage. In a Swedish census follow up, men with fathers in manual occupations had considerably higher coronary heart disease mortality risk than those whose fathers were in non-manual occupations.[40] For all cause mortality the association with father's social class was less clear, with mortality being dependent on adult social class to a considerably greater degree than childhood social class. The particular dependence of coronary heart disease risk in comparison with some other causes of death on childhood socioeconomic circumstances has also been observed in area based studies from Finland.[46,47]

The findings of such studies can be difficult to interpret, given the association of childhood social circumstances with social conditions and behavioural risk factors for cardiovascular disease in adulthood, despite statistical adjustment for these factors.[33] In this respect, the results from a cohort of male former students of Glasgow University, who would have experienced a relatively homogeneous and privileged adulthood social environment,[48] are of value. Men who had studied at the university between 1948 and 1968 were invited to participate in a medical examination carried out by the student health department.[49] Data collected included sociodemographic information, details of health behaviours, and measured blood pressure.[49] The social class of the fathers of the students was coded to the Registrar-General's classification, with a combined social class III grouping being used since the distinction between non-manual and manual classes was not introduced until near the end of the recruitment period. A strong trend of increasing risk of cardiovascular disease mortality moving from fathers' social class I to social class V is seen, with little trend evident for the other cause of death groups (Table 3.8).

This study has the advantage of having collected information on fathers' occupation at entry to further education (when most students would have been living at home), rather than relying on recall in middle age, which has been used in most studies of this issue. Furthermore, confounding by adulthood circumstances is unlikely to be as problematic as in most studies. Less than 5% of school leavers entered university over the period of this study,[50] and those who did so would generally have received educational credentials that placed them in a privileged social position in adult life. The association is specific for cardiovascular disease mortality; other broad cause of death groups—which would be equally influenced by adulthood social circumstances and health related behaviours—show no association with fathers' social class.

Social mobility and CHD risk

There is little evidence that upward social mobility from childhood social background to adulthood social position increases the risk of CHD through generating the stress of status incongruity. Similarly, there is little evidence that

Table 3.8 Father's social class and mortality among Glasgow University students.

Social class of fathers	Number of deaths				
	All cause mortality ($n = 866$)	CVD ($n = 339$)	Cancer ($n = 305$)	Other ($n = 222$)	CVD* ($n = 339$)
I	1·0	1·0	1·0	1·0	1·0
II	1·13	1·50	1·10	0·81	1·46
	(0·93–1·37)	(1·08–2·10)	(0·80–1·50)	(0·56–1·16)	(1·04–2·03)
III	1·21	1·62	1·06	1·00	1·65
	(1·00–1·47)	(1·16–2·26)	(0·77–1·45)	(0·71–1·43)	(1·18–2·30)
IV	1·25	1·82	1·12	0·85	1·89
	(0·91–1·72)	(1·10–3·02)	(0·65–1·92)	(0·44–1·63)	(1·14–3·13)
V	1·33	2·36	0·47	1·35	2·33
	(0·78–2·25)	(1·11–5·00)	(0·11–1·91)	(0·54–3·41)	(1·10–4·94)
p value for trend	0·036	0·002	0·91	0·67	0·001

Values are relative risks (95% confidence intervals). CVD, cardiovascular disease.
*Risk adjusted for systolic blood pressure and smoking.
Source: Davey Smith et al.[48]

downward social mobility—from a non-manual occupational background of father to a manual occupation in middle age—is associated with an elevated risk of CHD. This is of interest with respect to health related social selection models of the genesis of health inequalities.[51] The social selection argument suggests that people destined to be unhealthy in adulthood have characteristics in earlier life that influence both later social class membership and later health, and that this generates the social distribution of CHD risk in adulthood. These characteristics can either be childhood illnesses (which could clearly influence both later social class and later health), physical measures such as height or obesity, or behavioural factors such as smoking, illegal drug use, or drinking. Despite the theoretical plausibility of these mechanisms, the evidence suggests they make at most a modest contribution to socioeconomic differentials in CHD.[51] In a detailed analysis of social mobility from childhood through to middle age it was found that the main determinant of cardiovascular disease mortality risk was the cumulative influence of social position across the life course, rather than cardiovascular disease risk being a product of social mobility.[52] The only exception to this general pattern is related to the small percentage of the population who moved from non-manual jobs at labour market entry to manual jobs in middle age, who experienced a high rate of cardiovascular disease mortality. For this small group, it is possible that health status had an influence on future occupation trajectory. This is also consistent with data from Finland that showed downwardly mobile men to have higher cardiovascular disease risk.[43] The contribution of elevated CHD risk among the downwardly mobile to the overall pattern of socioeconomic differentials in the population is small, however.

Lifetime social circumstances and CHD risk factors

In the West of Scotland Collaborative Study other potential pathways between social position in childhood and CHD risk in adulthood were examined, by analysing conventional risk factors in relation to father's (childhood) and own (adulthood) social class. Men with fathers of manual social class had lower, rather than higher, serum cholesterol concentrations compared with men with fathers of non-manual social class. Behavioural risk factors—such as smoking and exercise—were more dependent on adulthood social position than on parental social class. The evidence from this Scottish cohort supports the notion that such activities are powerfully influenced by the social environment experienced during adult life, and that modifying such behaviours is dependent upon the presence of the social circumstances required for maintaining favourable health related behaviours. However, the influence of lifetime socioeconomic circumstances on CHD risk factors need not necessarily show precisely the same patterns in different countries or in different time periods. It is possible that lifetime socioeconomic patterning of behaviours such as smoking and exercise may show period and cohort effects that may be specific to particular countries, regions, and population subgroups. For example, in Britain there is evidence that early life social circumstances have a stronger influence on smoking among women than among men,[37,53–55] although this is not necessarily the case in other countries. Trends in adolescent smoking in the USA show that the highest initiation rates are found in poorer, non-Hispanic girls.[56] These examples serve to highlight the potential variability of early life disadvantage on health behaviours that may be dependent on gender, race or ethnic group, time period, and place.

An example of the potential complexity of the lifetime socioeconomic patterning of CHD risk factors can be seen in Table 3.9, which shows data on smoking, lack of exercise, overweight, alcohol consumption, and poor perceived health according to father's occupation and respondent's average income 1965–1974. The data are from the Alameda County study—a population based prospective investigation, started in 1965, of predictors of health and functioning in a representative sample of adults in Alameda County, California. Table 3.9 shows risk factor patterns at two points in time: first at the baseline examination in 1965, and then 29 years later among those cohort members who had not died or been lost to follow up. These data show the reversal in socioeconomic gradients in smoking that occurred in the latter half of the twentieth century. It is interesting that even though the adult socioeconomic pattern of smoking changed from being more common among the well off to being more common among lower socioeconomic groups, at every level of adult socioeconomic position those from poorer backgrounds had higher smoking exposures. Thus, if we look within the high income group in 1965, those from manual backgrounds had an average of 13.9 pack years of smoking compared with 12.0 pack years for those from non-manual backgrounds. The same is true in 1994,

Table 3.9 Father's occupation, adult income in 1965–1974 and age adjusted mean level of smoking, and odds ratios (95% confidence intervals) for lack of exercise, overweight, high alcohol consumption, and poor perceived health for women and men in the Alameda County study at baseline interview in 1965 ($n = 5707$, median age 35) and in 1994 ($n = 2381$, median age 64).

Father's occupation	Mean adult income 1965–1974	Smoking (pack yr)	Sedentary Low 25% physical activity	Overweight High 25% BMI	Alcohol consumption High 25%	Poor perceived health
At baseline interview (1965)						
Non-manual	High 25% (n = 467)	12·0	Reference	Reference	Reference	Reference
	Middle 50% (n = 400)	11·0	1·0 (0·82–1·21)	1·22 (1·0–1·50)	0·74 (0·61–0·90)	1·26 (0·98–1·62)
	Low 25% (n = 304)	8·8*	1·69 (1·39–2·06)	1·36 (1·1–1·67)	0·42 (0·33–0·53)	1·73 (1·36–2·21)
Manual	High 25% (n = 313)	13·9*	1·32 (1·08–1·1)	1·66 (1·35–2·4)	0·79 (0·64–0·96)	1·29 (1·0–1·66)
	Middle 50% (n = 368)	12·5	1·3 (1·07–1·58)	1·6 (1·31–1·95)	0·56 (0·46–0·69)	1·25 (0·97–1·60)
	Low 25% (n = 443)	9·9*	1·84 (1·52–2·21)	1·85 (1·52–2·25)	0·50 (0·41–0·62)	2·34 (1·86–2·94)
At follow up interview (1994)						
Non-manual	High 25% (n = 467)	12·9	Reference	Reference	Reference	Reference
	Middle 50% (n = 400)	16·2*	0·86 (0·63–1·17)	1·16 (0·84–1·61)	0·88 (0·66–1·18)	1·37 (0·94–2·0)
	Low 25% (n = 304)	14·8	1·14 (0·81–1·59)	1·53 (1·09–2·15)	0·3 (0·45–0·88)	1·57 (1·05–2·37)
Manual	High 25% (n = 313)	16·5*	1·2 (0·86–1·67)	1·59 (1·11–2·26)	0·58 (0·4–0·83)	1·73 (1·17–2·57)
	Middle 50% (n = 368)	16·9*	0·83 (0·61–1·14)	1·53 (1·12–2·10)	0·57 (0·42–0·78)	1·35 (0·92–1·98)
	Low 25% (n = 443)	19·3*	1·31 (0·95–1·79)	2·81 (2·06–3·85)	0·51 (0·37–0·71)	2·49 (1·71–3·61)

*Significantly different from reference category (non-manual + high income) in pairwise comparison ($p < 0.05$).

except by that time the adult socioeconomic patterning of smoking had completely reversed so that it was then more common among lower socioeconomic groups.

This is an illustration that having socioeconomic data from across the life course may provide useful information on heterogeneity of risk among adult socioeconomic groups, even under social conditions where powerful changes occur in the link between adult socioeconomic position and a risk factor. Those from poorer childhood backgrounds were at increased risk of smoking even under conditions where the adult socioeconomic patterning of smoking completely reversed. It is possible that family background and education may influence the initiation of smoking, while adult occupation and income may affect the age of stopping smoking. Similar effects have been observed for diet, where tastes for certain foods, such as consumption of fruit and salt, may be developed early in life but are subject to later modification based on adult socioeconomic influences.[57]

The results for other risk factors also reveal some life course socioeconomic effects. As the most advantaged socioeconomic group across the life course—the non-manual, high income group—are the reference category for the odds ratios (OR) presented, it is easy to compare this group with those from less advantaged backgrounds. Examining the high adult income group in 1965, there is evidence that those from manual homes had higher odds of being physically inactive (OR = 1.32), overweight (OR = 1.66), having poor perceived health (OR = 1.29), and of not being in the top 25% of alcohol consumers (OR = 0.79) in 1965. Similar patterns emerge in the 1994 data. It is also important to note that these patterns differ by sex. In data not shown here, the early life effects on overweight were especially strong among women, and the life course patterns of smoking somewhat more powerful among men.

Different patterns of association with lifetime socioeconomic conditions were also observed in a study of 13 854 people in the Netherlands.[58] In that study, lack of exercise and high body mass index showed both childhood and adult socioeconomic effects, while smoking was only influenced by adult socioeconomic position. Such direct international comparisons are potentially complicated by different time periods under study, the accuracy of the early life information (administrative records versus subject recall), selective survival, and the use of different socioeconomic indicators.

Evidence from the Kuopio Ischaemic Heart Disease Risk Factors Study in Finland (Table 3.10) shows very little overall socioeconomic variation in blood pressure and triglyceride levels among men aged 42–64 in 1989. It is only those men with the most disadvantaged lifetime socioeconomic position who have significantly higher blood pressure. Levels of fibrinogen showed strong patterning by current socioeconomic position (income) but no effects of father's occupation. For fibrinogen—a general acute phase inflammatory reactant—it might be expected that it would be most sensitive to contemporaneous socioeconomic position and underlying adult disease; however, in the Whitehall study fibrinogen was found to reflect both early and later life socioeconomic factors.[59] On the other hand, men with unskilled, manually employed fathers and high adult income had significantly higher levels of low density lipoprotein than men with similar adult incomes but from more advantaged homes.

Table 3.11 too presents data from the Kuopio study and shows how lifecourse socioeconomic indicators are associated with three important psychosocial risk factors: cynical hostility, hopelessness, and depression. The table gives β coefficients and standard errors estimated from a linear regression model with all socioeconomic indicators included in the model together and presented separately for each outcome. Cynical hostility, hopelessness, and depression have been associated with cardiovascular outcomes in population based samples.[60–63] The data presented here show how these important psychosocial risk factors are associated with an array of

35

Table 3.10   Father's occupation, adult income, and age adjusted mean levels of selected biological characteristics in 2549 men in the Kuopio Ischemic Heart Disease Risk Factor Study, 1989.

Father's occupation	Adult income	Systolic blood pressure (mmHg)	Plasma triglycerides mmol/L	LDL (mmol/L)	Fibrinogen (g/L)
Non-manual and skilled manual	High 25% ($n = 466$)	132·9	1·33	3·81	2·92
	Middle 50% ($n = 735$)	134·2	1·30	4·05*	3·02*
	Low 25% ($n = 343$)	134·7	1·33	4·13*	3·19*
Unskilled manual	High 25% ($n = 170$)	133·1	1·35	3·97*	2·92
	Middle 50% ($n = 531$)	133·4	1·27	4·10*	2·99*
	Low 25% ($n = 304$)	136·7	1·38	4·13*	3·17*

*Age adjusted means. (Different from reference category (non-manual and skilled manual/high) at $p < 0.05$.)
LDL, low density lipoprotein.

lifecourse socioeconomic indicators, including parental occupation and education, and the respondent's own education, occupation, and income. Variables cross-classifying mother's and father's occupation were hypothesised to represent "material resources" during childhood. Similarly, a variable cross-classifying maternal and paternal education was hypothesised to represent "intellectual resources" during childhood. Table 3.11 shows that adult levels of cynical hostility and hopelessness are both influenced by socioeconomic conditions at every stage of the life course. There are statistically independent effects of low parental education, the respondent's own low education, being a blue-collar worker, and having low income—even after simultaneously adjusting all these socioeconomic indicators. This suggests that these psychosocial risk factors (like some more traditional risk factors for CHD) may also have roots in early life. Furthermore, it clearly illustrates our earlier point about the potential for residual confounding. These analyses show that failure to adjust for each of these life course socioeconomic indicators may lead to residual socioeconomic confounding in an analysis focused on the association between cynical hostility or hopelessness on CHD that only adjusted for adulthood social circumstances. In contrast to the results for cynical hostility and hopelessness, the data for depression show that it is only associated with socioeconomic conditions in adulthood—current income and occupation.

In the West of Scotland study, blood pressure and lung function were associated with both current and parental social class, but more strongly with the former. This suggests that in this cohort, exposures—such as smoking and occupational exposures for lung function, or alcohol and

Table 3.11 Life course socioeconomic factors, cynical hostility, hopelessness, and depression in 2682 men in the Kuopio Ischemic Heart Disease Risk Factor Study, 1989.

	Cynical hostility (range = 23, median = 13, IQR = 5)	Hopelessness (Range = 8, median = 2, IQR = 3)	Depression (range = 13, median = 1, IQR = 3)
Parental occupation			
Father *Mother*			
High High	...	...	...
High Low	−0·213 (0·21)	0·029 (0·11)	−0·024 (0·11)
Low High	−0·580 (0·41)	0·269 (0·21)	0·160 (0·22)
Low Low	0·150 (0·19)	0·280 (0·10)**	0·063 (0·10)
Parental education			
Father *Mother*			
High High	...	...	...
High Low	0·293 (0·34)	0·292 (0·17)	0·133 (0·18)
Low High	−0·104 (0·26)	0·054 (0·13)	−0·050 (0·14)
Low Low	0·598 (0·20)**	0·401 (0·09)***	0·083 (0·10)
Individual education			
High	...	...	...
Low	0·425 (0·20)*	0·215 (0·09)*	−0·118 (0·10)
Individual occupation			
White-collar	...	...	...
Farmer	−0·328 (0·25)	0·377 (0·12)**	−0·118 (0·13)
Blue-collar	0·961 (0·20)***	0·698 (0·09)***	0·338 (0·10)**
Individual income			
Top 75%	...	...	...
Bottom 25%	0·882 (0·20)***	0·716 (0·10)***	0·593 (0·11)***

Values are age adjusted parameter estimates (standard error).
"High" parental occupation includes white collar and skilled manual workers, while "low" includes unskilled manual workers. "High" education includes those completing at least primary school, while "low" includes those not completing primary school.
IQR, inter-quartile range. $*p<0·05$, $**p<0·01$, $***p<0·001$.

other dietary factors for blood pressure—are more dependent upon adult than childhood social circumstances. Body mass index and triglyceride levels, on the other hand, were dependent on childhood social class rather than current social class: men with fathers of manual social class had higher body mass indices and higher triglyceride levels than men with non-manual fathers, and once father's social class was taken into account there was no association of current social class with body mass index and a reverse association for triglycerides—i.e. higher triglyceride levels among the men in non-manual rather than manual occupations in adulthood.[64] High body mass index and elevated triglyceride levels are components of the insulin resistance syndrome. This is compatible with some studies indicating that the concomitants of adverse childhood socioeconomic circumstances are

37

associated with an elevated risk of diabetes and impaired glucose tolerance in adulthood.[65,66] The components of insulin resistance syndrome cluster in childhood,[67,68] and this clustering tracks into adulthood. This suggests that a common factor, already active in young childhood, underlies the risk of insulin resistance syndrome from early life onwards.

There is evidence that some, but not all, conventional risk factors measured in adulthood are influenced by childhood socioeconomic circumstances and that this patterning may be subject to temporal and place variation. In the West of Scotland study the CHD differentials according to father's social class were attenuated, but not abolished, by adjustment for adult risk factors,[69] suggesting that outcomes of social environment in childhood could have a longterm influence on CHD risk in adulthood. In the Boyd Orr cohort, leg length in childhood—an indicator of growth and nutritional status—was inversely associated with risk of CHD mortality occurring over the subsequent 60 years.[70] Infections acquired in childhood could also increase the risk of CHD many years later.[71,72] Socioeconomic position in childhood is also related to birthweight, with there being lower birthweights on average among those born into a less favourable social environment, and several studies have found low birthweight to be related to increased CHD risk.[10] Childhood and gestational social circumstances could clearly contribute to socioeconomic differentials in CHD.

The development of CHD risk over the life course

The long incubation period for CHD has been recognised for many years,[73] and a life course approach to its aetiology is a natural extension of this view. In this discussion we have focused on studies for which the main focus is the social patterning of CHD risk. However, most of the important risk factors identified for CHD are socially patterned. The following factors are putative CHD risk factors or are of particular interest from a life course perspective, according to their period of influence:

- maternal health, development, and diet before and during pregnancy
- parental history of CHD
- Low birthweight
- socioeconomic deprivation from childhood onwards
- stress from childhood onwards
- poor growth in childhood
- short leg length in childhood
- obesity in childhood
- certain infections acquired in childhood
- diet from childhood onwards
- blood pressure in late adolescence
- serum cholesterol level in late adolescence
- smoking from late adolescence onwards
- little physical activity from late adolescence onwards

- blood pressure in adulthood
- serum cholesterol level in adulthood
- obesity in adulthood
- job insecurity and unemployment in adulthood
- short stature in adulthood
- binge alcohol drinking in adulthood
- diabetes and components of syndrome X in adulthood
- elevated levels of fibrinogen and other acute phase reactants in adulthood
- certain infections acquired in adulthood.

It is clear that CHD can be considered the archetype of diseases whose determinants should be sought across the entire life course: from conditions existing at the time of conception and during intrauterine development, through nutrition, growth and health in childhood, to social conditions, occupation, diet, physical activity and smoking throughout adult life. In Table 3.12 we combine a marker of early life circumstances 'father's social class' and behavioural and socioeconomic factors acting in adulthood, and demonstrate their joint influence on CHD mortality. If factors acting at different stages of life—such as childhood social circumstances, education, deprivation, level of area of residence in adulthood, adulthood occupational social class, and smoking and drinking in adulthood—are combined, then large differences in cardiovascular disease risk can be observed.[74] Socioeconomic inequalities in CHD can only be understood through consideration of how a variety of exposures that increase CHD risk are influenced by social circumstances; how this social dependence leads to them clustering across time, such that some individuals are adversely influenced by a wide array of risk factors; and thus how the accumulation of—and interaction between—influences acting at different stages of life determines the pattern of CHD within and between populations.

Table 3.12 Age adjusted relative rates of CHD mortality by father's social class and later life risk factors in the West of Scotland Collaborative Study.

	Father's social class	
	Non-manual	Manual
Smoking		
Other	1	1·56 (1·18–2·07)
Current cigarette	2·01 (1·46–2·77)	2·78 (2·12–3·63)
Alcohol		
< 15 units/wk	1	1·44 (1·18–1·75)
≥ 15 units/wk	1·17 (0·80–1·70)	1·86 (1·50–2·31)
Screening social class		
Non-manual	1	1·46 (1·18–1·82)
Manual	1·53 (1·06–2·21)	1·78 (1·45–2·17)

Reinterpreting explanations for CHD inequalities according to adulthood social position

The contribution of adult cardiovascular risk factors

A greater body of research has investigated the contribution of particular health related behaviours and physiological risk factors to CHD mortality differentials according to adult, as opposed to childhood, socioeconomic position. One of the first studies with objective data on coronary heart disease incidence, which demonstrated higher rates among men with lower income,[75] investigated this through comparing blood pressure levels, cholesterol concentrations, obesity, and smoking patterns of higher and lower income groups. Only small differences in these factors were found between income groups, and they did not appear able to account for the differences in disease incidence.[76] The risk factor data did not relate to the individuals experiencing coronary heart disease events in this study, however, so a direct assessment of their contribution to socioeconomic differentials could not be made.

In the first Whitehall study much of the large gradient in CHD mortality risk according to employment grade could not be accounted for by differences in smoking behaviour, blood pressure, plasma cholesterol, body mass index or CHD existing at the time of study entry.[77] Similarly a prospective study of a third of a million men screened for the Multiple Risk Factor Intervention Trial between 1970 and 1973, with 16 years of mortality follow up, found a strong inverse association between the income level of the area of residence of the men and their risk of mortality from coronary heart disease and stroke.[78,79] While adjustment for smoking, cholesterol levels, blood pressure, and diabetes somewhat attenuated these associations, it did not remove them. Prospective studies from Sweden, Finland, Denmark, and the USA, using a variety of indices of social position, have reached essentially the same conclusions for both men and women.[25]

It has been suggested that the residual associations seen between social class and coronary heart disease incidence are due to the inaccuracy inherent in using single measurements of risk factors as proxy measures of lifetime exposure.[80] While measurement imprecision in these factors renders the exploration of causes of differentials problematic,[81] it is also the case that the use of social class alone leads to a marked underestimation of the strength of the relationship between socioeconomic position and mortality.[27] Studies with more precise classification of socioeconomic circumstances demonstrate much greater differentials than those using cruder measures, such as occupational class in adulthood alone. Studies with precise measurement of life course socioeconomic position and risk factors are required to take this issue forward. In the West of Scotland study, for example, the substantial differentials in cardiovascular mortality according to lifetime social circumstances was little altered by adjustment for a wide range of behavioural and physiological risk factors measured in adulthood.[82]

A study of Finnish men constitutes the most detailed prospective investigation of factors contributing to the socioeconomic gradient in cardiovascular mortality undertaken to date.[83] The risk of all cause and cardiovascular disease mortality across quintiles of adulthood income showed two and a half to threefold differences. It was possible to adjust for 22 risk factors: plasma fibrinogen, serum high density lipoprotein cholesterol, serum apolipoprotein B, blood leucocytes, serum copper, mercury in hair, serum ferritin, blood haemoglobin, serum triglycerides, systolic blood pressure, body mass index, height, cardiorespiratory fitness, cigarette smoking, alcohol consumption, leisure time physical activity, depression, hopelessness, cynical hostility, participation in organisations, quality of social support, and marital status.[83] After adjustment, the association between social position and cardiovascular disease mortality was greatly attenuated, while the associations between social position and all (fatal and non-fatal) coronary heart disease incidence remained substantial. As the authors acknowledge, it is difficult to interpret such analyses, for several reasons. First, some of the factors adjusted for may be markers of disease presence (for example, blood leucocytes, fibrinogen), and statistical adjustment for these could, in essence, be adjusting for the presence of cardiovascular disease, which is itself produced by social factors. The reduction in relative risks in the lower income groups which occurs on adjustment for these factors cannot be taken as demonstrating the "explanation" of why the social distribution of cardiovascular mortality exists. Second, some factors (for example, height, body mass index, serum triglycerides) may be the outcome of socioeconomic processes that act in early life. Adjusting for them similarly fails to account for the reasons for the social distribution in cardiovascular mortality, since it automatically leads to questions as to how childhood social conditions may influence insulin resistance syndrome and thus coronary disease risk. Finally, as we have discussed earlier, the reasons for the social distribution of certain behaviours (for example, smoking and exercise) itself should become a target for explanation.

Adult socioeconomic position as a measure of life course social trajectories

An important implication of the life course perspective on the socioeconomic distribution of CHD in adulthood is that differences in disease rates between adulthood socioeconomic groups could, at least in part, be generated by their earlier life socioeconomic trajectories. This has important implications for the interpretation of the distribution of CHD risk in adulthood. In particular, the finding that CHD risk is not simply elevated among the poor but demonstrates a finely graded association with social position has been taken to suggest that material circumstances alone cannot underlie the differentials.[84,85] The Whitehall study has been particularly influential here. This study recruited civil servants in London to a prospective investigation of cardiovascular disease risk factors and found a strong inverse gradient between employment level and CHD mortality (Table 3.13). The mortality rate is lower in the administrative grade civil servants than in the professional/executive civil servants. Since professional/executive grade civil servants are clearly not suffering from the effects of contemporaneous poverty it has been suggested that psychological factors, generated by internalisation of position within the social hierarchy, must be the important determinants of differentials continuing into the higher end of the socioeconomic spectrum.[86] Table 3.13, however, demonstrates that there are clear differences in height by civil service employment grade, and since height is determined in childhood and is strongly influenced by socioeconomic factors, it is clear that the professional/executive group experienced more childhood deprivation than the administrators.

Another potential effect of early life is reflected in lung function measurements, with early life environment being known to influence adulthood lung function.[87] Obesity in adulthood is, as we have seen, a reflection of childhood social circumstances,[88] and car ownership was an indicator of wealth, accumulated across the life course in part from parental gifts and inheritance. A comprehensive survey of the social origins of civil servants was conducted around the time the Whitehall study was established.[89] This demonstrated that around three-quarters of administrative grade civil servants had fathers in social class I and II occupations, as opposed to 34% of executive grade and 23% of clerical grade civil servants. Conversely, virtually no administrative grade civil servants had fathers who were semiskilled or unskilled manual workers, whereas 15% of executive grade and 22% of clerical grade employees did so. Only around 1 in 10 administrative grade civil servants had skilled manual fathers, whereas a third of executive grade and nearly 40% of clerical grade civil servants had fathers in these occupations. It is clear that the social origins—and therefore the social

Table 3.13 Employment grade and associated factors in the Whitehall study.

	Administrators	Professional and executive	Clerical	Other
CHD mortality				
10 years (% dead)	2·2	3·6	4·9	6·6
25 years*	6·4	7·3	9·1	10·1
Smokers	28·8	37·3	53·0	60·9
Height (cm)	178·5	176·3	174·0	173·2
FEV$_1$ (height adjusted)	3·25	3·18	2·95	2·89
BMI > 28 kg/m^2(%)	10	12	14	17
Car ownership (%)	91	82	39	34
Stomach cancer*	0·16	0·29	0·46	0·57

* Mortality per 1000 person years.
BMI, body mass index; FEV$_1$, forced expiratory volume in 1 second.
Source: Marmot et al. (1984),[90] Davey Smith et al. (1990),[27] van Rossum CTM et al. (2000),[106] Davey Smith et al. (1991).[94]

circumstances in early life—of the administrative grade and other grades of civil servants vary considerably. Whereas very few administrative grade civil servants would have experienced deprivation in childhood, a higher proportion of executive and clerical grade civil servants would have done so.

The existence of a socioeconomic gradient in CHD mortality among predominantly middleclass groups, such as the civil servants in the Whitehall study,[90] has, as mentioned above, been widely cited as evidence that psychological factors, generated by internalisation of position within social hierarchies, must be important, since there is a low prevalence of material deprivation in adulthood among these groups.[84,91,92] While these adult psychosocial factors may well have a role, the socioeconomic gradient in cardiovascular disease among middleclass adults could also be generated by deprivation in childhood, which will have been almost entirely absent amongst the most privileged social groups (such as the administrative level civil servants) but will have been experienced by a proportion of other middleclass groups in less favoured adulthood social locations. This hypothesis is supported by the Glasgow University students' study, where childhood social circumstances strongly influenced CVD mortality in a relatively homogeneously affluent population.

In this regard, it is interesting that the several causes of death that show strong and graded associations with civil service employment grade, including lower rates among administrators than professional/executive civil servants, are causes of death known to be related to childhood deprivation. For example, stomach cancer mortality (Table 3.13) is strongly related to deprivation in childhood,[33,93] presumably because of *Helicobacter pylori* infection acquired in childhood, and is also strongly related to employment grade.[94]

The data showing that height is inversely related to CHD risk in the Whitehall study were interpreted as indicating a possible influence of childhood environment on adult cardiovascular disease risk.[77] Adjustment for socioeconomic measures in adulthood accounted for some, but not all, of this association.[27,77,90] Little of the socioeconomic gradient in cardiovascular disease was attributable to height.[27,90] The degree to which the indicators of exposure—on the one hand height as an indicator of a variety of potential early life exposures, and on the other hand employment grade and car ownership as indicators of socially patterned adult experiences—will influence the extent to which one or other measure appears more strongly associated to health outcomes.[21] This reinforces the need for studies with valid and detailed data collected at all stages of the life course. The specificity of associations between exposure measures and various health outcomes can also help here.[93] For example, height is inversely associated with CHD, stroke, respiratory disease, and stomach cancer risk,[95] all known to be related to early life exposures,[93] but not to lung cancer risk—even though the latter is strongly related to adult socioeconomic circumstances, mainly through a strongly socially patterned risk factor, smoking.

Childhood influences on adult socioeconomic differentials in health will, of course, include the outcomes of psychosocial experiences in childhood.

For example, smoking in adulthood is related to a group of childhood experiences including emotional, physical, and sexual abuse, parental separation or divorce, and growing up with a substance abusing, mentally ill, or incarcerated household member.[96] There is also evidence that such factors influence later health status,[97] including the health of future generations through adverse influences on birth outcomes among women. A life course approach to chronic disease in adulthood must consider the full range of material and psychosocial factors acting across the life course, which may be precursors of disease onset.

Conceptualising social inequalities within a life course perspective

The life course approach to chronic disease in adulthood—and therefore the life course approach to socioeconomic inequalities in the distribution of chronic disease in adulthood—attempts to move on from an epidemiology that concentrates on risk factors acting in a supposedly independent manner among individuals. This search for independent contributors to risk is in part an outcome of the underlying model of disease causation, captured in the well known metaphor of the "web of causation".[98] While the idea of a complex web of causal components is certainly useful, it is atemporal and ignores the fact that what we observe at any one point in time as an array of adult risk factors is the result of interlacing chains of biological and social exposures that have coevolved over time. In this way the life course approach addresses the recent debate regarding the individualistic focus of much epidemiology, which concentrates on the lifestyles or physiological risk factor profiles of people abstracted from their social context.[98–100] The many weaknesses of epidemiological approaches, which fail to locate exposure–disease associations within their historical, political, and social context, have been convincingly elaborated.[101] Perhaps less widely acknowledged is that the abstraction of such associations from their particular context can lead to severely misleading conclusions.

Consider the example mentioned earlier of the extensive research on β-carotene consumption and the risk of cardiovascular disease. Observational studies revealed strong apparently protective effects of β-carotene, but longterm randomised controlled trials found that, if anything, β-carotene increased cardiovascular disease risk (see Figure 3.1).[102] There are now a series of similar examples: hormone replacement therapy, vitamin E and vitamin C intake in relation to cardiovascular disease among them. What these examples have in common is that the groups of people who were apparently receiving protection from these substances in the observational studies were very different from the groups not using them, on a whole host of characteristics of their lives. Believing that these differences could be summed up in measures of a few "potential confounders" and adequately adjusted for in statistical analyses fails to recognise the complexity of the reasons why people differ with regard to particular and general characteristics

44

of their lives. It would be gratifying if the refutation of observational studies by randomised controlled trial evidence in these areas led to a critical evaluation of approaches that abstract single elements of people's lives—which are almost always behavioural, psychological, or therapeutic—from the complexity of the life and times of people, and relate these to single health outcomes. This would be preferable to the mobilisation of auxiliary hypotheses to explain each apparent "mistake" on a case by case basis.

A life course approach does not attempt to abstract individual life trajectories from their contexts[7]; indeed, the longterm and sometimes irreversible outcomes of social circumstances at different stages of life are seen as becoming literally embodied.[103] Human bodies and minds in different social locations become crystallised reflections of the social experiences within which they have developed. The socially patterned nutritional, health, and environmental experiences of parents and self influence birthweight, height, weight, and lung function, for example, which are in turn important indicators of future health prospects. These biological and psychological aspects of bodies (and the histories of bodies) should be viewed as frozen social relations, rather than as asocial explanations of health inequalities which, once accepted, exclude the social from consideration.[103] The life course approach to health inequalities views the physical and the social as being mutually constitutive, since aspects of bodily form can influence social trajectory in the same way as social experiences become embodied. Low birthweight, growth in childhood (and final adult height), persistent infections acquired in early life (with organisms such as *H. pylori*), or the failure to acquire certain infections (leading to immunological programming increasing the risk of atopy), lung function, degree of adiposity, a habitus that embraces particular dispositional characteristics (including attitudes, health related behaviours and mood), modes of self presentation, and ways of dealing with misfortune, may seem to fall within different categories, but they are all essential components of life trajectories that influence health. An epidemiology that appreciates the necessary interconnections between these different domains of life will avoid the dead ends to which research strategies based on abstraction and narrowing the focus of attention can lead.

Acknowledgements

John Lynch was supported by research grant HD35120-01A2 from the National Institute of Child Health and Development, and the National Institute of Ageing. Part of this work was facilitated by the European Science Foundation's Programme on Social Variations in Health Expectancy.

References

1 Marmot MG, Davey Smith G, Stansfeld S *et al*. Health inequalities among British civil servants: the Whitehall II study. *Lancet* 1991;**337**:1387–94.

2 Eachus J, Williams M, Chan P *et al.* Deprivation and Cause-Specific Morbidity: Evidence from the Somerset and Avon Survey of Health. *BMJ* 1996;**312**:287–92.

3 Lynch J, Kaplan GA, Salonen R, Cohen RD, Salonen JT. Socioeconomic status and carotid atherosclerosis. *Circulation* 1995;**92**:1786–92.

4 Lynch JW, Kaplan GA, Cohen RD, Salonen R, Salonen JT. Socioeconomic status and progression of carotid atherosclerosis: Prospective evidence from the Kuopio Ischemic Heart Disease Risk Factor Study. *Arteriosclerosis Thromb Vasc Biol* 1997;**17**:513–19.

5 Colhoun HM, Rubens MB, Underwood SR, Fuller JH. Cross sectional study of differences in coronary artery calcification by socioeconomic status. *BMJ* 2000;**321**:1262–3.

6 Ciocco A, Klein H, Palmer CE. Child health and the selective service physical standards. *Public Health Rep* 1941;**56**:2365–75.

7 Kuh D, Ben-Shlomo Y, eds. *A life course approach to chronic disease epidemiology.* Oxford: OUP, 1997.

8 Austin MA. Genetic epidemiology of dyslipidaemia and atherosclerosis. *Ann Med* 1996;**28**:459–63.

9 Davey Smith G, Hart C Ferrell C, *et al.* Birth weight of offspring and mortality in the Renfrew and Paisley Study: prospective observational study. *BMJ* 1997;**315**:1189–93.

10 Barker DJP. *Mothers, babies and health in later life.* Edinburgh: Churchill Livingstone, 1998.

11 Gunnell D, Davey Smith G, Frankel S, *et al.* Childhood leg length and adult mortality: follow up of the Carnegie (Boyd Orr) Survey of Diet and Health in Pre-War Britain. *J Epidemiol Community Health* 1998;**52**:142–52.

12 Davey Smith G, Hart C, Hole D, *et al.* Education and occupational social class: which is the more important indicator of mortality risk? *J Epidemiol Community Health* 1998;**52**:153–60.

13 Frankel S, Davey Smith G, Gunnell D. Childhood socioeconomic position and adult cardiovascular mortality: the Boyd Orr cohort. *Am J Epidemiol* 1999;**150**:1081–4.

14 McCarron P, Davey Smith G. Raised blood pressure, height, weight, blood lipid levels and other physiological measurements in children and adolescents and risk of CHD in adults. London: National Heart Forum, 2001.

15 DHSS. *Inequalities in health.* Report of a research working group chaired by Sir Douglas Black. London: DHSS, 1980.

16 Ebrahim S, Davey Smith G. Systematic review of randomised controlled trials of multiple risk factor interventions for preventing coronary heart disease. *BMJ* 1997;**314**:1666–74.

17 Ebrahim S, Davey Smith G. Health promotion for coronary heart disease: past, present and future. *Eur Heart J* 1998;**19**:1751–7.

18 Shaw GB. *The doctor's dilemma.* London: Constable, 1911.

19 Shaw GB. Everybody's *political what's what?* London: Constable, 1944.

20 Nyyssönen K, Parviainen MT, Salonen R, Tuomilehto J, Salonen JT. Vitamin C deficiency and risk of myocardial infarction: prospective population study of men from eastern Finland. *BMJ* 1997;**314**:634–8.

21 Phillips A, Davey Smith G. How independent are "independent" effects? Relative risk estimation when correlated exposures are measured imprecisely. *J Clin Epidemiol* 1991;**44**:1223–31.

22 Phillips AN, Davey Smith G. Bias in relative odds estimation owing to imprecise measurement of correlated exposures. *Stat Med* 1992;**11**:953–61.

23 Marmot MG, Bosma H, Hemingway H, Brunner E, Stansfeld S. Contribution of job control and other risk factors to social variations in coronary heart disease incidence. *Lancet* 1997;**350**:235–9.

24 Karasek R, Theorell T. *Healthy Work.* New York: Basic Books, 1990.

25 Davey Smith G. Socioeconomic differentials. In: Kuh D, Ben-Shlomo Y, eds. *A life course approach to chronic disease epidemiology.* Oxford: OUP, 1997.

26 Davey Smith G, Harding S. Is control at work the key to socioeconomic gradients in mortality? *Lancet* 1997;**350**:1369–70.

27 Davey Smith G, Shipley MJ, Rose G. Magnitude and causes of socioeconomic differentials in mortality: further evidence from the Whitehall study. *J Epidemiol Community Health* 1990;**44**:265–70.

28 Marks RU. A review of empirical findings. *Milbank Mem Fund Q* 1967;**45**:51–107.

29 Forsdahl A. Are poor living conditions in childhood and adolescents an important risk factor for arteriosclerotic heart disease? *Br J Prev Soc Med* 1977;**31**:91–5.

30 Forsdahl A. Living conditions in childhood and subsequent development of risk factors for arteriosclerotic heart disease. *J Epidemiol Community Health* 1978;**32**:34–7.

31 Barker DJP, Osmond C. Infant mortality, childhood nutrition, and ischaemic heart disease in England and Wales. *Lancet* 1986;**i**:1077–81.
32 Arnesen E, Forsdahl A. The Tromso heart study: coronary risk factors and their association with living conditions during childhood. *J Epidemiol Community Health* 1985;**39**:210–14.
33 Davey Smith G, Hart C, Blane D, Hole D. Adverse socioeconomic conditions in childhood and cause-specific adult mortality: prospective observational study. *BMJ* 1998;**316**:1631–5.
34 Burr ML, Sweetnam PM. Family size and paternal unemployment in relation to myocardial infarction. *J Epidemiol Community Health* 1980;**34**:93–5.
35 Notkola V, Punsar S, Karvonen MJ, Haapakaski J. Socioeconomic conditions in childhood and mortality and morbidity caused by coronary heart disease in adulthood in rural Finland. *Soc Sci Med* 1985;**21**:517–23.
36 Wannamethee SG, Whincup PH, Shaper G, Walker M. Influence of fathers' social class on cardiovascular disease in middle-aged men. *Lancet* 1996;**348**:1259–63.
37 Blane D, Hart CL, Davey Smith G, Gillis CR, Hole DJ, Hawthorne VM. The association of cardiovascular disease risk factors with socioeconomic position during childhood and during adulthood. *BMJ* 1996;**313**:1434–8.
38 Gliksman MD, Kawachi I, Hunter D, *et al*. Childhood socioeconomic status and risk of cardiovascular disease in middle aged US women: a prospective study. *J Epidemiol Community Health* 1995;**49**:10–15.
39 Kaplan GA, Salonen JT. Socioeconomic conditions in childhood and ischaemic heart disease during middle age. *BMJ* 1990;**301**:1121–3.
40 Vagero D, Leon D. Effect of social class in childhood and adulthood on adult mortality. *Lancet* 1994;**343**:1224–5.
41 Gillum RF, Paffenbarger RS. Chronic disease in former college students. XVII Sociocultural mobility as a precursor of coronary heart disease and hypertension. *Am J Epidemiol* 1978;**108**:289–98.
42 Hasle H. Association between living conditions in childhood and myocardial infarction. *BMJ* 1990;**300**:512–3.
43 Lynch JW, Kaplan GA, Cohen RD, *et al*. Childhood and adult socioeconomic status as predictors of mortality in Finland. *Lancet* 1994;**343**:524–7.
44 Marmot M, Shipley M, Brunner E, Hemingway H. Relative contribution of early life and adult socioeconomic factors to adult mortality in the Whitehall II study. *J Epidemiol Community Health* 2001;**55**:301–7.
45 Wamala SP, Lynch JW, Kaplan GA. Women's exposure to early and later life socioeconomic disadvantage and coronary heart disease risk. *Int J Epidemiol* 2001;**30**:275–84.
46 Valkonen T. Male mortality from ischaemic heart disease in Finland, relation to region of birth and region of residence. *Eur J Popul* 1987;**3**:61–83.
47 Koskinen S. *Origins of regional differences in mortality from ischaemic heart disease in Finland*. National Research and Development Centre for Welfare and Health Research Report 41. Helsinki: NAWH, 1994.
48 Davey Smith G, McCarron P, Okasha M, McEwen J. Social circumstances in childhood and cardiovascular disease mortality: prospective observational study of Glasgow university students. *J Epidemiol Community Health* 2001;**55**:340–1.
49 McCarron P, Davey Smith G, Okasha M, McEwen J. Life course exposure and later disease: a follow-up study based on medical examinations carried out in Glasgow University (1948-68). *Public Health* 1999;**113**:265–71.
50 *Higher Education* (Robbins Report; Cmnd. 2154). London: HMSO, 1963.
51 Blane D, Davey Smith G, Bartley M. Social selection: what does it contribute to social class differences in health? *Sociol Health Illness* 1993;**15**:1–15.
52 Hart CL, Davey Smith G, Blane D. Social mobility and 21 year mortality in a cohort of Scottish men. *Soc Sci Med* 1998;**47**:1121–30.
53 Brunner E, Shipley MJ, Blane D, Davey Smith G, Marmot MG. When does cardiovascular risk start? Past and present socioeconomic circumstances and risk factors in adulthood. *J Epidemiol Community Health* 1999;**53**:757–64.
54 Graham H, Hunt K. Socioeconomic influences on women's smoking status in adulthood: insights from the West of Scotland Twenty-07 study. *Health Bull* 1998;**56**:757–65.
55 Graham H, Der G. Influences on women's smoking status. The contribution of socioeconomic status in adolescence and adulthood. *Eur J Public Health* 1999;**9**:137–41.
56 Anderson C, Burns DM. Patterns of adolescent smoking initiation rates by ethnicity and sex. *Tobacco Control* 2000;**9**(suppl. 2):ii4–8.

57 Lynch JW. Socioeconomic factors in the behavioral and psychosocial epidemiology of cardiovascular disease. In: Schneiderman N, Gentry J, da Silva JM, Speers M, Tomes H, eds. *Integrating Behavioral and Social Sciences with Public Health.* Washington: APA Press, 2000.

58 Van de Mheen H, Stronks K, Looman CWN, Mackenbach J. Does childhood socioeconomic status influence adult health through behavioural factors? *Int J Epidemiol* 1998;**27**:431–7.

59 Brunner E, Davey Smith G, Marmot M, Canner R, Beksinska M, O'Brien J. Childhood social circumstances and psychosocial and behavioural factors as determinants of plasma fibrinogen. *Lancet* 1996;**347**:1008–13.

60 Everson SA, Goldberg DE, Kaplan GA, Cohen RD, Pukkala E, Tuomilehto J, Salonen JT. Hopelessness and risk of mortality and incidence of myocardial infarction and cancer. *Psychosom Med* 1996;**58**:113–21.

61 Everson SA, Kaplan GA, Goldberg DE, Salonen R, Salonen JT. Hopelessness and 4-year progression of carotid atherosclerosis: The Kuopio Ischemic Heart Disease Risk Factor Study. *Arteriosclerosis, Thromb Vasc Biol* 1997;**17**:1490–5.

62 Everson SA, Kauhanen J, Kaplan GA, *et al.* Hostility and increased risk of mortality and acute myocardial infarction: The mediating role of behavioral risk factors. *Am J Epidemiol* 1997;**146**:142–52.

63 Barefoot JC, Schroll M. Symptoms of depression, acute myocardial infarction, and total mortality in a community sample. *Circulation* 1996;**93**:1976–1980.

64 Davey Smith G, Hart C. Insulin resistance syndrome and childhood social conditions. *Lancet* 1997;**349**:284.

65 Lehingue Y. Fetal environment and coronary ischemia risk: review of the literature with particular reference to syndrome X. *Rev Epidemiol Sante Publique* 1996;**44**:262–77.

66 Alvarsson M, Efendic S, Grill VE. Insulin responses to glucose in healthy males are associated with adult height but not with birth weight. *J Intern Med* 1994;**236**:275–9.

67 Bao W, Srinivasan SR, Wattigney WA, Berenson GS. Persistence of multiple cardiovascular risk clustering related to syndrome X from childhood to young adulthood. *Arch Intern Med* 1994;**154**:1842–7.

68 Raitakari OT, Porkka KVK, Rdsdnen L, Rvnnemaa T, Viikari JSA. Clustering and six year cluster-tracking of serum total cholesterol, HDL-cholesterol and diastolic blood pressure in children and young adults. *J Clin Epidemiol* 1994;**47**:1085–93.

69 Davey Smith G, Hart C. Socioeconomic Factors and Determinants of Mortality. *JAMA* 1988;**280**:1744–5.

70 Gunnell DJ, Davey Smith G, Frankel S, *et al.* Childhood leg length and adult mortality: follow up of the Carnegie (Boyd Orr) Survey of Diet and Health in Pre-war Britain. *J Epidemiol Community Health* 1998;**52**:142–52.

71 Zhu J, Nieto J, Horne BD, Anderson JL, Muhlestein JB, Epstein SE. Prospective study of pathogen burden and risk of myocardial infarction or death. *Circulation* 2001;**103**:45–51.

72 Shah PK. Link between infection and atherosclerosis. Who are the culprits: viruses, bacteria, both, or neither? *Circulation* 2001;**103**:5–7.

73 Rose G. Incubation period of coronary heart disease. *BMJ* 1982;**284**:1600–1.

74 Davey Smith G, Hart C. Lifecourse socioeconomic and behavioural influences on cardiovascular disease mortality: the Collaborative study. *Am J Public Health* 2001 (in press).

75 Pell S, D'Alonzo CA, Del W. Myocardial infarction in a one-year industrial study. *JAMA* 1958;**166**:332–7.

76 Pell S, D'Alonzo CA. Blood pressure, body weight, serum cholesterol, and smoking habits among executives and non-executives. *J Occup Med* 1961;**3**:467–70.

77 Marmot MG, Rose G, Shipley M *et al.* Employment grade and coronary heart disease in British civil servants. *J Epidemiol Community Health* 1978;**32**:244–9.

78 Davey Smith G, Neaton JD, Wentworth D, Stamler R, Stamler J. Socioeconomic Differentials in Mortality Risk among Men Screened for the Multiple Risk Factor Intervention Trial: I. White Men. *Am J Public Health* 1996;**86**:486–96.

79 Davey Smith G, Wentworth D, Neaton JD, Stamler R, Stamler J. Socioeconomic Differentials in Mortality Risk among Men Screened for the Multiple Risk Factor Intervention Trial: II. Black Men. *Am J Public Health* 1996;**86**:497–504.

80 Pocock SJ, Shaper AG, Cook DG, Phillips AN, Walker M. Social class differences in ischaemic heart disease in British men. *Lancet* 1987;**ii**:197–201.

81 Davey Smith G, Phillips AN. Confounding in epidemiological studies: why "independent" effects may not be all they seem. *BMJ* 1992;**305**:757–9.

82 Davey Smith G, Hart C, Blane D, Gillis C, Hawthorne V. Lifetime socioeconomic position and mortality: prospective observational study. *BMJ* 1997;**314**:547–52.
83 Lynch JW, Kaplan GA, Cohen RD, Tuomilehto J, Salonen JT. Do known risk factors explain the relation between socioeconomic status, risk of all-cause mortality, cardiovascular mortality and acute myocardial infarction? *Am J Epidemiol* 1996;**144**:934–42.
84 Syme SL. To prevent disease: the need for a new approach. In: Blane D, Brunner E, Wilkinson R, eds. *Health and Social Organisation.* London: Routledge, 1996.
85 Marmot M. The social pattern of health and disease. In: Blane D, Brunner E, Wilkinson R, eds. *Health and Social Organisation.* London: Routledge, 1996.
86 Stewart-Brown S. What causes social inequalities in health and why is the question taboo? *Crit Public Health* 2000;**10**:233–42.
87 Mann SL, Wadsworth MEJ, Colley JRT. Accumulation of factors influencing respiratory illness in members of a national birth cohort and their offspring. *J Epidemiol Community Health* 1992;**46**:286–92.
88 Parsons TJ, Power C, Logan S, Summerbell CD. Childhood predictors of adult obesity: a systematic review. *Int J Obesity* 1999;**23**(suppl. 8):S1–107.
89 Kelly MP. *White-collar proletariat: the industrial behaviour of British civil servants.* London: Routledge & Kegan Hall, 1980.
90 Marmot MG, Shipley MJ, Rose G. Inequalities in death-specific explanations of a general pattern? *Lancet* 1984;**i**:1003–6.
91 Wilkinson RG. *Unhealthy societies: the afflictions of inequality.* London: Routledge, 1996.
92 Marmot MG, Bobak M. International comparators and poverty and health in Europe. *BMJ* 2000;**321**:1124–8.
93 Davey Smith G, Gunnell D, Ben-Shlomo Y. Life-course approaches to socioeconomic differentials in cause-specific adult mortality. In: Leon D, Walt G. *Poverty, Inequality and Health.* Oxford: OUP, 2000.
94 Davey Smith G, Leon D, Shipley MJ, Rose G. Socioeconomic differentials in cancer among men. *Int J Epidemiol* 1991;**20**:339–45.
95 Davey Smith G, Hart C, Upton M *et al.* Height and cause-specific mortality: aetiological implications of associations with cardiorespiratory and cancer mortality. *J Epidemiol Community Health* 2000;**54**:97–103.
96 Anda RF, Croft JB, Felitti VJ, *et al.* Adverse childhood experiences and smoking during adolescence and adulthood. *JAMA* 1999;**282**:1652–8.
97 Taylor SE, Repetti RL. Health Psychology: What is an unhealthy environment and how does it get under the skin? *Annu Rev Psychol* 1997;**48**:411–47.
98 Krieger N. Epidemiology and the web of causation: has anyone seen the spider? *Soc Sci Med* 1994;**39**:887–903.
99 Koopman JS, Lynch JW. Individual causal models and population system models in epidemiology. *Am J Public Health* 1999;**89**:1170–4.
100 Diez-Roux AV. Bringing context back into epidemiology: variables and fallacies in multilevel analysis. *Am J Public Health* 1998;**88**:216–22.
101 Schwartz S, Carpenter KM. The right answer for the wrong question: consequences of type III error for public health research. *Am J Public Health* 1999;**89**:1175–80.
102 Egger M, Schneider M, Davey Smith G. Spurious precision? Meta-analysis of observational studies. *BMJ* 1998;**316**:140–4.
103 Najman JM, Davey Smith G. The embodiment of class-related and health inequalities: Australian policies. *Aust NZ J Public Health* 2000;**24**:3–4.
104 Enos WF, Holmes RH, Beyer J. Coronary disease among United States soldiers killed in action in Korea. *JAMA* 1953;**152**:1090–3.
105 McNamara JJ, Molot MA, Stremple JF, Cutting RT. Coronary artery disease in combat casualties in Vietnam. *JAMA* 1971;**216**:1185–7.
106 Van Rossum CTM, Shipley MJ, van de Mheen H, Grobbee DE, Marmot MG. Employment grade differences in cause specific mortality. A 25 year follow up of civil servants from the first Whitehall study. *J Epidemiol Community Health* 2000;**54**:178–84.

4: Work and coronary heart disease

MICHAEL MARMOT, TORES THEORELL, AND
JOHANNES SIEGRIST

There is good evidence that psychosocial factors at work are related to risk of coronary heart disease and may play an important part in contributing to the social gradient in coronary heart disease. There have been a number of different approaches to measurement of work stress, and research more recently has tended to focus on a few explicit theoretical concepts. Among these, the models of job demand–control[1,2] and effort–reward imbalance[3,4] have received special attention.

A number of different diseases have been related to psychosocial conditions in the workplace, most notably coronary heart disease, musculoskeletal disorders, and mental illness. This chapter deals with two types of question: the relation between conditions at work and coronary heart disease; and the contribution this relationship may make to variations in disease in society.

Work and socioeconomic differences in coronary heart disease

Coronary heart disease in most industrialised countries is now more common in lower socioeconomic groups (reviewed by Marmot and Bartley in Chapter 2). The evidence suggests that this is a change and that formerly coronary heart disease was more common in high status groups. Indeed, writing in 1910, Osler noted coronary heart disease to be common in his patients of high socioeconomic status. He made reference to "pressure working the machine to its maximum capacity" and he talked of the typical coronary patient as one "the indicator of whose engine is always at full speed ahead".[5]

Osler's view was consistent with the common notion that people in high status jobs had more heart disease because such jobs were stressful. As stated above, the first part of this proposition may have been true: namely that coronary heart disease was more common in higher socioeconomic groups, although it is no longer. It is doubtful whether it was ever true that people in high status jobs were under more stress than people of low status. As this chapter will show, the modern concept of stress is, in general, more likely to be found lower down the social hierarchy.

Osler appeared to have been struck by this paradox. He wondered why coronary heart disease was apparently more common in men of high status if work and worry were major causes, as "worry and work are the lot and portion of the poor".

There is now a widely validated body of knowledge on risk factors for coronary heart disease that relates to development of atherosclerosis, and a somewhat less secure body of knowledge relating to predisposition to thrombosis. The major risk factors are high levels of blood pressure and plasma total cholesterol, and smoking. Although smoking, in particular, shows a strong social gradient,[6] these risk factors account for no more than a third of the social gradient in cardiovascular disease.[7,8] Similarly, smoking is high in many countries of central and eastern Europe and may relate to the high rates of cardiovascular disease,[9] but data from the international MONICA studies show that international variations in smoking, high blood pressure, and raised plasma cholesterol levels account for less than half of the international variation in coronary heart disease mortality rates.[10]

We are left then with two types of question. First, what accounts for the social and international variation in unhealthy behaviours such as atherogenic diet, smoking, and sedentary lifestyle? Second, given that these factors appear to be inadequate explanations of social and international variations in cardiovascular mortality, what else could account for the observed differences? We have argued elsewhere that one must look for explanations in the nature of social and economic organisation of societies.[11] One particular feature is the nature of working life, both because what happens in the workplace may be important for health, and because work and the operation of the labour market play a central role in the organisation of social and economic life, which in turn are important in the social determinants of health. The evidence that supports the importance of work for cardiovascular and other diseases is presented below.

The changing nature of work

There are at least four important reasons for the centrality of work and occupation in advanced industrialised societies. First, having a job is normally a prerequisite for a regular income. Level of income determines a wide range of life chances. Second, training for a job and achievement of occupational status are the most important goals of primary and secondary socialisation. It is through education, job training, and status acquisition that personal growth and development are realised, that a core social identity outside the family is acquired, and that intentional, goal directed activity in human life is shaped. Third, occupation defines a most important criterion of social stratification in advanced societies. Amount of esteem and social approval in interpersonal life largely depend on the type of job, professional training, and level of occupational achievement. Furthermore, type and quality of occupation, and especially the degree of self direction at work, strongly influence personal attitudes and behavioural patterns in areas that are not directly related to work, such as leisure, family life, education, and political activity.[12] Finally, occupational settings produce the most pervasive and continuous demands during one's lifetime, and they absorb the largest amount of active time in adult life. Exposure to adverse job conditions carries the risk of illness by virtue of the amount of time spent and the quality of demands faced at the workplace. At the same time, occupational settings provide unique opportunities to experience reward, esteem, success, and satisfaction. To understand the impact of working life on health in general, it is important to realise the profound changes that have taken place in the nature of work in established market economies. Among these are the following:

- fewer jobs are defined by physical demands; more by psychological and emotional demands
- fewer jobs are available in mass production, more in the service sector
- more jobs are concerned with information processing due to computerisation and automation.

These changes in the nature of work have gone along with changes in the nature of the labour market. There has been increasing participation of women in the labour market, an increase in short term and part-time working, and—most importantly—an increase in job instability and structural unemployment. For instance, Hutton describes Britain as the 40–30–30 society: 40% of the male population of working age have secure jobs, 30% are not working, and 30% are in insecure jobs.[13] The figure of 30% not working may cause some surprise, given that the official unemployment rate is around 8%. The 30% includes the officially unemployed, those no longer seeking work, those prematurely retired, and people with disabilities. If 30% of the male population of working age are in insecure jobs, this must have an effect on the rest of the working population, who must wonder if their job is next. This is a change. In Europe until relatively recently, there were national commitments to security of employment. Now, the rhetoric extols labour market flexibility.[14] The other side of flexibility is job insecurity.

The high percentage of people not working is not unique to Britain. In Finland, for example, the mean age of entry to the labour market is now 27 years and mean age of exit is 53. When the Finnish social contract was nationally agreed, the assumption was that working life would last 40 years. If it lasts 26 years on average, this has a profound importance for the costs of the welfare state. It also changes attitudes to work if a job for life is no longer a realistic expectation for large sections of the labour market. Research on work and health has to take this job insecurity into account, especially since loss of job was shown to be associated with elevated risk of mortality in independent prospective studies both in Britain and in Finland.[15,16]

This changing nature of work and the labour market has occurred at the same time as substantial increases in income inequalities in many countries.[17] Wilkinson has shown that, internationally, life expectancy is related more closely to income distribution than to overall wealth as measured by gross national product.[18] This has now been documented in two independent studies for the states of the USA.[19,20] If inequality, rather than absolute level of deprivation, is an important driver of health differentials, it may, as Wilkinson has suggested, be a reflection of the quality of the social environment. It may also suggest that discontent related to unfavourable social comparison (relative social deprivation) and associated stress reactions may have important health consequences.

The scientific challenge, then, consists of identifying the stress-eliciting conditions related to the nature of work, the structure of salaries (income distribution), and labour market constraints that may account for differences in morbidity and mortality that are reported within and between populations.

The psychosocial work environment

Research on psychosocial work-related stress differs from traditional biomedical occupational health research by the fact that stressors cannot be identified by direct physical or chemical measurements. Rather, theoretical concepts are needed to analyse the nature of work in order to identify particular stressful job characteristics at a level of generalisation that allows for their identification in a wide range of different occupations.

These theoretical concepts are operationalised using methods derived from the social and behavioural sciences such as systematic observation, structured interviews, and standardised questionnaires (the so-called "paper and pencil" tests). Therefore, measuring stressful working conditions provides a theoretical and methodological challenge. In theoretical terms, those components of working life need to be identified that produce intense, recurrent, and longlasting stressful experiences at least in a substantial proportion of those exposed. Moreover, researchers have to argue whether they should restrict their formulations to particular job characteristics, or whether they should analyse stressful work experience in terms of an interaction of work characteristics and of coping characteristics of the working person.

At a methodological level, measures of work stress are expected to be reliable, sensitive to change, and valid. Two theoretical models, the demand–control model and effort–reward imbalance model, fulfil these methodological criteria and identify stressful working conditions that are widely prevalent in advanced marked economies, such as changes in task profiles, work control, structure of salaries, and occupational stability. These two models have been tested in a number of studies, and a substantial body of knowledge has been generated, strengthening the assumption that stressful experiences at work are associated with elevated risk of coronary heart disease and other diseases.

The demand–control model

In the 1960s, research into job conditions and coronary heart disease explored working demands and working hours.[21] In the 1970s, several research traditions found evidence for a favourable effect on mental health produced by skill development[22] and autonomy at work.[12,23] Karasek's original contribution was to formulate a two-dimensional concept of work stress, in which a high level of psychological demands combined with a low level of decision latitude (low level of decision authority and low level of skill utilisation) was predicted to increase the risk of stressful experience and subsequent physical illness (in particular, coronary heart disease).[1] In 1981, Karasek first found evidence of a predictive role of high demand–low control conditions in coronary heart disease, using data on a representative Swedish sample.[24] Since then, many prospective and cross-sectional studies on associations of stressful work, as defined by high demand and low control (job strain), with cardiovascular risk and disease have been conducted (for overviews see references 2, 25–28). A number of these studies have focused on methodological considerations and have used new outcome measures, the majority of which have revealed positive findings.

Karasek's original hypothesis that excessive psychological demands interact with lack of decision latitude in generating increased risk of cardiovascular disease was supplemented by a second hypothesis, which concerned the learning of new patterns of behaviour and skills on the basis of psychosocial job experience. According to this, learning for adults accrues over a lifetime of work experience. It may contribute to workers' ability to exert control over their working situation and thus have an impact on broader conditions of adult life. According to this hypothesis, the "active" situation is associated with the development of a feeling of mastery, which inhibits the perception of strain during periods of overload, for instance. This makes it likely that "active" jobs may stimulate healthy functioning. Epidemiological studies in Sweden indicated that "active" jobs are associated with high rates of participation in socially active leisure and political activities,[2] and, conversely, the daily residual strain arising in "strain" jobs gives rise to accumulated feelings of frustration which may inhibit learning attempts. It is obvious that some of the classic high strain jobs are found in mass production, especially under conditions of piecework and machine-paced assembly line work. Nevertheless, a number of "strain" jobs have also been identified in the service sector. The concept, therefore, proves to be relevant in different employment sectors, and will remain important in the foreseeable future owing to changing patterns of employment. For example, the rate of temporary employment is increasing in western Europe, particularly for those with low education. It is in these kinds of employment that lack of control will be a major problem. Even in those with a high level of education, the increasing demands for flexibility will create new problems of decision latitude. The ever increasing demands for effectiveness from the workforce are raising the levels of psychological demands for all workers. This is particularly reflected in Swedish national welfare statistics.

The original demand–control concept has now been modified to include social support at work as a third dimension,[29] and to assess work control in a life course perspective "total job control exposure".[30] Another important innovation concerns the exploration of health effects produced by intervention studies based on the theoretical concept.[31–33] Theorell and colleagues are currently evaluating the effects of a case–control study aimed at improving the psychosocial skills of managers. Preliminary results suggest an improved work environment for employees of managers enrolled in the study, with higher reported decision latitude and lower cortisol levels after 1 year (T. Theorell, personal communication, 2000).

Evidence from studies

The importance of work related psychosocial factors to the development of ill health and disease can be illustrated from the Whitehall studies of British civil servants. The finding of dramatic differences in mortality by grade of employment in the first Whitehall study, which could not be explained by conventional risk factors alone,[8] led to the initiation of a second longitudinal study of civil servants—the Whitehall II study of 10 308 male and female civil servants. A major aim of this second study was to investigate occupational and other social influences on health and disease in a white-collar, office based population. In pursuing the work environment as a source of possible explanations, we have examined characteristics of the demand–control model. One hypothesis is that the lower the grade of employment in the civil service, the lower the level of control over the job, the lower the use of skills, and the higher the level of monotony. These may be related to the higher rate of cardiovascular and other diseases in lower employment grades. Initial analyses of the psychosocial work environment confirmed the above, with men and women in lower employment grades reporting lower levels of control, less varied work and use of skills, and a slower pace of work. Overall, fewer of the lower grades expressed themselves as satisfied with their work situation.[6]

The Whitehall II study has been studying psychosocial factors in relation to a range of health problems such as sickness absence, musculoskeletal and psychiatric disorders, and coronary heart disease. In analysing these health problems, the crucial task has been to separate the effects of work from those of other influences on health.

Psychosocial work characteristics and coronary heart disease

The design of the Whitehall II study is longitudinal, permitting assessment of the psychosocial work environment over a period of time and also its relationship to the development of new coronary heart disease. In addition to self reported measures, independent measures of the psychosocial work environment were used to address the question of whether job stress is influenced by subjective perceptions or by more objective appraisals of the work, or both. Both men and women with low control, either self reported or independently assessed, had a higher risk of new self reported coronary heart disease during a mean follow up period of 5 years (Figure 4.1). This association could not be explained by employment grade, negative affectivity, or classical coronary risk factors. Using the job strain model, it was found that job demands, social supports, and the interactions between work characteristics were not related to the risk of new coronary heart disease. Specific characteristics of this sample of white-collar workers may have contributed to this negative finding: high job demands were more common in higher employment grades, and high job demands and high job control were positively associated, resulting in comparatively few high strain jobs.[34]

In addition to Whitehall II, other studies have looked at the association of characteristics of the work environment to heart disease. The Swedish case–control study of over 2000 men and women, the Stockholm Heart Epidemiology Programme (SHEEP) has investigated the role of psychosocial and other factors in the development of myocardial infarction.

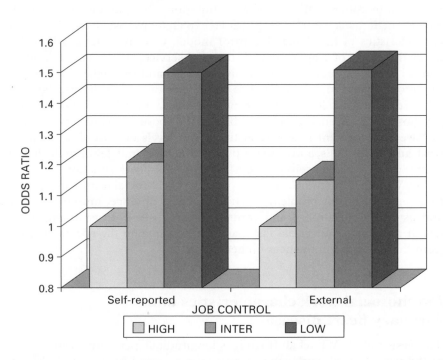

Figure 4.1 Five-year coronary heart disease incidence by self-reported and external job control for men and women in the Whitehall II study. From Bosma et al. (1997).[34]

Men who reported high demands and low control in their job were at greater risk of developing a myocardial infarction. This relationship was more pronounced for manual workers.[35] An investigation of the psychosocial work environment in the 10 years preceding myocardial infarction also showed that a decrease in the amount of control at work was associated with an increased risk of myocardial infarction. Again, this effect was stronger in manual workers and in men under 55 years of age (Figure 4.2).[36] Data from both the SHEEP and Whitehall II studies regarding loss of control and its possible effect on future risk of myocardial infarction illustrate that the increased risk does not develop rapidly after reported loss of control, but increases gradually over time. Thus, there may be a possibility of preventing myocardial infarction if individuals at risk can be identified within a specified period.

The different associations between aspects of the psychosocial work environment and coronary heart disease correspond to the review by Schnall and Landsbergis, in which 17 out of 25 studies found significant associations between job control and cardiovascular outcome, whereas associations with job demands were significant in only 8 out of 23 studies.[25] A further review of the role of psychosocial work characteristics and coronary heart disease has been conducted, using a quality filter to identify the best available evidence.[28] The filter included:

- a prospective population based design
- at least 500 participants (aetiological studies in healthy populations) or 100 participants (prognostic studies in coronary heart disease patient populations)

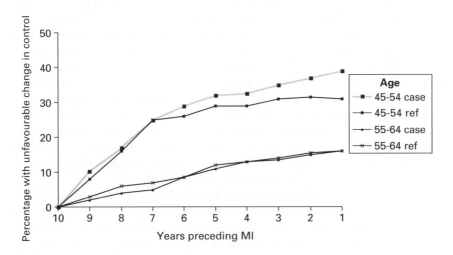

Figure 4.2 Percentage change in work control in years preceding myocardial infarction (MI) in the SHEEP Swedish case–control study. The vertical axis indicates the percentage in the least favourable quartile of change in control from 10 years to 1 year preceding MI. From Theorell et al. (1998).[36]

- instruments for exposure measurement used in two or more study populations
- fatal or validated non-fatal coronary heart disease as outcomes.

Table 4.1 shows that 6 of the 10 studies showed a positive association between aspects of the job strain model and coronary heart disease. The negative associations were possibly due to factors specific to the populations studied. For example, the studies by Reed et al.[37] and Suadicani et al.[38] studied men who were relatively old, particularly at the end of the follow up period when a large proportion had retired. The study by Hlatky et al.[39] was not a representative sample and there may have been other selection factors in operation in determining who underwent coronary angiography. Finally, the bus drivers studied by Netterstrom and Suadicani might have more reason than other workers to deny difficulties at work.[40] Other studies using observational techniques instead of self reports have confirmed this possibility.[41] It is likely that these results will influence the subsequent use and development of this theoretical model in future research studies. Improved measurement of the psychosocial work environment will lead to further methodological refinement of the model, and in particular for job demands, the issue of interaction within the job strain model warrants further investigation.[35]

Biological pathways linking job strain with coronary heart disease

Possible mechanisms behind the association between job strain and risk of myocardial infarction have been discussed extensively in several publications.[27,42] One biological finding which may prove to be consistent is that low job control is associated with elevated concentrations of plasma fibrinogen. The initial finding in the Whitehall I study has been replicated in the Whitehall II study.[43,44] An interesting aspect of the findings in the latter study was that the results were particularly strong after adjustment for several risk factors, and when job assessments based upon expert judgements were used. They were less strong when subjective assessments were used. These findings are similar to a case–control study in the SHEEP study in Stockholm.[45] After adjustments had been made, a clear relationship was observed between indirect assessments of (high) psychological demands and (low) control, and high plasma fibrinogen level.

One interpretation of these findings may be that job strain (in particular low control) is associated not so much with coronary atherosclerosis, but more with sudden triggering mechanisms (within seconds or minutes) such as clotting, which could give rise to a sudden block in a coronary artery or with mechanisms that cause semiacute deterioration of the condition of the myocardium (within weeks or months). It has been known for some time in physiology that longlasting energy mobilisation may inhibit the anabolic activities of the endocrine system, which may in turn affect the myocardium

Table 4.1 Psychosocial work characteristics and coronary heart disease.

Reference	Country	Total sample (% women)	Age at entry (yr)	Exposure	Follow up (yr)	Events (n)	Events: type	Adjustments	Relative risk	Summary +−
Prospective aetiological studies										
60	USA	876 (37)	45–64	Job control/demands (individual and ecological)	10	Not stated	Fatal CHD + non-fatal MI + coronary insufficiency + angina	Age, smoking, blood pressure, cholesterol	2·9 all women (clerical women RR = 5·2) No association in men Ecological exposure was associated with risk in men and women	+
61	Sweden	958 096 (51)	20–64	Hectic work and few possibilities for learning (ecological)	1	1201	Non-fatal MI (hospitalisation)	Age, 10 sociodemographic factors, smoking, heavy lifting	1·5*	+
62	Finland	902 (33) factory workers	20–62	Job control, physical strain, variety (individual)	10	60	Fatal CHD + and Non-fatal CHD	Age, smoking, blood pressure, cholesterol, alcohol, relative weight	4·95* for low control, low variety, high physical strain	+ +
37	Hawaii (Japanese ancestry)	4737 (0)	45–65	Job control, demands and their interaction (ecological)	18	359	Fatal CHD and non-fatal MI	Age	No effect of control, demands or their interaction (NS trend for lower strain men to have higher CHD)	0

continued

Table 4.1 *continued*

Reference	Country	Total sample (% women)	Age at entry (yr)	Exposure	Follow up (yr)	Events (n)	Events: type	Adjustments	Relative risk	Summary +−
40	Denmark	2045 (0) bus drivers	21–64	Job variety, satisfaction	10	59	Fatal CHD	Age	2·1 *high* job variety and satisfaction associated with CHD risk	0
38	Denmark	1752 (0)	59 (mean)	Job influence, pace, monotony, satisfaction, ability to relax	3	46	Fatal CHD + non-fatal MI	None	Only inability to relax after work associated with CHD	0
63	USA	1683 (0)	38–56	Job control, demands and their interaction (ecological)	25	283	Fatal CHD	Age	1·4 for job strain	0
34	UK	10308 (33) civil servants	35–55	Job control, demands (individual, assessed twice 3 yr apart, and ecological)	5	654	Angina + doctor diagnosed ischaemia	Age, smoking, blood pressure, cholesterol, body mass index, employment grade	1·93 self reported or externally assessed low job control predicted CHD	+
54	Finland	1727 (0)	42–60	Job demands, resources, income	8·1	89	Fatal CHD + non-fatal MI	Age, behavioural, biological and psychosocial covariates	1·57 for the effect of high demands, low resources and low income; 2.59 when adjustment made for age only	+

64	USA	3575 (0)		Job control demands (ecological)	519	Fatal CHD +non-fatal MI		1·41* for low control	+
Prognostic studies									
39	USA	1489 (24) employed patients undergoing coronary angiography	41–59	Job control, demands (individual)	5	Fatal CHD + non-fatal MI prevalence of coronary artery disease	Ejection fraction, extent of coronary atherosclerosis, myocardial ischaemia	0·96 for effect of job strain on events. Job strain was associated with normal coronary arteries	–
65	Switzerland	222 (0) after first MI	30–60	Job work load, locus of control, social supports	1	All cause mortality, reinfarction, severe symptoms or poor exercise capacity	Age, severity of MI, exercise	High workload and low external locus of control associated with outcome	+

CHD, coronary heart disease; MI, myocardial infarction; NS, not significant.

From Hemingway and Marmot (1998).[28]

*p value for relative risk <0.05

+0=no association; +=moderate (relative risk ≤2.0) association; + +=strong (relative risk >2.0) association.

itself, making it more vulnerable to damage. Immune mechanisms could be important. A study in Stockholm has shown that men who report low job control have higher serum levels of interleukin 6, which is part of the communication between the immune system and the brain.[46] Increased interleukin 6 activity is a reflection of either increased inflammatory activity or energy mobilisation or both.

The mechanisms behind the observed relationships between job conditions and coronary heart disease risk need to be elucidated, since these will have important applications in both occupational medicine and law.

Effort–reward imbalance model

Earlier in this chapter we emphasised the growing importance of job insecurity in the modern worldwide economy. "Job control" in this perspective implies more than the original concept, which was directed towards characteristics of work tasks. A related concept, the model of effort–reward imbalance, focuses more explicitly on links between work tasks and labour market dynamics. This model maintains that the work role defines a crucial link between the self regulatory needs of the individual (for example, self esteem, self efficacy) and the social opportunity structure. In particular, conferment of occupational status is associated with recurrent options of contributing and performing, of being rewarded or esteemed, and of belonging to some significant group (work colleagues). Yet these potentially beneficial effects are contingent on a prerequisite of exchange in social life: reciprocity. Effort at work is spent as part of a socially organised exchange process to which society at large contributes in terms of rewards. Rewards are distributed by three transmitter systems: money, esteem, and career opportunities including job security. The model of effort–reward imbalance claims that lack of reciprocity between costs and gains (i.e. high cost, low gain conditions) defines a state of emotional distress, which can lead to the arousal of the autonomic nervous system and associated strain reactions. For instance, having a demanding but unstable job, achieving at a high level without being offered any promotion prospects, are examples of high cost–low gain conditions at work. In terms of current developments of the labour market in a global economy, the emphasis on occupational rewards including job security reflects the growing importance of fragmented job careers, of job instability, underemployment, redundancy, and forced occupational mobility, as well as their financial consequences.[3,4] The model of effort–reward imbalance applies to a wide range of occupational settings, most markedly to groups that suffer from growing segmentation of the labour market, and to groups exposed to structural unemployment and rapid socioeconomic change. Effort–reward imbalance is frequent in the service occupations and professions, in particular those dealing with person to person interactions.

It is important to note that the two models mentioned, the demand–control and the effort–reward imbalance models, differ in a number of respects.

First, while the demand–control model focuses on situational characteristics of the work environment, an explicit distinction is made between situational and personal characteristics in the effort–reward imbalance model. A specific personal pattern of coping with demands, termed "overcommitment", has been included in the model to estimate more accurately individuals' stressful experiences. Overcommitment defines a set of attitudes, behaviours, and emotions reflecting excessive striving in combination with a strong desire to have approval and be respected. People characterised by overcommitment are exaggerating their efforts beyond levels usually considered appropriate. There is evidence that excessive efforts result from perceptual distortion (in particular an underestimation of challenges and an overestimation of coping resources) which in turn may be triggered by an underlying motivation to experience respect and approval.[4] Second, components of the effort–reward imbalance model (salaries, career opportunities, job security) are linked to more distant macroeconomic labour market conditions, while the demand–control model's major focus is on workplace characteristics. Finally, in stress theoretical terms, the range of control over one's environmental situation at work is the core dimension of the demand–control model, whereas in the second model threats to—or violation of—legitimate rewards based on the assumption of reciprocity and fairness in social exchange represent the core dimensions. Despite these differences, there is promise in studying the combined effects of these two models in future research.

Evidence from studies

So far, six studies have reported findings with partial or full confirmation of the model's basic assumptions about cardiovascular risk or disease. An overview of the major studies is given in Table 4.2. Three of these studies are prospective: a German study of blue-collar workers, covering some 2000 person-years;[47] the Whitehall II study mentioned above;[48] and a Swedish cohort study of some 5720 healthy employed men and women (baseline data only).[49] Two studies are cross-sectional, one analysing associations of psychosocial work stress with cardiovascular risk factors in a group of 179 male middle managers,[50] and one representing a large case–control study of 951 male and female coronary heart disease patients and 1147 controls.[51] Finally, a follow up study of 106 coronary patients who underwent coronary angioplasty was conducted to explore the role of effort–reward imbalance in predicting coronary restenosis.[52]

With regard to future incident coronary heart disease, effort–reward imbalance at work was associated with a relative risk two to six times higher than in those who were free from chronic work stress.[47,48] This excess risk could not be explained by established biomedical and behavioural risk factors, as these variables were taken into account in multivariate statistical analysis. Yet additional evidence derived from cross-sectional investigations shows that chronic psychosocial work stress is also associated with relevant coronary risk factors, for example, high blood pressure, high levels of blood lipids, or a joint manifestation of these two risk factors.[49,50,53] These findings

Table 4.2 Adverse health outcomes of effort–reward imbalance at work.

Reference	Country	Total sample (% women)	Type of study	Exposure	Health measure	Adjustment	Relative risk	Summary+−
48	UK	10 308 (33) civil servants	Prospective mean 5·3 yr	High effort, low reward (proxy measures)	Angina, doctor diagnosed ischaemia	Age, smoking, blood pressure, cholesterol, BMI, employment grade, negative affectivity, job control	2·15	+
47	Germany	416 (0) blue-collars	Prospective mean 6·5 yr	High effort, low reward	Incident fatal or non-fatal CHD	Age, smoking, blood pressure, cholesterol, BMI	6·15	+
49	Sweden	5720 (44)	Prospective (baseline data)	High effort, low reward (ratio and score over-commitment)	Hypertension, total cholesterol, LDL and HDL cholesterol	Age, smoking, BMI, physical exercise	1·62 for hypertension (ratio in men) 1·39 for LDL cholesterol (overcommitment in women)	+ (partial) + (partial)
50	Germany	179 middle managers	Cross-sectional	High effort, low reward	Hypertension, LDL cholesterol	Age, BMI, exercise, smoking, alcohol	5·77 3·57	+ +

Ref	Country	Sample	Study design	Measure	Outcome	Adjusted for	Result	Association
56, 57	UK	10 308 (33) civil servants	Prospective mean 5·3 yr	High effort, low reward (proxy measures)	New reports of psychiatric disorders	Age, employment grade, baseline mental health	2·57 for men, 1·67 for women	+
					Subjective health functioning	Age, employment grade, baseline ill health, negative affectivity	All significant, ranging from 1·44 to 2·33	+
55	Germany	1337 (12) transport workers	Cross-sectional	High effort, low reward (proxy measures)	Level of reported symptoms	Reported health, physically demanding work, occupational hazards	Ranging from 1·99 to 3·06	+
52	Germany	106 (0) coronary patients	Follow up 1 yr	High effort, low reward	Coronary restenosis, based on angiographic measures	Age, cholesterol, hypertension, smoking, multivessel disease	2·86	(partial)

BMI, body mass index; CHD, coronary heat disease; HDL, high density lipoprotein; LDL, low density lipoprotein. +0=no association; +=moderate (relative risk ≤2.0) association; ++=strong (relative risk >2.0) association.

demonstrate that the explanatory power of the model goes beyond disease manifestation by enabling a more comprehensive definition of people at risk at an earlier stage of disease development. Even in those suffering from manifest coronary heart disease, the model is useful in predicting the further course of disease. For example, one study found a powerful independent effect of the intrinsic component of the model, overcommitment, on the risk of coronary restenosis following successful angioplasty treatment.[52]

Further evidence is derived from recent findings of the case–control study mentioned above: male coronary heart disease patients were more often exposed to high effort–low reward conditions at work compared with their healthy controls, whereas female disease patients more often suffered from high levels of overcommitment.[51] Moreover, in a Finnish prospective study that did not provide an explicit measure of the model, significantly elevated hazards of cardiovascular mortality were observed among men whose work was defined by high demands, low resources, and low income, a finding that the authors interpreted in the framework of the effort–reward imbalance model.[54]

Further validation of the model is provided by studies that document adverse health effects of effort–reward imbalance using health measures other than those related to the cardiovascular system, for example, gastrointestinal problems,[55] psychiatric disorders,[56] and poor subjective health.[57]

In conclusion, there is substantial support for the stress-theoretical assumptions linking high cost–low gain conditions at work, in combination with specific personal characteristics, to the development of cardiovascular risk and disease. Research is needed to link these associations with the more traditional occupational hazards that adversely affect the cardiovascular system, such as noise, exposure to toxic substances, and shift work. Preliminary evidence indicates that psychosocial work stress, as measured by the effort–reward imbalance model, mediated effects of shift work on cardiovascular health.[58]

Comparison of models in predicting future coronary heart disease

In the Whitehall II study, an attempt to compare the two models with respect to the prediction of future coronary heart disease has been made. The results show that both effort–reward imbalance and low job control were independently related to coronary heart disease outcomes. There was a doubling of risk of developing new coronary heart disease when each model was controlled for the other and for potential confounders (Figures 4.3 and 4.4).[48] Similarly, in the large case–control study of coronary heart disease patients, a combination of information on the models resulted in an improved risk estimation of myocardial infarction.[51] These findings suggest the potential advantages in devising job stress models that combine both personal and environmental factors to help explain differences in coronary heart disease and other diseases.

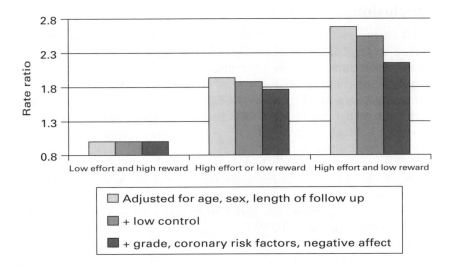

Figure 4.3 Effort–reward imbalance and coronary heart disease incidence for men and women in the Whitehall II study. From Bosma *et al.* (1998).[48]

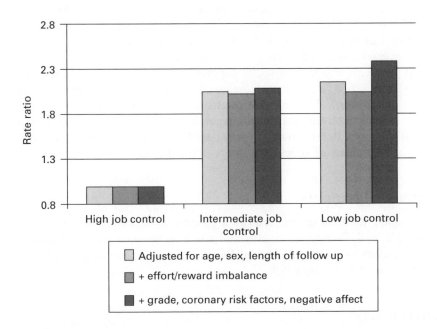

Figure 4.4 Job control and coronary heart disease incidence for men and women in the Whitehall II study. From Bosma *et al.* (1998).[48]

Conclusion

In this chapter, we have argued that two theoretical models hold particular promise in explaining at least part of the variation in coronary heart disease—a variation that may be attributed in part to work stress as defined by the demand–control and effort–reward imbalance models. High demand–low control conditions and high cost–low gain conditions at work are unequally distributed both between and within societies, and potentially provide a framework in which to understand the contribution of psychosocial factors at work to the development of disease.

The conceptual differences between the models have direct implications for the design of intervention measures to improve health; whereas the emphasis of the demand–control model is on changes of the task structure (such as job enlargement, job enrichment, and increasing the amount of support within the job), the reduction of high cost–low gain conditions includes action at three levels: the individual level (for example, reduction of excessive need for control), the interpersonal level (for example, improvement of esteem reward), and the structural level (for example, adequate compensation for stressful work conditions by improved pay and related incentives, opportunities for job training, learning new skills, and increased job security).

Despite the central role of work in the above models, an exclusive focus on working life carries the risk of underestimating the true health costs of adverse stressful circumstances unrelated to work. This becomes dramatically clear if we consider the evidence on the health burden of longterm unemployment.[16] The characteristics of family life and leisure activities are also of crucial importance in reducing the stresses and strains of working life. Conversely, stressful events in an individual's personal life, such as marital problems and lack of social support, can exacerbate the burden of work-related stress and may increase a person's disposition towards developing disease.[59] The study of the work–family interface points to the need to extend the framework of reference in stress research by taking into account the social determinants of coronary heart disease. These and other factors are the focus of specific chapters in this book.

Acknowledgements

This chapter is based on material in a chapter by Marmot M, Siegrist J, Theorell T and Feeney A, Health and the Psychosocial Environment at Work, in: Marmot M and Wilkinson RG eds. *Social Determinants of Health*, Oxford University Press, 1999.

References

1 Karasek RA. Job demands, job decision latitude and mental strain: implications for job design. *Admin Sci Q* 1979;**24**:285–308.

2 Karasek R, Theorell T. *Healthy work: stress, productivity, and the reconstruction of working life.* New York: Basic Books, 1990.

3 Siegrist JS, Weber K. Sociological concepts in the etiology of chronic disease: the case of ischaemic heart disease. *Soc Sci Med* 1986;**22**:247–53.

4 Siegrist J. Adverse health effects of high-effort/low-reward conditions. *J Occup Health Psychol* 1996;**1**:27–41.

5 Osler W. The Lumleian Lectures on angina pectoris. *Lancet* 1910;**i**:839–44.

6 Marmot MG, Davey Smith G, Stansfeld SA *et al.* Health inequalities among British Civil Servants: the Whitehall II study. *Lancet* 1991;**337**:1387–93.

7 Marmot MG, Adelstein AM, Robinson N, Rose G. The changing social class distribution of heart disease. *BMJ* 1978;**2**:1109–12.

8 Marmot MG, Shipley MJ, Rose G. Inequalities in death – specific explanations of a general pattern. *Lancet* 1984;**i**:1003–6.

9 Bobak M, Marmot MG. East-West mortality divide and its potential explanations: proposed research agenda. *BMJ* 1996;**312**:421–5.

10 MONICA. The World Health Organisation MONICA Project. Ecological analyses of the association between mortality and major risk factors of cardiovascular diseases. *Int J Epidemiol* 1994;**23**:505–16.

11 Marmot MG. Social differentials in health within and between populations. *Daedalus* 1994;**123**:197–216.

12 Kohn MS, Schooler C. Occupational experience and psychological functioning: An assessment of reciprocal effects. *Am Sociol Rev* 1973;**38**:97–118.

13 Hutton W. High risk. *The Guardian* October 30 1995;2–3.

14 Beatson M. *Labour market flexibility.* London: Department of Employment, 1995.

15 Morris JK, Cook DG, Shaper AG. Loss of employment and mortality. *BMJ* 1994;**308**:1135–9.

16 Martikainen PT, Valkonen T. Excess mortality of unemployed men and women during a period of rapidly increasing unemployment. *Lancet* 1996;**348**:909–12.

17 Joseph Rowntree Foundation. Inquiry into income and wealth chaired by Sir Peter Barclay. York: Joseph Rowntree Foundation, 1995.

18 Wilkinson RG. Income distribution and life expectancy. *BMJ* 1992;**304**:165–8.

19 Kaplan GA, Pamuk ER, Lynch JW, Cohen RD, Balfour JL. Inequality in income and mortality in the United States: analysis of mortality and potential pathways. *BMJ* 1996;**312**:999–1003.

20 Kawachi I, Kennedy BP. Health and social cohesion: why care about income inequality? *BMJ* 1997;**314**:1037–40.

21 Hinkle LE, Whitney LH, Lehman EW *et al.* Occupation, education and coronary heart disease. *Science* 1968;**161**:238–46.

22 Hackman JR, Lawler EE. Employee reactions to job characteristics. *J Appl Psychol* 1971;**55**:259–86.

23 Gardell B. Alienation and mental health in the modern industrial environment. In: Levi L, ed. *Society, stress and disease. The psychosocial environment and psychomatic diseases.* London: Oxford University Press, 1971.

24 Karasek R, Baker D, Marxer F, Ahlbom A, Theorell T. Job decision latitude, job demands and cardiovascular disease: a prospective study of Swedish men. *Am J Public Health* 1981;**71**:694–705.

25 Schnall PL, Landsbergis PA. Job strain and cardiovascular disease. *Annu Rev Public Health* 1994;**15**:381–411.

26 Kristensen TS. The demand-control-support model: Methodological challenges for future research. *Stress Med* 1995;**11**:17–26.

27 Theorell T, Karasek RA. Current issues relating to psychosocial job strain and cardiovascular disease research. *J Occup Health Psychol* 1996;**1**:9–26.

28 Hemingway H, Marmot M. Psychosocial factors in the aetiology and prognosis of coronary heart disease: systematic review of prospective cohort studies. *BMJ* 1999;**318**: 1460–7.

29 Johnson JV, Hall EM. Job strain, work place social support, and cardiovascular disease: a cross-sectional study of a random sample of the Swedish working population. *Am J Public Health* 1988;**78**:1336–42.

30 Johnson JV, Stewart W, Fredlund P *et al. Psychosocial Job Exposure Matrix: An Occupationally Aggregated Attribution System for Work Environment Exposure Characteristics.* Stockholm, Sweden: National Institute for Psychosocial Factors and Health, 1990.

31 Theorell T. Health promotion in the workplace. In: Badura B, Kickbusch I, eds. *Health promotion research. Towards a new social epidemiology.* Copenhagen: WHO, 1992.

32 Orth-Gomer K, Eriksson I, Moser V, Theorell T, Fredlund P. Lipid lowering through work stress reduction. *Int J Behav Med* 1994;3:204–14.

33 Karasek R. Stress prevention through work organisation. Conditions of work digest. Preventing stress at work. International Labour Office, Geneva, 1992;11:23–40.

34 Bosma H, Marmot MG, Hemingway H, Nicholson A, Brunner EJ, Stansfeld S. Low job control and risk of coronary heart disease in the Whitehall II (prospective cohort) study. *BMJ* 1997;314:558–65.

35 Hallqvist J, Diderichsen F, Theorell T, Reuterwall C, Ahlbom A, SHEEP study group. Is the effect of job strain on myocardial infarction due to interaction between high psychological demands and low decision latitude? Results from the Stockholm Heart Epidemiology Program (SHEEP). *Soc Sci Med* 1998;46:1405–15.

36 Theorell T, Hallqvist A. Decision latitude, job strain, and myocardial infarction: a study of working men in Stockholm. *Am J Public Health* 1998;88:382–88.

37 Reed DM, Lacroix AZ, Karasek RA, Miller D, MacLean CA. Occupational strain and the incidence of coronary heart disease. *Am J Epidemiol* 1989;129:495–502.

38 Suadicani P, Hein HO, Gynetelberg F. Are social inequalities as associated with the risk ischaemic heart disease a result of psychosocial working conditions? *Atherosclerosis* 1993;101:165–75.

39 Hlatky MA, Lam LC, Lee KL et al. Job strain and the prevalence and outcome of coronary artery disease. *Circulation* 1995;92:327–33.

40 Netterstrom B, Suadicani P. Self-assessed job satisfaction and ischaemic heart disease mortality: a 10 year follow up of urban bus drivers. *Int J Epidemiol* 1993;22:51–6.

41 Greiner BA, Ragland DR, Krause N, Syme SL, Fisher JM. Objective measurement of occupational stress factors—an example with San Francisco urban transit operators. *J Occup Health Psychol* 1997;4:325–42.

42 Theorell T, Karasek R. The demand-control-support model and CVD. In: Schnall PL, Belkic K, Landsbergis P, Baker D, eds. *The Workplace and Cardiovascular disease.* Occupational Medicine. Philadelphia: Hanley & Belfus, 2000.

43 Markowe HLJ, Marmot MG, Shipley MJ, et al. Fibrinogen: a possible link between social class and coronary heart disease. *BMJ* 1985;291:1312–14.

44 Brunner EJ, Marmot MG, White IR et al. Gender and employment grade differences in blood cholesterol, apolipoproteins and haemostatic factors in the Whitehall II study. *Atherosclerosis* 1993;102:195–207.

45 Tsutsumi A, Theorell T, Hallqvist J, Reuterwall C, de Faire U. Association between job characteristics and plasma fibrinogen in a normal working population: a cross sectional analysis in referents of the SHEEP study. *J Epidemiol Community Health* 1999;53:348–54.

46 Theorell T, Hasselhorn HM, Vingard E, Andersson B, MUSIC Norrtalje Study Group. Interleukin 6 and cortisol in acute musculoskeletal disorders: results from a case-referent study in Sweden. *Stress Med* 2000;16:27–35.

47 Siegrist J, Peter R, Junge A, Cremer P, Seidel D. Low status control, high effort at work and ischemic heart disease: prospective evidence from blue-collar men. *Soc Sci Med* 1990;31:1127–34.

48 Bosma H, Peter R, Siegrist J, Marmot MG. Alternative job stress models and the risk of coronary heart disease. *Am J Public Health* 1998;88:68–74.

49 Peter R, Alfredsson L, Hammar N, Siegrist J, Theorell T, Westerholm P. High effort, low reward and cardiovascular risk factors in employed Swedish men and women—baseline results from the WOLF study. *J Epidemiol Community Health* 1998;52:540–7.

50 Siegrist J, Peter R. Chronic work stress is associated with atherogenic lipids and elevated fibrinogen in middle-aged men. *J Intern Med* 1997;242:149–56.

51 Peter R, Hallqvist J, Reuterwall C, Siegrist J, Theorell T, SHEEP Study Group. Psychosocial work environment and myocardial infarction: improving risk estimation by combining two alternative job stress models in the SHEEP study. Submitted.

52 Joksimovic L, Siegrist J, Meyer-Hammar M et al. Overcommitment predicts restenosis after successful coronary angioplasty in cardiac patients. *Int J Behav Med* 1999;6:356–69.

53 Peter R, Siegrist J. Chronic work stress, sickness absence and hypertension in middle managers: general or specific sociological explanations? *Soc Sci Med* 1998;45:1111–20.

54 Lynch J, Krause N, Kaplan GA, Tuomilehto J, Salonen JT. Workplace conditions, socioeconomic status and the risk of mortality and acute myocardial infarction: the Kuopio Ischaemic Heart Disease Risk Factor Study. *Am J Public Health* 1997;87:617–22.

55 Peter R, Geissler H, Siegrist J. Associations of effort-reward imbalance at work and reported symptoms in different groups of male and female public transport workers. *Stress Med* 1998;**14**:175–82.
56 Stansfeld S, Fuhrer R, Shipley MJ, Marmot M. Work characteristics predict psychiatric disorder: prospective results from the Whitehall II study. *Occup Environ Med* 1999;**15**:302–7.
57 Stansfeld S, Bosma H, Hemingway H, Marmot M. Psychosocial work characteristics and social support as predictors of SF-36 functioning: the Whitehall II study. *Psychosom Med* 1998;**60**:247–55.
58 Peter R, Alfredsson L, Knutsson A, Siegrist J, Westerholm P. Does a stressful psychosocial work environment mediate the effects of shift work on cardiovascular risk factors. *Scand J Work Environ Health* 1999;**25**:376–81.
59 Brown GW, Harris T. *Social Origins of Depression.* London: Tavistock, 1978.
60 Lacroix A, Haynes S. Occupational exposure to high demand/low control work and coronary heart disease incidence in the Framingham cohort. *Am J Epidemiol* 1984;**120**:481.
61 Alfredsson L, Spetz CL, Theorell T. Type of occupation and near-future hospitalization for myocardial infarction and some other diagnoses. *Int J Epidemiol* 1985;**14**:378–88.
62 Haan MN. Job strain and ischaemic heart disease: an epidemiologic study of metal workers. *Ann Clin Res* 1988;**20**:143–5.
63 Alterman T, Shekelle RB, Vernon SW, Burau KD. Decision latitude, psychologic demand, job strain, and coronary heart disease in the Western Electric study. *Am J Epidemiol* 1994;**139**:620–7.
64 Steenland K, Johnson J, Nowlin S. A follow up study of job strain and heart disease among males in the NHANES1 population. *Am J Ind Med* 1997;**31**:256–60.
65 Hoffmann A, Pfiffner D, Hornung R, Niederhauser H. Psychosocial factors predict medical outcome following a first myocardial infarction. Working Group on Cardiac Rehabilitation of the Swiss Society of Cardiology. *Coron Artery Dis* 1995;**6**:147–52.

5: Social relations and coronary heart disease

STEPHEN STANSFELD AND REBECCA FUHRER

There is now considerable evidence that high levels of social support are protective against coronary heart disease, while social isolation is related to increased mortality risk. However, it is not clear whether social relations primarily influence the aetiology of coronary heart disease, or only have an effect in people with established disease, thus influencing prognosis.

Epidemiological studies of social relations and mortality, as distinct from studies of morbidity, form the largest body of convincing evidence on the association between social relations and coronary heart disease.[1,2] In these studies, lack of social networks and social isolation predict increased mortality risk in comparison with those who are not socially isolated, the influence often operating over long periods of time. There is also evidence of the specificity of this risk to increased cardiovascular disease mortality and deaths from accident and suicide, but not to other causes of death (namely cancer), from a study of male health professionals.[3,4] Nevertheless, the mechanism of this effect and the detail of the pathways through which social relations influence health have yet to be worked out.

There are two ways in which social relations might act on health to influence mortality. First, social relations might be implicated in the aetiology of disease, particularly coronary heart disease, with social isolation being a risk factor for the onset of coronary heart disease. Second, social relations might influence the prognosis among people with established disease, with good support being related to greater longevity and poor support being related to increased mortality risk. In this way, social relations might influence the progression of disease or the development of complications (for example, development of arrhythmias). The evidence seems to be stronger for the pathway linking social support and prognosis, but no systematic attempt has been made to distinguish between the effect on aetiology and the effect on prognosis in the available literature. Effects on aetiology and prognosis are necessarily confounded in studies examining social relations at baseline and linking support to future mortality. This chapter will attempt to distinguish between these two pathways and their effect on mortality.

Two modes of action for social relations have been suggested within each of the areas of aetiology and prognosis. Relations may either have a direct effect on health through several different pathways, or they may operate by buffering the impact of acute stressors, such as life events, or chronic stressors, sometimes referred to as chronic strains.[5] In the second case, it is postulated that social relations do not influence health in the absence of stressors and only operate to modify and reduce the otherwise noxious influence of stressors on health.

Direct effects may occur through neurohumoral responses to social relations. Positive social relations may boost self esteem, reduce anxiety, increase perceptions of control over the environment, increase the meaningfulness of the social and physical environment, fulfil needs for attachment, and increase physical enjoyment and wellbeing.[6] In these ways—although it is not clear which of these pathways may be most important—positive relations may dampen neurophysiological arousal, leading to lower levels of circulating catecholamines and cortisol. On the other hand, social isolation or negative interaction may lead to increased anxiety and depression and a heightening of physiological arousal, potentially with secondary metabolic disturbance. Such metabolic disturbance might increase the likelihood of atherogenesis, increase the tendency to clotting, or increase the possibilities of arrhythmias. There is evidence to support this from both human and non-human primate studies. Depression has been identified as a risk factor for coronary heart disease in many studies, described in Chapter 7. It is possible that depression could be a mediating factor between social relations and coronary heart disease. Lack of social relations, or negative characteristics of close relationships may lead to depression,[7] which in itself may be associated with neurohumoral and metabolic disturbance on the pathway to coronary heart disease. On the other hand, depression may not be a mediating factor, and inadequate social relations and depression may directly and independently affect the risk of coronary heart disease.[4]

Buffering may also occur in different ways. Discussion of stressors with a supportive person may reduce feelings of threat through a process of reappraisal. This might lead to a reduction in anxiety and an alternative approach to coping with the stressor. The provision of practical aid and support may lessen the impact of a stressor. Similarly, emotional support following a stressor such as an acute life event (for example, the death of a close friend) can help to reduce distress, relieve anxiety and depression, and may thus also reduce concomitant physiological arousal. One life event may often precipitate another event, each contributing to a cumulative impact on health. Social support may help in coping with the initial life event, and thus avert further events.

Social relations, social support, social networks: distinguishing the concepts

We are here using "social relations" as an umbrella term to describe both social networks and social support. It is important when attempting to understand these mechanisms to distinguish between social networks and functional aspects of support.[7] The latter refers to the quality and type of support that is provided by the network members, whereas the social network itself refers to the social contacts (and structure of those contacts) in a group of people, and can be described in terms of number and frequency of contacts.

Social support has been defined as "resources provided by other persons".[8] It has also been seen as "information leading the subject to believe he is cared for and loved, is esteemed and valued and belongs to a social network of communication and mutual obligation".[9] Weiss identified five functions of support: indication of personal value, group membership, provision for attachment and intimacy, opportunity for nurturance, and availability of help (informational, emotional, and material).[10]

Social support research has now recognised that close relationships can have negative as well as positive aspects. There is increasing evidence to suggest that these negative aspects of close relationships may have a very powerful effect on both physical and mental health.[11-13] It also appears that different aspects of support may influence different manifestations of coronary heart disease. Perhaps the most definitive and long established evidence links social support and mortality. This is described below as the first evidence of the association between support and coronary heart disease.

Social network measures can be further broken down by separating them into the number of contacts with the primary group, or group of persons to whom the person is most attached, and those with more distant network members, less likely to provide meaningful support. Other useful indices include the density of the network—an estimate of how much each network member is in contact with each other; this gives some idea of how integrated the network members are. The advantage of network measures in research on social relations is that they are easy to measure, easy for respondents to recall reliably in surveys, and verifiable by external assessment.[14] Such measures are also probably less susceptible to the reporting of socially desirable responses than are assessments of quality of support. Network measures can provide an index of social integration: how much the individual is a part of a community of mutual obligation and exchange.

The major disadvantage of network measures is that they do not provide any indication of the quality of interaction taking place in social contacts. This means that while a gross lack of social support, such as social isolation, might be identified, a more finely graded appreciation of the types of social support transacted in relationships is not available. Richer information is potentially available by examining quality of support as well as social networks.[15] In general, types of support may be divided into "emotional" and "practical or instrumental" support. Emotional support has been operationalised into various linked subtypes, including "informational" support, where support sources provide information which may help the respondent in problem solving and "self appraisal", thereby promoting self esteem. Practical support may be manifested in many forms, including practical help and financial support.

Model

Pathway 1: a model of the pathways between social relations and coronary heart disease

A model of the alternative pathways between social relations and coronary heart disease is shown in Figure 5.1. The effect of social networks on the aetiology of coronary heart disease may be mediated through social support, in that larger networks would increase the probability of having better support (path 1). Recent analyses in the Whitehall II study support this: larger numbers of close network members were associated with higher ratings on the types of support provided per person.[16] However, larger numbers could also increase the likelihood of negative interactions, which may be harmful to health owing to the stress response elicited by negative interactions.[16] Alternatively, lack of social contacts may act directly, as social isolation is predictive of poor health outcomes and mortality.[18] Paths 6 and 2 exemplify the latter two pathways. Social isolation, possibly mediated through decreased social support, may also affect the progression of disease, increasing the duration of illness and/or the risk of mortality (paths 4 and 5). Social isolation may not be the same as a mere lack of social contacts.

Although social networks are a foundation of social support as mentioned above, social support also operates at a different level through individual relationships which may be independent of the network structure. Therefore, the quality and nature of social support may influence the occurrence of disease (path 3), the prognosis of disease (path 4), and the risk of mortality (path 5). This schematic representation will serve as a framework for the following review. The pathways.

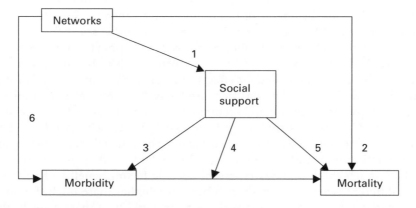

Figure 5.1 Pathways between social networks, social support and coronary heart disease morbidity and mortality.

75

Pathway 2: social networks and mortality

Some of the earliest evidence, bearing on the relationship of social relations and health, relates to the effect of social networks on mortality (pathway 2). This evidence has come from a number of large, prospective community studies. One of the earliest reports was that of the Alameda County study in which a social network index was devised, combining social contacts composed of marital status, number of contacts with friends and relatives, church and group membership. Low scores on this index (those with the least social connections) were predictive of 1.9 to 3 times greater mortality over a 9 year period.[1] Furthermore, social ties were still predictors of mortality in this study at 17 year follow up.[19] A major strength of this study was to adjust for potential confounding factors such as socioeconomic status, health related behaviours, and particularly prior ill health which might lead to reduction in social contacts and give a spurious relationship between social networks and subsequent illness. This and subsequent studies[4] successfully disprove the theory that ill health is the primary cause of the social network–mortality relationship. Nevertheless, it could be argued that this does not eliminate a positive health/ energy or fitness effect due to constitutionally based levels of fitness or vitality, which may predict both level of social networks and mortality independently.

A disadvantage of the social network index is its inability to separate qualitative and quantitative aspects of social relations. For instance, marital status may be an indirect indicator of quality of support. Additionally, marital status is an indicator of a socially favoured role that confers health benefits irrespective of social support. This means that the evidence from the Alameda County study does not contradict pathway 2. Further analysis in the Alameda County study suggested that types of ties had different effects at different ages: marital status was more important for those aged less than 60 years at baseline, while ties with close friends and relatives were more important in those who were more than 60 years old at baseline.[19] The specificity of the effects of ties on mortality depending on life stage is shown among older people in the Durham County study,[20] in which contacts with children and siblings as well as support from the social network had independent effects on mortality risk. In the Tecumseh study,[21] there were independent effects of marital status and attendance at meetings on mortality among men; probably both formal and informal relationships are important and seem not to be substitutable. This is echoed in a large US study of middleaged professional men where independent effects on total mortality were found for not being married, not belonging to a church group, and the absence of close relatives.[3] A question arises as to how much these findings represent specific health benefits of contacts with different types of network members, or whether there might be other explanations. For instance, network contacts could be a marker for health promoting behaviours such as physical activity.

In the Tecumseh study there were weaker associations between contacts with relatives and friends and mortality among men, but stronger associations with other types of community involvement, such as leisure activities that involved meeting other people, including attending sporting events, classes, films, plays, and meetings of voluntary organisations.[21] It may be that these activities are associated with social class and education, which may be the underlying determinant of coronary risk. On the other hand, such leisure activities may be the pathway through which the influences of social class and education on health are mediated. In the Swedish study of men born in 1913 and 1923, those with the lowest degree of home activities had the highest mortality. Mortality was also related to the degree of outside home activities and social activities.[22] In the men aged 60, parties at home, organised sport, visiting friends, and trade union meetings all contributed significantly to the social activity–mortality relationship. It is not clear what the health effect here might be due to. It could be either a direct effect of social contact, or due to the health benefit of physical activity involved in these social activities, the material resources available to be able to undertake these activities, the more general benefit of being integrated in a social group, or to some combination of these. Significant correlations between the social network measures suggest that men who are active in one field tend to be active in others.[22] House suggests that social networks have a positive influence on health through providing people with a sense of belonging, with reasons for living beyond themselves, with incentives to engage in more preventive and thera-peutic behaviours, and a sense of coherence to their lives.[21] Hence, health related behaviours such as physical activity may be encouraged by social contacts and be intermediate on the pathway between social contacts and health.

In general, the effects of social relations were weaker in women in the Tecumseh study, stronger for coronary heart disease as a cause of death, and in the same direction as for men. In women, only church attendance was significantly associated with mortality. One reason for the weaker association between social networks and mortality in the Tecumseh study compared with the Alameda County study may be to do with the social context and the different meanings of social contacts in these two settings. Alameda County is a semiurban setting, whereas Tecumseh is a rural farming area. Questions on social contacts with relatives and friends may be less differentiating in rural areas where they are part of the fabric of everyday life and less notable as special events, unlike urban areas where social contacts may be rarer among people living away from their areas of origin. In a study in Evans County Georgia, social network interaction was found to have only a fairly weak protective effect on morbidity in white men, and no effect in white women or in black men and women.[23] Some of the inconsistencies between large community studies may relate to the different characteristics of the populations studied, and their different patterns of social networks, health behaviours, and illness. Thus, finding associations between social networks and mortality in large studies representative of the total population strengthens the evidence base, as in a study linking social network interactions and Swedish national mortality data in 17 433 Swedish men and women, where an increased total mortality risk of 3.3 was found comparing the lowest with the highest network group.[18]

One finding common to the Tecumseh study and to the Evans County study is that mortality rates seem to be especially high at very low levels of contacts.[23] This suggests that the effects of social networks on mortality are not linear and that risk is much greater in those who are socially isolated. This was also the case in a large, random sample of the Swedish population where the increased mortality risk was confined to the most isolated 20–30% of the population.[18] It may be that, as House suggests, a "minimal level of relationship or activity is somehow more critical than the quality of those relationships" (page 138).[21] This is in favour of the path 2 hypothesis. Alternatively, the level of social contacts may not be the crucial variable influencing health, but something about the characteristics of the socially isolated that makes them vulnerable to ill health. For instance, extreme social isolation may be associated with adversely health related behaviours such as alcohol abuse. Such behaviours may be predictive of mortality independently of social networks.

A study of a random sample of American Health Maintenance Organisation members followed for 15 years suggested that social network measures—particularly "network scope", the number of different domains in which people had contacts—were more strongly associated with coronary mortality than morbidity. On this basis, the authors suggested that social networks might be more effective in supporting recovery after illness has occurred, than in preventing the incidence of new disease.[24]

Pathway 3: social support and coronary heart disease aetiology

Most studies in the area of social relations and coronary heart disease have measured social networks rather than types of social support, so there is less evidence to substantiate this pathway. Nevertheless, if the association between social networks and mortality represents an effect of social relations on health, rather than social networks being a proxy for some other variable influencing health, it would seem surprising if quality of social contacts was not important in the protective effect of social relations on mortality. If this is the case, then quality of social relationships might influence the onset of disease or its progression. This section focuses on the onset of disease.

In men, there is evidence that functional aspects of support predict the onset of acute myocardial infarction. In a series of 736 fifty year old Swedish men, high levels of availability of attachment (including support to boost self esteem, security, comfort, and love) and social integration (including appraisal, tangible support, and "belongingness") were associated with a lower incidence of acute myocardial infarction.[25] One problem of this and other studies is the difficulty of fully separating out the effect of network size from the support given by network members. On the whole, this study does lend credence to the view that acknowledging type and quality of support increases the association between social relations and health.

What might the mechanism be for an association between quality of social support and coronary heart disease aetiology? Low levels of social integration, defined as appraisal, tangible support, and "belongingness", were associated with higher rates of smoking, higher levels of plasma fibrinogen, and lower levels of leisure time physical activity. Low levels of attachment were associated with lower levels of leisure time physical activity, but also, paradoxically, lower systolic blood pressure and cholesterol. Thus, part of the effects of social support on coronary heart disease aetiology may be mediated through health related behaviours. In another study of young, healthy women, the perception that they were frequently undermined by individuals in their social network was related to higher fibrinogen levels, independent of the perceived frequency of support.[26] However, in multivariate analysis in the study of Swedish men, both social integration (odds ratio 3·8, 95% confidence interval 1·1–13·9) and availability of attachment (OR = 3·1, 95% CI 1·3–7·6) were associated with acute myocardial infarction independently of hyperlipidaemia, obesity, hypertension, diabetes mellitus, and physical inactivity.[25] This suggests that the effects of quality of social relations is either mediated through other unmeasured factors or is exerting a more direct effect on the cardiovascular system. Evidence for these direct effects in men, if not in women, is supplied by a study of men aged 70–79 years from the MacArthur Community Study of Aging.[27] Men with higher levels of emotional support had lower levels of norepinephrine (noradrenaline), epinephrine (adrenaline), and cortisol in overnight urine samples than men with low support. A similar effect was found for high levels of network ties on norepinephrine, and high instrumental support on lower norepinephrine and cortisol levels. As the authors remark, these cross-sectional findings are "intriguing but not definitive".[27] Clearly, these findings need longitudinal confirmation, but they point to larger effects of quality of social support on potentially mediating stress-related hormone levels than network variables indicating number of contacts. There is also evidence of chronic physiological arousal in relation to low levels of social support at work: elevated heart rate during work, sleep, and leisure taken from 24 hour electrocardiograms among 148 men and women from seven occupations was associated with low levels of social support from colleagues and supervisors.[28]. Chronic autonomic dysfunction may be associated with increased coronary risk. Of course, in such a cross-sectional study, it is unclear whether low social support at work has a causal role on elevated heart rates or whether people who are already physiologically highly aroused are likely to experience more conflict at work or report it more negatively.

Pathway 4: social support and the progression of coronary heart disease

Could a low degree of social support influence the progression of existing coronary heart disease? According to this pathway, the effects of low social support would occur in the presence of existing disease and social support would not be involved in aetiology. Most studies have not examined progression of disease, which is rather difficult, but have settled for a more definitive endpoint such as mortality. These studies are discussed below. There have been several studies of patients undergoing coronary angiography to examine the association between social support and severity of progression of coronary atherosclerosis. In general, social network membership does not seem to have been related to degree of atherosclerosis.[29] However, a significant inverse association was found between levels of instrumental support provided by others and atherosclerosis. A significant inverse association has also been found between levels of emotional support and the extent of atherosclerosis, particularly in patients classified as showing the type A behaviour pattern.[30] Thus, although structural features of social integration, as assessed by social network measures, do not appear to be associated with disease severity, more qualitative features such as levels of social support do exhibit a negative association with disease severity and favour a role for social support in the progression of coronary heart disease. Angiography studies examining quantitative evidence of coronary atherosclerosis have demonstrated that lack of social integration is associated with both the severity and extent of coronary disease in women, even after adjustment for standard coronary risk factors.[31] Perhaps surprisingly, lack of attachment was not associated with the degree or severity of disease. It could be that severe disease had led to impairment of social as well as physical functioning and that deficits in support were secondary to illness. The authors examined this by adjusting their findings according to the physician's appraisal of the severity of angina symptoms and the patients' perception of their general health, and found that the effects of low social support were maintained. However, the results of angiography studies need to be viewed cautiously because of the possibility of selection bias in such samples on the basis of how people are referred for angiography.

Social support and mortality risk in people with existing coronary heart disease

Some of the strongest evidence of the effects of low social support relate to subsequent mortality risk in patients with existing coronary heart disease. The association between social support and the prognosis for patients following myocardial infarction is strong and consistent. Ruberman and colleagues were the first to report that more socially isolated men were at increased risk of death after myocardial infarction.[32] This has been confirmed in several subsequent studies. Williams *et al.* found that individuals who were not married and had no confidant had significantly poorer survival following myocardial infarction over the subsequent 5 year period.[33] In another study, relative risk of mortality was increased among those with low social support even after adjustment for sex, ethnicity, education, employment, smoking, diabetes mellitus, hypertension, and hypercholesterolaemia.[34] In addition, social integration has been found to have an effect on mortality risk in men, but only in those with type A rather than type B personalities.[35] This is similar to an earlier finding that type A behaviour and social support are inversely associated. Lack of participation in social or community groups has also been found to predict mortality in a 6 month period following cardiac surgery.[36] Berkman *et al.* suggested that low levels of emotional support may be the reason why social isolation conveys greater mortality risk in patients following myocardial infarction.[37] In her study, emotional support was measured prior to the myocardial infarction, as all patients were participating in a longitudinal study. Diagnosis of myocardial infarction was identified through hospital monitoring and chart review for all cohort members. In analyses adjusting for age, the severity of the myocardial infarction, and other morbidity, subjects who reported no sources of emotional support experienced a nearly threefold higher mortality rate at 6 months than those reporting one or more sources of support.

It is possible that the effects of lack of social support on mortality following myocardial infarction are mediated through the development of depression. Depression, especially recurrent depression, has been associated with increased mortality risk after myocardial infarction.[38] It is possible that depression could increase the risk of sudden death from ventricular arrhythmias by increased sympathetic activation influencing a susceptible damaged heart.[39] However, among women who had already had an acute coronary event, lack of social integration and depression independently predicted recurrent cardiac events including acute myocardial infarction and cardiovascular mortality.[40] This is reminiscent of the results of a community based French study which also found independent effects of depression and social relations on mortality (see Chapter 7).[4] Neither of these two studies suggested that the effects of low levels of social relations on coronary heart disease are mediated through depression.

Intervention studies providing social support in patients with coronary heart disease might be expected to demonstrate an ameliorative effect on depression. A randomised control study suggested that monthly supportive and educational interventions by a nurse therapist to patients following myocardial infarction, who were identified by questionnaire to be under stress, were associated with greater longevity than in subjects who did not receive such intervention.[41] In addition, stress scores were also reduced in the intervention group. However, in a subsequent intervention this favourable response was not replicated and, if anything, women fared less well in the intervention group.[42] These interventions are further discussed in Chapter 16.

Pathway 5: social support and coronary heart disease mortality

Most community studies of social relations and mortality have measured only social networks, not the functional aspects of support. Kaplan et al. reported from the Kuopio study in eastern Finland of 2682 men followed up for just under 6 years, that men were at increased risk of death if they reported few persons to whom they gave or from whom they received support, and low quality of social relationships.[43] Lack of participation in organisations, having few friends, and not currently being married, were also associated with greater overall mortality risk. These findings were not confounded by baseline health status, smoking, alcohol intake, coffee consumption, physical activity, body mass index, or income.

Functional aspects of social support are likely to have a stronger association with mortality than social networks because they capture more of the social interaction, as shown in the results of the Kuopio study, as opposed to the Swedish National Study.[18] Frequency of interaction and use of emotional support when troubled were not associated with mortality risk in the Kuopio study, although use of instrumental or practical support when troubled was associated with increased risk. It may be the case that the heavy use of instrumental support is associated with existing illness, loss of functioning in everyday activities and hence additional need of support. There is also a suggestion from the Whitehall II study that high levels of practical support provided may indicate that high levels of support were required because of existing illness or low physical or social functioning.[16]

Overall, Kaplan et al. argue that social support does not appear to be a proxy for baseline health status,[43] in fact associations between social support and mortality appear to be stronger in the healthy subgroup at baseline. This study strongly supports the position of the earlier cohort studies that the predictive power of low social support on mortality cannot be explained as merely occurring in people with existing coronary disease. The fact that the effect of social support is stronger in those who are healthy at baseline favours an effect on incident disease rather than an effect on the prognosis of existing disease. Of course, an effect on prognosis of unrecognised disease cannot be ruled out, but seems unlikely. If the effect was largely on prognosis rather than aetiology, then these results would require that low social support had a greater effect on progression of illness in those who were initially healthy than in those who were initially ill, which seems unlikely.

Overall synthesis of results

Do social relations influence the aetiology or prognosis of coronary heart disease? The effects on prognosis seem fairly clear. Lack of emotional support increases the mortality risk in patients after myocardial infarction even after adjustment for the severity of the myocardial infarction. Such an adjustment might be expected to control for the effects of social support prior to the onset of the acute myocardial infarction. The effect of social relations on an undisputed outcome such as mortality is endorsed by angiography studies, which (despite their limitations in terms of sampling) add associations between social relations and quantifiable evidence of atherosclerotic progression. If there is good evidence that social relations influence the prognosis of coronary heart disease, what about aetiology?

First, can aetiology and prognosis be separated? Postmortem studies suggest that the development of atherosclerosis in Western countries may begin as early as adolescence. Nevertheless, overt coronary heart disease is unusual before the fourth and fifth decades in men. Thus, although any putative effect of social relations in the first three decades of life may be operating in the presence of atherosclerosis, this is likely still to be prior to clinically detectable coronary heart disease. This has relevance to many of the large epidemiological field studies that have examined the association of social relations and coronary heart disease events, and in which there is a long interval between the baseline measurement of social support and the coronary heart disease outcome. This result supports an effect on aetiology rather than prognosis—although an effect on prognosis cannot be altogether ruled out. The distinction between effects on aetiology and prognosis may be particularly blurred if lack of social relations is influencing the development of existing atherosclerosis. Morover, the association between social relations and coronary heart disease is present even after adjustment for baseline illness,[1,43] and in one study was even stronger in the sample free of illness at baseline. If there is an effect of social relations on aetiology, it may be partially mediated by health related behaviours, such as physical activity and diet, both of which have been implicated in the aetiology of coronary heart disease. Lack of support and negative characteristics of close relationships may also have direct effects on bodily systems mediated through chronic hormonal responses that might lead to the development of atherosclerosis. Such longterm influences would also be in keeping with an effect on aetiology.

Finally, is it the quality or the quantity of support that matters? Many studies have suggested that there is specificity in the protectiveness of different sources of support by sex, and particularly by age. They argue that the mere presence of social contacts is insufficient, and that the type of support provided is important. Nonetheless, there are many more studies of social networks than of social support—and social networks do show clear effects on aetiology and prognosis of coronary heart disease. It may be that, although it is suggestive that functional aspects of support have more powerful effects than networks, further confirmation using detailed measures of both are needed. If quality rather than quantity is important, this does not explain why many large epidemiological studies find powerful negative effects for social isolation. It could be that there is a spectrum of increasing protective effect across social contacts enhanced by quality of support, which is mediated by dampening the effects of stressor-related hormones. Risk of coronary heart disease could be much increased in those who are extremely socially isolated by a different additional mechanism such as poor health-related behaviours.

Altogether, there seems to be evidence for effects of social relations on both aetiology and prognosis of coronary heart disease. Moreover, type of support and quality of support seem to confer additional protection over and above the effects of simple social contacts.

References

1 Berkman LF, Syme SL. Social networks, host resistance and mortality: a nine year follow-up study of Alameda county residents. *Am J Epidemiol* 1979;**109**:186–204.
2 House JS, Landis KR, Umberson D. Social relationships and health. *Science* 1988; **241**:540–5.
3 Kawachi I, Willett WC, Colditz GA, Stampfer MJ, Speizer FE. A prospective study of coffee drinking and suicide in women. *Arch Intern Med* 1996;**156**:521–5.
4 Fuhrer R, Dufouil C, Antonucci TC, Shipley MJ, Helmer C, Dartigues JF. Psychological disorder and mortality in French older adults: do social relations modify the association? *Am J Epidemiol* 1999;**149**:116–26.
5 Pearlin LI, Schooler C. The structure of coping. *J Health Soc Behav* 1978;**19**:2–21.
6 Cohen S. Psychosocial models of the role of social support in the etiology of physical disease. *Health Psychol* 1988;7:269–97.
7 Stansfeld SA, Fuhrer R, Shipley MJ. Types of social support as predictors of psychiatric morbidity in a cohort of British Civil Servants (Whitehall II Study). *Psychol Med* 1998; **28**:881–92.
8 Cohen AS, Syme L. *Social Support and Health*. New York: Academic Press, 1985.
9 Cobb S. Social support as a moderator of life stress. *Psychosom Med* 1976;**38**:300–13.
10 Weiss RS. The provisions of social relationships. In: Rubin Z, ed. *Doing Unto Others*. Englewood Cliffs: Prentice Hall, 1974.
11 Coyne JC, Downey G. Social factors and psychopathology: stress, social support and coping processes. *Annu Rev Psychol* 1991;**42**:401–5.
12 Stansfeld SA, Rael EGS, Head J, Shipley M, Marmot M. Social support and psychiatric sickness absence: a prospective study of British civil servants. *Psychol Med* 1997;**27**:35–48.
13 Fuhrer R, Stansfeld SA, Chemali J, Shipley MJ. Gender, social relations and mental health: prospective findings from an occupational cohort (Whitehall II study). *Soc Sci Med* 1999; **48**:77–87.
14 Orth-Gomer K, Unden AL. The measurement of social support in population surveys. *Soc Sci Med* 1987;**24**:83–94.
15 Stansfeld S, Marmot M. Deriving a survey measure of social support: the reliability and validity of the Close Persons Questionnaire. *Soc Sci Med* 1992;**35**:1027–35.
16 Fuhrer R, Stansfeld SA. How gender affects patterns of social relations and their impact on health: a comparison of one or multiple sources of support from close persons. *Soc Sci Med* (in press).
17 Seeman TE. Social ties and health: the benefits of social integration. *Ann Epidemiol* 1996; **6**:442–51.
18 Orth-Gomer K, Johnson JV. Social network interaction and mortality. A six year follow-up study of a random sample of the Swedish population. *J Chron Dis* 1987;**40**:949–57.
19 Seeman TE, Kaplan GA, Knudsen L, Cohen R, Guralnik J. Social network ties and mortality among the elderly in the Alameda County Study. *Am J Epidemiol* 1987;**126**:714–23.
20 Blazer DG. Social support and mortality in an elderly community population. *Am J Epidemiol* 1982;**115**:684–94.
21 House JS, Robbins C, Metzner HL. The association of social relationships and activities with mortality: prospective evidence from the Tecumseh Community Health Study. *Am J Epidemiol* 1982;**116**:123–40.
22 Welin L, Tibblin G, Svardsudd K *et al*. Prospective study of social influences on mortality. The study of men born in 1913 and 1923. *Lancet* 1985;**i**(8434):915–18.
23 Schoenbach VJ, Kaplan BH, Fredman L, Kleinbaum DG. Social ties and mortality in Evans County, Georgia. *Am J Epidemiol* 1986;**123**:577–91.

24 Vogt TM, Mullooly JP, Ernst D, Pope CR, Hollis JF. Social networks as predictors of ischaemic heart disease, cancer, stroke and hypertension: incidence, survival and mortality. *J Clin Epidemiol* 1992;**45**:659–66.

25 Orth-Gomer K, Rosengren A, Wilhelmsen L. Lack of social support and incidence of coronary heart disease in middle-aged Swedish men. *Psychosom Med* 1993;**55**:37–43.

26 Davis MC, Swan PD. Association of negative and positive social ties with fibrinogen levels in young women. *Health Psychol* 1999;**18**:131–9.

27 Seeman TE, Charpentier PA, Berkman LF *et al*. Predicting changes in physical performance in a high-functioning elderly cohort: MacArthur studies of successful aging. *J Gerontol* 1994;**49**:M97–108.

28 Unden AL, Orth-Gomer K, Elofsson S. Cardiovascular effects of social support in the work-place: twenty-four hour ECG monitoring of men and women. *Psychosom Med* 1991;**53**:50–60.

29 Seeman TE, Syme SL. Social networks and coronary artery disease: a comparison of the structure and function of social relations as predictors of disease. *Psychosom Med* 1987;**49**:341–54.

30 Blumenthal JA, Burg MM, Barefoot J, Williams RB, Haney T, Zimet G. Social support, type A behaviour, and coronary heart disease. *Psychosom Med* 1987;**49**:331–40.

31 Orth-Gomer K, Horsten M, Wamala SP *et al*. Social relations and extent and severity of coronary artery disease. The Stockholm Female Coronary Risk Study. *Eur Heart J* 1998; **19**:1648–56.

32 Ruberman W, Weinblatt E, Goldberg JD, Chaudhary BS. Psychosocial influences on mortality after myocardial infarction. *N Engl J Med* 1984;**311**:552–9.

33 Williams RB, Barefoot JC, Califf RM *et al*. Prognostic importance of social and economic resources among medically treated patients with angiographically documented coronary artery disease. *JAMA* 1992;**267**:520–4.

34 Farmer IP, Meyer PS, Ramsey DJ, Goff DJ, Wear ML. Higher levels of social support predict survival following acute myocardial infarction: the Corpus Christi Heart Project. *Behav Med* 1996;**22**:59–66.

35 Orth-Gomer K, Unden AL. Type A behavior, social support, and coronary risk: interaction and significance for mortality in cardiac patients. *Psychosom Med* 1990;**52**:59–72.

36 Oxman TE, Freeman DH, Manheimer ED. Lack of social participation or religious strength and comfort as risk factors for death after cardiac surgery in the elderly. *Psychosom Med* 1995;**57**:5–15.

37 Berkman LF, Leo-Summers L, Horwitz RI. Emotional support and survival after myocardial infarction. A prospective, population-based study of the elderly. *Ann Intern Med* 1992;**117**:1003–9.

38 Lesperance F, Frasure-Smith N, Talajic M. Major depression before and after myocardial infarction: its nature and consequences. *Psychosom Med* 1996;**58**:99–110.

39 Cameron O. Depression increases post-MI mortality: how? *Psychosom Med* 1996; **58**:111–12.

40 Horsten M, Mittleman MA, Wamala SP, Schenck-Gustafsson K, Orth-Gomer K. Depressive symptoms and lack of social integration in relation to prognosis in middle-aged women. The Stockholm Female Coronary Risk Study. *Eur Heart J* 2000;**21**:1043–5.

41 Frasure-Smith N, Prince R. The ischemic heart disease life stress monitoring program: impact on mortality. *Psychosom Med* 1985;**47**:431–45.

42 Frasure-Smith N, Lesperance F, Prince RH *et al*. Randomised trial of home-based psychological nursing intervention for patients recovering from myocardial infarction. *Lancet* 1997;**350**:473–9.

43 Kaplan GA, Wilson TW, Cohen RD, Kauhanen J, Wu M, Salonen JT. Social functioning and overall mortality: prospective evidence from the Kuopio Ischemic Heart Disease Risk Factor Study. *Epidemiol* 1994;**5**:495–500.

6: Hostility, psychosocial risk factors, changes in brain serotonergic function, and heart disease

REDFORD WILLIAMS

Our understanding of the role of hostility in heart disease—and the role of a broad range of other, related, psychosocial factors in human disease—owes much to two cardiologists, Meyer Friedman and Ray Rosenman. They were the very first to document, using accepted epidemiological methodology, that a psychosocial factor, type A behaviour (comprising two major components, time urgency and free floating hostility), is prospectively associated with increased risk of a particular disease—coronary heart disease.[1] Indeed, by the early 1980s, the research establishment was close to declaring type A behaviour an "established" CHD risk factor.[2]

The failure to replicate Friedman and Rosenman's type A findings in another well designed, largescale prospective study,[3] along with several other negative studies,[4] raised serious concerns about the type A hypothesis. A Medline search on type A behaviour in the late 1970s would elicit scores of citations; one in the late 1990s elicits only a few. Despite the decline of interest in the type A construct, the seeds that Friedman and Rosenman planted have sprouted and grown into a flourishing field of research on psychosocial risk factors "beyond type A".

Beginning with a study showing an association between one of the type A components, hostility, and angiographically documented coronary atherosclerosis,[5] this field has matured to the point where hostility is now broadly accepted as a risk factor, not only for coronary heart disease but for a wide range of other life threatening and minor illnesses. In this chapter I shall review the epidemiological evidence documenting the impact of hostility on disease risk, but that is only the first part of the story. A comprehensive review of this field must also take into account the following points:

- The scope of research has been extended beyond a focus on single factors such as hostility to include a range of psychosocial characteristics.

- The emphasis has shifted away from the earlier obsession with identifying factors that make an "independent" contribution to risk, to an approach that takes into account the tendency for psychosocial risk factors to cluster in the same individuals and groups, where their effect on health is compounded.

- Further epidemiological research combined with sophisticated laboratory research using the tools of cellular and molecular biology has made good progress toward identifying biobehavioural mechanisms whereby the psychosocial risk factors contribute to the development of disease.

- The role of early childhood experiences in predisposing to the development of hostility and other psychosocial risk factors is a growing focus of research, as are the neurobiological mechanisms whereby early experience is translated into adult psychosocial and biobehavioural characteristics that increase risk of disease.

All the progress in the foregoing areas has led clinical researchers in behavioural medicine to begin the process of developing and testing behavioural treatment interventions aimed at ameliorating the ill effects of hostility and other psychosocial risk factors.

Hostility and clustering of psychosocial risk factors

Epidemiological evidence

The initial study documenting an association between hostility and coronary atherosclerosis used the Cook–Medley hostility scale from the Minnesota Multiphasic Personality Inventory (MMPI) to measure hostility.[5] This made it possible for researchers to go back to archival MMPI data that had been collected in the past, rescore for the Cook–Medley hostility scale, and determine whether there was a prospective association between these hostility scores and the subsequent development of disease.

Two studies of this sort, one using MMPI data collected from male medical students in the 1950s,[6] and one using MMPI data from the Western Electric study of middleaged men in the 1950s,[7] both found increases in coronary heart disease incidence over follow up periods of 20–25 years among the men who had high Cook–Medley hostility scores. The effect size for these scores was smaller in the middleaged Western Electric study subjects than in the 25-year-old medical students, consistent with the same "hardy survivor" effect that also reduces the impact of smoking and cholesterol levels on coronary heart disease risk with increasing age.

Both studies also found that all cause mortality was predicted by the Cook–Medley hostility scores and that effect sizes were larger than for prediction of coronary heart disease. This suggests that whatever is being measured by the Cook–Medley hostility scale is not a specific risk factor for

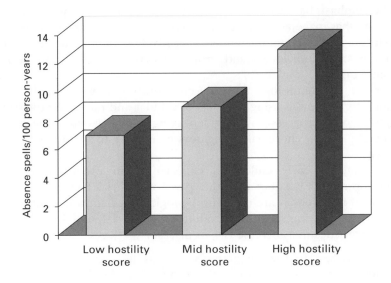

Figure 6.1 Hostility and long-term absences from work due to injury on the job among male Finnish municipal workers. Adapted from Vahtera *et al.*[8]

coronary heart disease but a *general risk factor* that lowers resistance or increases vulnerability to a wide range of pathogenic processes. One good example of the broad impact of hostility on health comes from a study of Finnish municipal workers, which found increasing rates of long work absences due to injury among men with high hostility scores.[8]

As shown in Figure 6.1, those with high hostility scores had twice the rate of long absences. Numerous other studies have also found Cook–Medley hostility scores to predict a wide range of diseases. One that made an important methodological contribution to the measurement of hostility was a study that followed up lawyers who had completed the Minnesota Multiphasic Personality Inventory while in medical school in the 1950s.[9] In addition to finding a nearly fivefold higher death rate over the ensuing 25 years among those with higher Cook–Medley hostility scores, this study used content analysis to group the 50 MMPI items comprising the Cook–Medley hostility scale into rational content clusters. Six clusters were identified, but only three were predictive of mortality. These three had good construct validity and reflected an attitudinal component (cynical mistrust), an affective component (anger), and a behavioural component (aggression). When these three clusters were combined into a single scale comprising 27 of the 50 Cook–Medley hostility scale items, they were a stronger predictor of mortality than the overall Cook–Medley hostility scale.

Just as a Medline search comparing the late 1990s with the late 1970s would show a decline in type A citations, a similar search using "hostility" as the keyword would document a striking increase in the number of citations. Despite some negative studies, a meta-analysis of the body of research on the physical health consequences of hostility concluded that the psychological trait of hostility—cynical mistrust, anger, and aggression—is a risk factor not only for coronary heart disease but also for virtually any physical illness.[10]

It has become increasingly clear that hostility is not the only psychosocial factor that predisposes to coronary heart disease or to poor health in general. Thus, depression predicts increased coronary heart disease risk and all cause mortality in healthy people,[11,12] as well as increased risk of dying in coronary heart disease patients.[13] Although the evidence is less extensive, anxiety has also been found to predict increased coronary heart disease risk (see Chapter 7).[14]

In addition to these psychological risk characteristics, research has also identified aspects of the social environment that are prospectively associated with increased risk of coronary heart disease and other major illnesses. Social isolation (the lack of relationships that provide tangible or emotional support) predicts increased disease risk in healthy populations,[15] as well as a poorer prognosis in coronary heart disease patients (see Chapter 5).[16] Stress at work, whether defined as demand–control or effort–reward imbalance, has also been shown to predict increased coronary heart disease rates in healthy people,[17] although an impact on prognosis in coronary heart disease patients has not been confirmed (see Chapter 4).[18] Finally, lower socioeconomic status also predicts increased risk of coronary heart disease and all cause mortality in healthy people,[19,20] as well as a poorer prognosis in coronary heart disease patients (see Chapter 2).[16]

Other chapters in this book deal with these other psychosocial risk factors in greater detail, but there is an important point to be made here: hostility and other psychosocial risk factors do not occur (or act to affect health) independently of one another. Rather, they tend to cluster in the same individuals and groups. Thus, working women who report high job strain are also characterised by increased levels of hostility, anger, depression, anxiety, and social isolation,[21] and lower socioeconomic status groups score higher on measures of hostility, depression, and social isolation.[22,23] When these psychosocial risk factors occur together, as they tend to do, especially in people of lower socioeconomic status, their adverse impact on health is compounded. In the Kuopio Ischaemic Heart Disease Risk Factor study, for example, those with one or two psychosocial risk factors had subsequent mortality rates that were twice those of participants with no psychosocial risk factors; but those with three psychosocial risk factors were *four times* more likely to die over the follow up period.[24]

This clustering of psychosocial risk factors has important implications for any efforts to understand and mitigate the health damaging effects of psychosocial risk factors. First, it leads to the suspicion that, like the psychosocial risk factors themselves, the biobehavioural characteristics responsible for the development of disease (or a poorer prognosis once disease is present) might occur together in the same individuals or in certain groups. The clustering of both psychosocial and biobehavioural characteristics suggests that there may be common antecedents to account for the clustering, indicating that a developmental perspective might be useful in guiding research on psychosocial risk factors. Finally, all of the foregoing suggests that behavioural interventions aimed at ameliorating the health damaging effects of psychosocial risk factors should not be focused on single factors, but rather should be targeted to reduce the entire cluster—for example, hostility, depression, and social isolation, which tend to occur together in workers with high levels of job strain.[21]

Biobehavioural pathways to disease

Before considering how psychosocial risk factors might affect the gradual development of coronary atherosclerosis and other pathogenic processes over the course of years, it is worth noting that the low threshold for negative emotions such as anger, anxiety, and sadness in persons with psychosocial risk factors could contribute to the acute precipitation of cardiac events over the space of a few minutes to hours. Anger, for example, is just as potent a trigger of acute ischaemic episodes as strenuous physical exertion during ambulatory electrocardiographic monitoring of coronary heart disease patients.[25,26] Angina develops sooner and lasts longer during exercise testing in patients who are depressed.[27] The risk of suffering a myocardial infarction is doubled during the 2 hours following an episode of intense anger,[28] and trebled in people of lower educational attainment,[29] suggesting the compounding of acute risk by the combination of psychosocial risk factors. It has been estimated that episodes of intense anger are responsible for triggering 36 000 acute myocardial infarctions in the USA each year.[30]

The toll due to chronic action of biobehavioural characteristics over periods of years in people with psychosocial risk factors is likely to be far greater. Induction of anger in laboratory settings produces greater cardiovascular responses mediated by the sympathetic nervous system in people scoring higher on the Cook–Medley hostility scale.[31–33] This increased activation of the sympathetic nervous system in hostile individuals generalises to the naturalistic environment, as documented by larger increases in daytime urinary epinephrine (adrenaline) excretion and downregulation of lymphocyte β-adrenergic receptors.[34,35] Increased sympathetic nervous system outflow has also been documented in patients with major depression.[36] Also common to both hostility and depression is decreased parasympathetic function, whether indexed as acute parasympathetic antagonism of sympathetic nervous system effects on myocardial function in laboratory studies,[37] or by heart rate variability during ambulatory electrocardiographic monitoring.[38,39] Major depression has long been known to be associated with increased and dysregulated function of the pituitary–hypothalamic–adrenal axis.[40] More recently, people scoring high on the Cook–Medley hostility scale have been found to have larger cortisol increases to stress in both ambulatory and laboratory studies.[33,41]

Although less studied with respect to biobehavioural mechanisms, both social isolation and job stress show changes similar to those just described for hostility and depression. Low levels of social support have been associated with increased urinary catecholamine excretion.[42] Increases in ambulatory blood pressure and left ventricular mass in people in high strain jobs are probably the result of chronically increased sympathetic nervous system input to the heart.[43] A study of women employed outside the home found that those with young children still living in the home—clearly a high demand–low control life situation—excreted higher levels of cortisol in the urine across the entire 24 hour period.[44]

In addition to the biological characteristics just described, increased levels of behavioural and physical risk factors have been found to accompany the psychosocial risk factors. Two large studies, one prospective and one cross-sectional, found hostility to be associated with increased cigarette smoking, alcohol consumption, body mass index, 24 hour energy intake, waist–hip ratio, and total cholesterol–high density lipoprotein ratio.[45,46] Hostility also predicts an increased incidence of hypertension.[6] Increased smoking and alcohol consumption are also well documented in depression.[47,48] People reporting low levels of social support are less likely to succeed in stopping smoking,[49] or to adhere to a prescribed medical regimen.[50]

It is highly likely that the biobehavioural accompaniments of psychosocial risk factors just described participate in pathogenesis through several biologically plausible pathways. Excessive sympathetic nervous system arousals could, over time, promote atherogenesis through mechanical injury of the arterial endothelium.[51] The biobehavioural characteristics described above could also affect the cellular and molecular biology of the monocyte–macrophage system to promote the development of atheromatous arterial lesions and impair the immune system's ability to destroy cancer cells.[52]

Before considering how the research reviewed thus far might serve as a guide to the development of behavioural interventions aimed at ameliorating the health-damaging effects of psychosocial risk factors and their accompanying biobehavioural characteristics, it will be instructive to consider how and why the clustering of this broad range of harmful characteristics might come about. In contrast to the progress just reviewed regarding the "downstream" biological mechanisms whereby hostility and other psychosocial risk factors contribute to pathogenesis, as Kaplan notes,[24] little attention has been given to the factors involved in the *development* of psychosocial (and associated biobehavioural) risk factors. I have proposed that reduced brain serotonergic function could account for the clustering of biobehavioural characteristics in people with hostile personality types.[53] Such a mechanism leads to a further question: how and why could reduced brain serotonergic function come about? To address this important question, we need to take a developmental perspective.

The developmental perspective

It is clear that adverse early life experiences can influence the development of *psychosocial* characteristics such as hostility, depression, and social isolation by direct effects on the learning history of the individual. Hamburg noted that poor children are more likely than those who are better off to be exposed to a wide range of adverse life experiences, including having a young and socially isolated mother, an absent father, and increased stress and violence.[54] In a longitudinal observational study of parent–child interaction patterns, Hart and Risley found that by the third year of life the average child of parents on welfare has heard fewer than 100 000 positive communications, in contrast to over 500 000 for the average child of professional class parents.[55] Considering the conditions in which lower socioeconomic status groups live, Kaplan concludes: "It is certainly not hard to believe that patterns of hostility, distrust, isolation, and despair are born in such environments."[24] Evidence of the impact of early experience on hostility levels comes from a prospective study in which Matthews *et al.* found that more negative and fewer positive parent–child interactions predicted increased hostility over a 3 year follow up period among adolescent boys.[56] There is also evidence that harsh childhood environments can affect *biobehavioural* risk factors. Danish studies find increased obesity in young adulthood among those who, as children, lived in poor quality housing or experienced parental neglect.[57,58]

In addition to this direct impact of harsh environments—"learning" that the world is an unpredictable, dangerous, depressing, and alienating place—evidence showing that adverse life experiences can lead to reduced central nervous system serotonin function provides another, complementary, causal pathway from lower socioeconomic status to increased expression of adverse psychosocial and biobehavioural characteristics. A review of extensive evidence from both animal and human studies, suggesting that low central nervous system serotonin function is a potential mediator of *each* of the psychosocial and biobehavioural characteristics found to cluster in certain individuals and low socioeconomic status groups, has led me to the hypothesis that reduced central nervous system serotonin function is one *neurobiological* mechanism that could account for this clustering.[53] The case for the involvement of reduced central nervous system serotonin in the clustering of psychosocial and biobehavioural risk factors is strengthened by a consideration of research showing the impact of early environmental factors on central nervous system serotonin function.

While genetic factors clearly influence central nervous system serotonin function,[59] it is equally clear that environmental factors also have an important role. Rhesus monkeys separated from their mothers at birth and reared with age matched peers showed modest reductions at 6 months of age of cerebrospinal fluid levels of the major serotonin metabolite, 5-hydroxyindoleacetic acid (5-HIAA), indicative of decreased brain serotonin turnover, in comparison with maternally reared monkeys.[60] The separated monkeys also exhibited more aggressive and fewer affiliative behaviours and larger hypothalamic–pituitary–adrenal axis responses to stress. By 5 years of age, the serotonin depletion in the separated monkeys is even more profound.[61] The continuing stress associated with their maladept social behaviours from 6 months to 5 years of age could be responsible for the larger serotonin depletion and concomitant persistence of the earlier noted biobehavioural effects.

In contrast to the effects of decreased early maternal attention just described, Meaney and coworkers found that an intervention (brief daily separations of 20 minutes) that *increased* the total daily amount of maternal care received by rat pups was associated with enhanced central nervous system serotonin function that had behavioural (decreased fearfulness) and biological (decreased hypothalamic–pituitary–adrenal axis response to stress) effects that persisted into adulthood.[62] Rats subjected to the brief separations showed an increase in hippocampal serotonin turnover that causes—through increased intracellular cyclic adenosine monophosphate (AMP) and phosphokinase A—an increase in expression of the gene that encodes the glucocorticoid receptor. This increase in hippocampal glucocorticoid receptors persisted into adulthood and was responsible for a smaller and more rapidly terminated corticotrophin and corticosterone response to stress among rats who underwent the brief separations, compared with control animals. When the separations were extended to 3 hours or longer, however, the benefits seen with brief separations were reversed.[63] Compared with control animals, the separated animals showed increases in both fearfulness and hypothalamic–pituitary–adrenal axis responses to stress, as well as increased alcohol preference—effects likely to be mediated by decreased serotonin turnover.

In the light of the foregoing, it now appears that there are at least two plausible pathways by which harsher and more adverse living conditions could account for the clustering of psychosocial and biobehavioural risk factors in individuals and groups. As noted earlier, simply experiencing these harsher conditions could teach that the world is unpredictable, dangerous, depressing, and alienating. Similarly, people experiencing such conditions could learn to use food, alcohol, and nicotine to ameliorate the distress they experience as the result of such living conditions. *In a parallel and complementary pathway*, as documented in the animal research just reviewed, these harsh conditions could also have the effect of reducing central nervous system serotonin function, which could add (either independently or synergistically) to the clustering of psychosocial and biobehavioural risk factors that occurs via learning mechanisms.

The case that altered brain serotonergic function is an important mediator of this clustering is strengthened by new research exploring the effects of a polymorphism of the promoter region (*5HTTLPR*) of the gene that encodes for the serotonin transporter. This polymorphism, consisting of long or short *5HTTLPR* alleles, is functional—the long allele is associated with increased synthesis of the serotonin transporter compared with the short allele.[64] Moreover, people with one or more long alleles have been found to score lower on measures of neuroticism than people who are homozygous for the short allele.[64] Compared with the maternally reared group, peer reared rhesus monkeys—who as noted above display many biobehavioural characteristics similar to those that cluster in humans with psychosocial risk factors—with two long *5HTTLPR* alleles have higher 5-HIAA levels in cerebrospinal fluid than those with one or more short alleles.[65] This remarkable finding demonstrates what promises to be an important gene–environment interaction: the *5HTTLPR* genotype regulates brain serotonin turnover, but only in monkeys subjected to early adversity. Among monkeys with a more nurturing early environment, the *5HTTLPR* genotype is unrelated to serotonin turnover.

The impact of *5HTTLPR* polymorphism on brain serotonin turnover and related biological characteristics has recently been documented in humans, where it has been found that people with one or two long alleles have significantly higher levels of 5-HIAA in cerebrospinal fluid than those with two short alleles.[66] Thus, it appears that the long allele acts as an autosomal dominant in regulating brain serotonin turnover in humans. In this study, both cerebrospinal fluid level of 5-HIAA and *5HTTLPR* genotype are correlated with sympathetic nervous system and cardiovascular responses to stress.

These findings, documenting the impact of early adversity on the development of psychosocial risk factors and accompanying biobehavioural characteristics, make a strong case for early interventions aimed at ameliorating this impact.[67] The case to begin in childhood with primary prevention of psychosocial risk factors such as hostility is only strengthened by consideration of further research showing that early adversity can lead to reduced brain serotonin function, especially, it is beginning to appear, in people with certain genotypes—for example, short *5HTTLPR* alleles. Indeed, it is possible to envision use of *5HTTLPR* genotyping as a means of identifying people at particularly high risk of stress-induced cardiovascular disease, in whom preventive measures might be especially beneficial. In the meantime, however, there is already ample evidence supporting the use of behavioural interventions as a means of secondary prevention in coronary heart disease and other major medical disorders.

Behavioural approaches to prevention, treatment, and rehabilitation

Group behavioural interventions to reduce psychosocial risk factors have been shown in randomised trials to improve prognosis in both coronary heart disease and cancer.[68-71] These encouraging results have helped to make the case for largescale clinical trials of behavioural interventions in both these conditions.[72] The National Heart, Lung, and Blood Institute is currently supporting such a trial—the ENhancing Recovery in Coronary Heart Disease (ENRICHD) study—the first largescale, multicentre, randomised clinical trial of a behavioural intervention, in this case targeting depression and social isolation, with the goal of not only reducing emotional distress but also improving the medical prognosis (see Chapter 16).[73]

Additional research suggests that structured and focused behavioural interventions provided in group format to patients with chronic medical conditions can also help reduce the need for (and hence cost of) medical services. In the Hawaii Medicaid study, Cummings and coworkers randomised patients with chronic medical conditions who were high utilisers of medical services to one of three groups: no mental health treatment; traditional one on one psychotherapy for up to 1 year (the then current Hawaii Medicaid benefit); or a highly structured group intervention involving no more than eight sessions of training in various coping skills. Compared with the other two groups, both of which showed 20–40% *increases* in medical costs during the year following randomisation, the patients receiving coping skills training experienced a 20% *decrease* in medical costs.[74]

The behavioural interventions that have been found effective in randomised clinical trials have a number of elements in common:

- Group settings are more efficient than individual approaches and have the added benefits of enabling patients to learn from each other and providing each other with social support.
- Proven principles of cognitive behaviour therapy and behaviour therapy along with social skills training enable patients to gain "hands on" practice in the use of skills that will help them manage stressful situations and the resulting negative emotions that arise.[75]
- Some form of reducing autonomic arousal, such as meditation or breathing exercises, combines with the increased awareness of negative emotions that comes with use of cognitive behavioural therapy skills to enable patients to decrease distressing thoughts and emotions while blunting potentially dangerous physiologic hyperarousal.
- Treatment is usually limited to a fixed number of sessions, often no more than six to ten, during which each skill is presented in a manualised, protocol driven format that helps patients learn to practise and apply the skill in real life situations.

Williams and Williams have developed the Life Skills Workshop incorporating the elements outlined above to train people to reduce psychosocial risk factors, using of a set of coping skills that will help them to increase awareness of negative thoughts and feelings; evaluate and manage negative thoughts and feelings; use assertion and problem solving when the evaluation calls for action; and use communication skills and empathy to help build and maintain positive and supportive relationships with others.[76,77] People who have attended these workshops show significant decreases in measures of hostility and depression and an increase in social support.

A hostility reduction intervention based on the Life Skills approach was used in a small but carefully conducted randomised clinical trial of patients who had suffered a myocardial infarction.[78] Compared with those randomised to usual care, patients receiving hostility reduction training

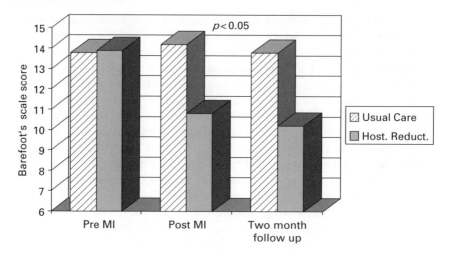

Figure 6.2 Effect of hostility reduction training in patients recovering from myocardial infarction (MI): hostility levels assessed using the 27 item hostility scale of Barefoot et al.[9] which includes the three critical components of cynical mistrust, anger, and aggression. Adapted from Gidron et al.[78]

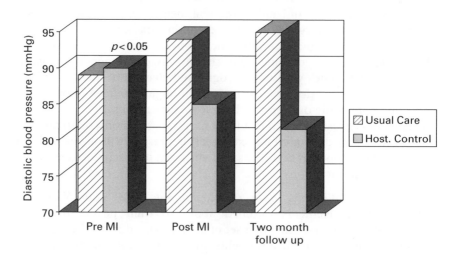

Figure 6.3 Effect of hostility reduction training on diastolic blood pressure in patients following myocardial infarction (MI). Adapted from Gidron et al.[78]

showed significant decreases in both hostility and blood pressure at the end of the eight session workshop, benefits that were maintained or enhanced at follow up 2 months later (Figures 6.2 and 6.3). A longer follow up found that patients who received hostility reduction training spent an average of

0.6 days in hospital during the 6 months following treatment, a significant reduction from the average of 2.5 days for patients in usual care.

Final thoughts

Since the late 1970s, when we were on the verge of declaring type A behaviour an established coronary heart disease risk factor, and the early 1980s, when it appeared that type A had failed to fulfil its promise, we have come a long way. It is now clear that the type A construct did contain a critical component, hostility, that was, indeed, coronary prone. However, so much more has emerged since that time. We have moved beyond the "guild" approach in which each group of researchers zealously guarded "their" risk factor—whether it was hostility, social isolation, job strain, depression, or socioeconomic inequality—against encroachments from the others, in some kind of zero sum game. There is a growing appreciation of the need to move beyond the "independent effects" mentality and focus our efforts on understanding the basis for clustering of psychosocial risk factors and their accompanying, health damaging, biobehavioural characteristics. Exciting new research employing the tools of molecular and cellular biology, molecular genetics, and neurobiology is increasing our understanding of the pathways whereby psychosocial risk factors contribute to (or may be markers for) risk of developing coronary heart disease and other life threatening illnesses.

All this progress has led us to the point where it is clearly time to use our understanding to guide the development of behavioural interventions that will reduce the risk of disease and improve health and wellbeing. This process has already begun, with encouraging results in hand from trials including patients with heart disease, cancer, and other chronic medical conditions. The research pointing to early childhood as a critical period for the development of psychosocial risk factors and accompanying biobehavioural characteristics has important implications for the primary prevention of disease. The emerging awareness of the critical role of brain serotonin—as influenced by both genes and environment—in driving the clustering of psychosocial and biobehavioural characteristics that are damaging to health will strengthen the case for early intervention.

References

1 Friedman M, Rosenman R. *Type A behavior and your heart*. New York: Knopf, 1974.
2 Review Panel on Coronary-Prone Behavior and Coronary Heart Disease. Coronary-prone behavior and coronary heart disease: A critical review. *Circulation* 1981;**63**:1199–215.
3 Shekelle RB, Hulley S, Neaton J *et al*. The MRFIT behavioral pattern study: II. Type A behavior and the incidence of coronary heart disease. *Am J Epidemiol* 1985;**122**:559–70.
4 Matthews KA, Haynes SG. Type A behavior pattern and coronary risk: Update and critical evaluation. *Am J Epidemiol* 1986;**123**:23–96.
5 Williams RB, Haney TL, Lee KL, Blumenthal JA, Kong Y. Type A behavior, hostility, and coronary atherosclerosis. *Psychosom Med* 1980:**42**:539–49.
6 Barefoot JC, Dahlstrom WG, Williams RB. Hostility, CHD incidence, and total mortality: A 25-year follow-up study of 255 physicians. *Psychosom Med* 1983;**45**:59–63.

7 Shekelle RB, Gale M, Ostfeld AM, Paul O. Hostility, risk of coronary disease, and mortality. *Psychosom Med* 1983;**45**:219–28.

8 Vahtera J, Kivimaki M, Koskenvuo M, Pentti J. Hostility and registered sickness absences: A prospective study of municipal employees. *Psychol Med* 1997;**27**:693–701.

9 Barefoot JC, Dodge KA, Peterson BL, Dahlstrom WG, Williams RB. The Cook-Medley Hostility Scale: Item content and ability to predict survival. *Psychosom Med* 1976;**51**:46–57.

10 Miller TQ, Smith TW, Turner CW, Guijarro ML, Hallet AJ. A meta-analytic review of research on hostility and physical health. *Psychol Bull* 1996;**119**:322–48.

11 Anda R, Williamson D, Jones D *et al*. Depressed affect, hopelessness, and the risk of ischemic heart disease in a cohort of U.S. adults. *Epidemiology* 1993;**4**:285–94.

12 Barefoot JC, Schroll M. Symptoms of depression, acute myocardial infarction and total mortality in a community sample. *Circulation* 1996;**93**:1976–80.

13 Frasure-Smith N, Lesperance F, Talajic M. Post-myocardial infarction depression and 18-month prognosis. *Circulation* 1994;**90**:I614–20.

14 Kawachi I, Sparrow D, Vokonas PS, Weiss ST. Symptoms of anxiety and risk of coronary heart disease. The normative aging study. *Circulation* 1994;**90**:2225–9.

15 House JS, Landis KR, Umberson D. Social relationships and health. *Science* 1988; **241**:540–5.

16 Williams RB, Barefoot JC, Califf RM *et al*. Prognostic importance of social and economic resources among medically treated patients with angiographically documented coronary artery disease. *JAMA* 1992;**267**:520–4.

17 Bosma H, Peter R, Siegrist J, Marmot M. Two alternative job stress models and the risk of coronary heart disease. *Am J Public Health* 1998;**88**:68–74.

18 Hlatky MA, Lam LC, Lee KL *et al*. Job strain and the prevalence and outcome of coronary artery disease. *Circulation* 1995;**92**:327–33.

19 Adler NE, Boyce T, Chesney MA, Folkman S, Syme SL. Socioeconomic inequalities in health: No easy solution. *JAMA* 1993;**263**:3140–5.

20 Marmot MG, Rose G, Shipley M *et al*. Employment grade and coronary heart disease in British civil servants. *J Epidemiol Community Health* 1978;**3**:244–9.

21 Williams RB, Barefoot JC, Blumenthal JA *et al*. Psychosocial correlates of job strain in a sample of working women. *Arch Gen Psychiatry* 1997;**54**:543–8.

22 Barefoot JC, Peterson BL, Dahlstrom WG, Siegler IC, Anderson NB, Williams RB. Hostility patterns and health implications: Correlates of Cook-Medley Hostility scale scores in a national survey. *Health Psychol* 1991;**10**:18–24.

23 Matthews KA, Kelsey SF, Meilahn EN *et al*. Educational attainment and behavioral and biologic risk factors for coronary heart disease in middle-aged women. *Am J Epidemiol* 1989;**129**:1132–44.

24 Kaplan GA. Where do shared pathways lead? Some reflections on a research agenda. *Psychosom Med* 1995;**57**:208–12.

25 Gabbay FH, Krantz DS, Kop WJ *et al*. Triggers of myocardial ischemia during daily life in patients with coronary artery disease: Physical and mental activities, anger, and smoking. *J Am Coll Cardiol* 1996;**27**:585–92.

26 Krantz DS, Hedges SM, Gabbay FH *et al*. Triggers of angina and ST-segment depression in ambulatory patients with coronary artery disease: Evidence for an uncoupling of angina and ischemia. *Am Heart J* 1994;**128**:703–12.

27 Krittayaphong R, Light KC, Golden RN, Finkel JB, Sheps DS. Relationship among depression scores, beta-endorphin, and angina pectoris during exercise in patients with coronary artery disease. *Clin J Pain* 1996;**12**:126–33.

28 Mittleman MA, Maclure M, Sherwood JB *et al*. Triggering of acute myocardial infarction onset by episodes of anger. *Circulation* 1995;**92**:1720–5.

29 Mittleman MA, Maclure M, Nachnani M, Sherwood JB, Muller JE. Educational attainment, anger, and the risk of triggering myocardial infarction onset. *Arch Intern Med* 1997;**157**:769–75.

30 Verrier RL, Mittleman MA. Life-threatening cardiovascular consequences of anger in patients with coronary artery disease. *Cardiol Clin* 1996;**14**:289–307.

31 Smith TW, Allred KD. Blood pressure reactivity during social interaction in high and low cynical hostile men. *J Behav Med* 1989;**11**:135–43.

32 Suarez EC, Williams RB. Situational determinants of cardiovascular and emotional reactivity in high and low hostile men. *Psychosom Med* 1989;**51**:404–18.

33 Suarez EC, Kuhn CM, Schanberg SM, Williams RB, Zimmermann EA. Neuroendocrine, cardiovascular, and emotional responses of hostile men: The role of interpersonal challenge. *Psychosom Med* 1998;**60**:78–88.

98

34 Suarez EC, Williams RB, Peoples MC, Kuhn CM, Schanberg SM. Hostility-related differences in urinary excretion rates of catecholamines. Paper presented at the Annual Meeting of the Society for Psychophysiological Research, Chicago, 1991.

35 Shiller AM, Suarez EC, Kuhn CM, Schanberg SM, Williams RB, Zimmermann EA. The relationship between hostility and beta-adrenergic receptor physiology in healthy young males. *Psychosom Med* 1997;**59**:481–7.

36 Veith RC, Lewis N, Linares OA *et al.* Sympathetic nervous system activity in major depression: Basal and desipramine-induced alterations in plasma norepinephrine kinetics. *Arch Gen Psychiatry* 1994;**51**:411–22.

37 Fukudo S, Lane JD, Anderson NB *et al.* Accentuated vagal antagonism of beta adrenergic effects on ventricular repolarization: differential responses between Type A and Type B men. *Circulation* 1992;**85**:2045–53.

38 Sloan RP, Shapiro PA, Bigger JT, Bagiella E, Steinman RC, Gorman JM. Cardiovascular autonomic control and hostility in healthy subjects. *Am J Cardiol* 1994;**74**:298–300.

39 Carney RM, Rich M, teVelde A, Saini J, Clark K, Freedland KE. The relationship between heart rate, heart rate variability and depression in patients with coronary artery disease. *J Psychosom Res* 1988;**32**:159–64.

40 Holsboer F, van Bardeleben U, Gerken A, Stallag K, Muller OA. Blunted corticotrophin and normal response to human corticotrophin-releasing factor in depression. *N Engl J Med* 1984;**311**:1127–30.

41 Pope MK, Smith TW. Cortisol excretion in high and low cynically hostile men. *Psychosom Med* 1991;**53**:386–92.

42 Fleming R, Baum A, Gisriel MM, Gatchel RJ. Mediating influences of social support on stress at Three Mile Island. *J Hum Stress* 1982;**8**:14–22.

43 Schnall P, Pieper C, Schwartz JE *et al.* The relationship between job strain, workplace diastolic blood pressure, and life ventricular mass. *JAMA* 1990;**263**:1971–2.

44 Luecken LJ, Suarez EC, Kuhn CM *et al.* Stress and employed women. I. Impact of marital status and children at home on neurohormone output and home strain. *Psychosom Med* 1997;**59**:352–9.

45 Siegler IC, Peterson BL, Barefoot JC, Williams RB. Hostility during late adolescence predicts coronary risk factors at midlife. *Am J Epidemiol* 1992;**136**:146–54.

46 Scherwitz KW, Perkins LL, Chesney MA, Hughes GH, Sidney S, Manolio TA. Hostility and health behaviors in young adults: the CARDIA study. Coronary Artery Risk Development in Young Adults Study. *Am J Epidemiol* 1992;**136**:136–45.

47 Glassman AH, Helzer JE, Covey LS *et al.* Smoking, smoking cessation, and major depression. *JAMA* 1990;**264**:1546–9.

48 Hartka E, Johnstone B, Leino EV, Motoyoshi M, Temple MT, Fillmore KM. A meta-analysis of depressive symptomatology and alcohol consumption over time. *Br J Addict* 1991;**86**: 1283–98.

49 Mermelstein R, Cohen S, Lichtenstein E, Baer JS, Kamarck T. Social support and smoking cessation and maintenance. *J Consult Clin Psychol* 1986;**54**:447–53.

50 Williams CA, Beresford SA James SA *et al.* The Edgecombe County High Blood Pressure Control Program, III: Social support, social stressors, and treatment dropout. *Am J Public Health* 1985;**75**:483–6.

51 Kaplan JR, Petterson K, Manuck SB, Olsson G. Role of sympathoadrenal medullary activation in the initiation and progression of atherosclerosis. *Circulation* 1991;**94** (suppl. VI):VI-23–32.

52 Adams DO. Molecular biology of macrophage activation: A pathway whereby psychosocial factors can potentially affect health. *Psychosom Med* 1994;**56**:316–27.

53 Williams RB. Neurobiology, cellular and molecular biology, and psychosomatic medicine. *Psychosom Med* 1994;**56**:308–15.

54 Hamburg DA. *Today's children: Creating a future for a generation in crisis.* New York: Times Books, 1992.

55 Hart T, Risley TR. *Meaningful differences in the everyday experience of young American children.* Baltimore: Paul H. Brookes, 1995.

56 Matthews KL, Woodall KL, Kenyon K *et al.* Negative family environment as a predictor of boys' future status on measures of hostile attitudes, interview behavior, and anger expression. *Health Psychol* 1996;**15**:30–7.

57 Lissau-Lund-Sorensen I, Sorensen TIA. Prospective study of the influence of social factors in childhood on the risk of overweight in young adulthood. *Int J Obes* 1992;**16**:169–75.

58 Lissau I, Sorensen TIA. Parental neglect during childhood and increased risk of obesity in young adulthood. *Lancet* 1994;**343**:324–7.

59 Higley JD, Thompson WW, Champoux M *et al.* Paternal and maternal genetic and environmental contributions to cerebrospinal fluid monoamine metabolites in Rhesus monkeys *(Macaca mulatta)*. *Arch Gen Psychiatry* 1993;**50**:615–23.

60 Higley JD, Suomi SJ, Linnoila M. A longitudinal assessment of CSF monoamine metabolites and plasma cortisol concentrations in young rhesus monkeys. *Biol Psychiatry* 1992;**32**:127–45.

61 Higley JD, Linnoila M. Low central nervous system serotonergic activity is traitlike and correlates with impulsive behaviour. A nonhuman primate model investigating genetic and environmental influences on neurotransmission. *Ann NY Acad Sci* 1997;**29**:39–56.

62 Meaney MJ, Bhatnagan S, Dioria J *et al.* Molecular basis for the development of individual differences in the hypothalamic-pituitary-adrenal stress response. *Cell Mol Neurobiol* 1993;**13**:321–47.

63 Plotsky PM, Eisler JA, Anand KJS. Neonatal pain and stress: Neural adaptations and long-term consequences. Paper presented at the Annual Meeting of the American College of Neuropsychopharmacology, San Juan, 15 December 1995.

64 Lesch KP, Bengel D, Heils A *et al.* Association of anxiety-related traits with a polymorphism in the serotonin transporter gene regulatory region. *Science* 1996;**274**:1527–31.

65 Bennett AJ, Lesch KP, Heils A *et al.* Serotonin transporter gene variation and early environment interact to affect CSF 5HIAA concentrations in Rhesus monkeys. *Mol Psychiatry* (in press).

66 Williams RB, Marchuk DA, Gadde KM, Siegler IC *et al.* Central nervous system serotonin function and cardiovascular response to stress. *Psychosom Med* 2001;**63**:300–5.

67 Williams RB. Lower socioeconomic status and increased mortality. Early childhood roots and the potential for successful interventions. *JAMA* 1998;**279**:1745–6.

68 Friedman M, Thoresen CE, Gill JJ. Alteration of type A behavior and its effect on cardiac recurrences in post myocardial infarction patients: Summary results of the Recurrent Coronary Prevention Project. *Am Heart J* 1986;**112**:653–65.

69 Blumenthal JA, Jiang W, Babyak M *et al.* Stress management and exercise training in cardiac patients with myocardial ischemia. *Arch Intern Med* 1997;**157**:2213–23.

70 Fawzy FI, Fawzy NW, Hyun CS *et al.* Malignant Melanoma: Effects of an early structured psychiatric intervention, coping, and affective state on recurrence and survival 6 years later. *Arch Gen Psychiatry* 1993;**50**:681–9.

71 Spiegel D, Bloom JR, Kraemer HC, Gottheil E. Effect of psychosocial treatment on survival of patients with metastatic breast cancer. *Lancet* 1989;**2**:888–90.

72 Williams RB, Chesney MA. Psychosocial factors and prognosis in established coronary artery disease. The need for research on interventions. *JAMA* 1993;**270**:1860–1.

73 Blumenthal JA, O'Connor C, Hinderliter A *et al.* Psychosocial factors and coronary disease. A National Multicenter Clinical Trial (ENRICHD) with a North Carolina focus. *NC Med J* 1997;**58**:802–8.

74 Cummings NA, Pallak MS, Dorken H, Henke CW. The impact of psychological intervention on health care costs and utilization: The Hawaii Medicaid Project. *HCFA Contract Report 11-C-983344/9*, 1991.

75 Beck J. *Cognitive therapy: Basics and beyond* New York: Guilford Press, 1995.

76 Williams RB, Williams VP. *Anger kills: Seventeen strategies for controlling the hostility that can harm your health*. New York: Times Books/Random House, 1993.

77 Williams VP, Williams RB. *LifeSkills: Eight Simple Ways to Build Stronger Relationships, Communicate More Clearly and Improve Your Health*. New York: Times Books/Random House, 1997.

78 Gidron Y, Davidson K, Bata I. The short-term effects of a hostility-reduction intervention in CHD patients. *Health Psychol* 1999;**18**:416–20.

7: Depression and coronary heart disease

STEPHEN STANSFELD AND REBECCA FUHRER

An association between psychological distress and heart disease has been recognised for many years.[1-4] This has partly arisen from the recognition that a sudden trauma or shock may precipitate myocardial infarction in a susceptible person. It has also arisen from the observation that prolonged exposure to stressors may be associated with chest pain, breathlessness, and exhaustion. Additionally, psychiatric disorder has frequently been observed among patients attending cardiac clinics, some of which may be explained as a reaction to cardiac disease and some by a greater tendency to refer to secondary cardiac care patients who have comorbid psychiatric disorder as well as coronary heart disease symptoms.

In a prescientific Western understanding of bodily function, the heart has been seen as the seat of the emotions: possibly because of bodily awareness of a rapidly beating heart in states of high emotional excitement. Linguistically, this association has been acknowledged in the phrase "broken-hearted", implying both an emotional disappointment and damage to the heart.

Increasing attention is being paid to this association in scientific investigations. Initially this focused on depression as a consequence of coronary heart disease, particularly myocardial infarction.[5,6] This is a clinical problem with implications for functioning and recovery. However, perhaps of more importance is the association of depression following myocardial infarction with increased mortality risk.[7]

In the late 1980s it was suggested that depression might be an important factor in the aetiology of incident coronary heart disease. In the wake of the failure of type A behaviour pattern to consistently predict coronary heart disease, reviewers began to report associations between measures of depression and coronary heart disease.[8] In a meta-analysis, depression related more strongly than type A behaviour pattern to coronary heart disease, leading the authors to comment:

These results strongly suggest that depression is importantly related to coronary heart disease and may play a role in its development. When one considers the vast amount of research performed on type A behaviour and the very small amount performed on depression (in relation to coronary heart disease), the finding that depression relates about as strongly to disease as does the [type A behaviour pattern] seems remarkable.[8]

This chapter discusses the evidence for the proposition that depression is an aetiological factor in coronary heart disease, and two of the possible pathways by which this might occur: one in which social factors predict coronary heart disease, and depression and its associated psychophysiological changes are an intervening step; and the second in which social factors predict coronary heart disease and depression, but depression is not on the pathway (Figure 7.1). This is followed by a discussion of anxiety as an aetiological factor in coronary heart disease.

Depression and the aetiology of coronary heart disease

First, it is necessary to define what is meant by "depression", as the term is used somewhat loosely in the available literature. Most studies employ self report rating scales of depression measuring "depressive symptoms" and this is how they are referred to here. Some studies have used clinical interviews to measure depression to which clinical diagnoses can be assigned: these are classified as "depressive illness". Anxiety states and phobic anxiety are included and referred to as described in the individual papers, while (as for depression) making the distinction between symptoms and clinically defined illnesses. A further condition to consider is "vital exhaustion".[9] This is considered by its proponents to be separate from depression, although the conditions share many symptoms.

Measurement of coronary heart disease

One issue to be considered is whether depression may have different associations dependent on the coronary heart disease outcome studied.

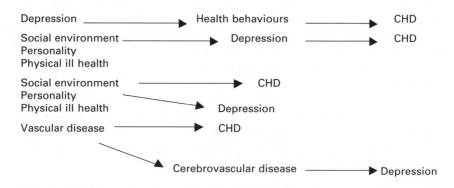

Figure 7.1 Mechanisms for the association of depression and coronary heart disease (CHD).

The task is not made easier by almost every study having its own idiosyncratic cardiac endpoints—and some combination of these comprising a total coronary heart disease score.

One concern about studies relying entirely on self report endpoints is that reporting style linked to high levels of negative affectivity may bias associations, leading to spurious associations between depression and self reported cardiac outcomes. This may contribute to the strong associations between depression and angina pectoris observed in some studies,[10] and may drive some of the associations between depression and total coronary heart disease when it includes angina pectoris. While the assessment of depression is dependent on self report measures, the assessment of coronary heart disease need not be. This emphasises the importance of selecting objectively verifiable cardiac endpoints in order to be certain of establishing a true association.

Depressive illness and coronary heart disease

In many of the earlier cross-sectional reports of depression and coronary disease, the direction of causation could not be easily ascertained as depression was often assessed either after a cardiac event or at the same time as a cardiac event.[11–14] Thus depression occurring secondary to coronary heart disease could not be ruled out. Since that time, a number of longitudinal studies of depressive illness and depressive symptoms have provided stronger evidence for depression as an antecedent of coronary heart disease (Table 7.1). Some of the most powerful longitudinal evidence comes from the Johns Hopkins Precursors Study, in which 1190 medical students were followed up for a median period of 37 years with an annual mailed questionnaire.[15] Depressive illness was measured by the responses to "direct questions concerning the occurrence of depression and associated treatment" rated by a panel of independent experts.[16] During follow up 132 men reported an episode of clinical depression with a cumulative incidence rate at 40 years of 12%, which is in line with general population rates. Depressive illness was associated with an almost doubled risk of coronary heart disease (myocardial infarction, angina pectoris, chronic ischaemic heart disease, requirement for angioplasty or bypass surgery) in men. The risk was also markedly increased in women, although less reliance could be placed on this finding because of the small number of female medical students in the cohort.

In order to counter the possibility that the results were explained by depression secondary to coronary heart disease, a reanalysis was carried out excluding all coronary events occurring within 2 years of the experience of depression; this did not alter the relative risks for coronary heart disease associated with depression. Depressive illness being the prior event is also supported by the median interval between the first episode of depression and the first coronary event being 15 years. This suggests that the effect of depression on coronary heart disease risk may operate over a long period,

Table 7.1 Prospective studies of the association between depression and coronary heart disease.

Study	Total sample	Age at entry (yr)/ sample	Depression measure	CHD measure	Follow up (yr)	Number of non-fatal and fatal events	Adjustments*	Relative risk (95% CI)	Summary
Anda et al. (1993)[45]	2832	45–77 Community sample	G W BS	Non-fatal/ fatal IHD	16	205 NF IHD 189 F IHD	Age, sex, race MS SMK CHOL SBP BMI ALC PA	NF 1·6 (1·10–2·40) F 1·5 (1·00–2·30)	Depressed affect and hopelessness predict fatal, non-fatal IHD
Ariyo et al. (2000)[30]	5888	65+ Community sample	CES-D	CHD MI Angina All cause mortality	6	606 F/NF CHD 270 F/NF MI 298 NF angina 614 deaths	Age, sex, race ED DIAB HYP SMK CHOL TGC PA HF	CHD 1·11 (1·01–1·22) MI 1·12 (0·97–1·29) Angina 1·13 (0·99–1·29) Death 1·13 (1·03–1·23)	Depressive symptoms an independent risk for CHD and mortality
Barefoot and Schroll (1996)[19]	730	60 Community sample		Acute MI All cause morality	10	122 NF 290 F	Age, sex SBP TGC SMK SW SL	MI 1·7 (1·23–2·34) Death 1·6 (1·29–2·11)	Depressive symptoms predict MI and mortality
Ferketich et al. (2000)[22]	7893	30–70+ Community sample	CES-D	Fatal, non-fatal CHD	11	Men 187 NF, 137 F Women 187 NF, 129 F	Age, race SMK HYP PI BMI DIAB NF-CHD	Men NF CHD 1·71 (1·14–2·56) F 2·34 (1·54–3·56) Women NF CHD 1·73 (1·11–2·68) F 0·74 (0·40–1·48)	Depression associated with increased risk of CHD in men and women and CHD death in men

Ford and Mead (1998)[15]	1190	26 (Avg) Male medical student	Self report of treatment of depression	CHD MI	40	163 NF	SMK COF CHOL HYP DIAB PA PMI	CHD 2·1 (1·24-2·63) MI 2·1 (1·11-4·06)	Depression. Independent longterm predictor of MI and CHD
Mendes de Leon and Krumholz (1998)[31]	2391	65-99 Community sample	CES-D	Non-fatal MI CHD Mortality	9	208NF 255 F	Age, DIAB EDUC ANG SMK SBP DBP	Men 0·99 (0·67-1·02) Women 1·03 (1·01-1·05)	Depressive symptoms independent predictors of CHD only in women
Sesso et al. (1998)[10]	1305	21-80 Community sample	MMPI-2-DEP SCL-90	Fatal/ non-fatal CHD	14	30 NF 20 F	Age, BMI SMK ALC SBP DBP FH	CHD 1·5 (0·82-2·58) MMPI 1·6 (0·93-2·64) SCL-90	Depressive symptoms possibly related to CHD

*Adjustments: SMK, smoking; ALC, alcohol; PA, physical activity; SL, sedentary leisure; MS, Marital status; SW, sedentary work; SBP, DBP, systolic diastolic BP; BMI, body mass index; CHOL, cholesterol; HYP, hypertension; DIAB, diabetes; ANG, angina; FH, family history; PMI, parental myocardial infarction; COFF, coffee; HF, heart failure; PI, poverty; Index NF-CHD, non-fatal CHD events.

CES-D, Center for Epidemiologic Studies Depression Scale; CHD, coronary heart disease; CI, confidence interval; F, fatal; GWBS, General Well-Being Schedule; IHD, ischaemic heart disease; MI, myocardial infarction; MMPI, Minnesota Multiphasic Personality Inventory; MMPI-2-DEP, Revised Minnesota Multiphasic Personality Inventory Depressive Thought Content Scale; NF, non-fatal; SCL-90, Symptom Checklist 90.

although the recurrent nature of depression may indicate that the first episode of depression is merely an indicator of proneness to multiple spells of depression with a much shorter time course of action on the heart. The generalisability of these results is limited because of the specific nature of the sample in terms of occupation, education, and income. If anything, however, these constraints should weaken the associations. This study also has little to say with regard to risk in women. Another limitation is the measurement of depression which, although it includes clinical criteria, is reliant on self report rather than standardised interview. It is more than a list of symptoms because it includes details of treatment. However, the fact that only 23% of participants reported no treatment for clinical depression during the follow up period means a very high prevalence of treated depression. This suggests that—as this figure is considerably higher than usual estimates of community prevalence—it is likely to include many less severe cases.

The association between depressive illness and coronary heart disease (inclusion criteria: angina, myocardial infarction, coronary artery surgery, use of nitrates) has been confirmed among men in a representative population in a case–control study of 5623 British general practice attenders.[17] Men with a diagnosis of depression based on Read codes taken from general practice records were three times more likely to develop coronary heart disease than control subjects, the risk persisting after adjustment for smoking, diabetes mellitus, hypertension, and deprivation score. This study did not find a similarly increased risk for depressed women. It is likely that depressive illness in this primary care sample was milder than that treated in secondary psychiatric care. Depression experienced within the 10 year period before the cardiac event was more likely to be associated with increased coronary risk than depression that occurred earlier. In contrast to the Johns Hopkins Precursors Study, this suggests that recency of depression is associated with increased coronary heart disease risk. Further work is required to understand this aspect of the association. These two studies find that the association between depression and coronary heart disease is stronger in men than in women and that there is likely to be some inconsistency over the length of the latent period between depression and the coronary event. A longer latent period suggests that depression is influencing longterm pathological processes leading to coronary heart disease. This might mean chronic sympathoadrenal hyperactivity, metabolic disturbance influencing the development of atherosclerosis, or hypothalamic–pituitary–adrenal axis stimulation leading to chronically elevated cortisol levels.[18]

Depressive symptoms and coronary heart disease

Do studies of depressive symptoms parallel the findings observed for clinical depression? Some of the first evidence on depressive symptoms and coronary heart disease came from the Glostrup study in which men and women born in 1914 were interviewed with the Minnesota Multiphasic

Personality Inventory (MMPI) and underwent a physical examination in 1964.[19] Higher depressive symptom scores on a scale extracted from the MMPI were prospectively associated with increased risk of acute myocardial infarction in men and women. Exclusion of participants with disease at baseline had very little influence on risk, and although removal of the items dealing with somatic complaints from the depression scale reduced the effect size, it still remained significant. The stability of the depression scale over the 10 year interval in this study (test–retest reliability 0.67) suggests that this scale may be tapping something more enduring than depressed mood. However, studies of personality traits such as neuroticism, which may be predictors of depression and anxiety, do not show the same prediction of coronary heart disease or all cause mortality.[20,21] Depressive symptoms, indicators of depressive illness (albeit often mild), are likely to have underlying physiological correlates that differ from those related to chronic anxiety indexed by neuroticism. The question remains, however, whether these depressive symptoms are a marker of an enduring chronic condition influencing coronary risk, or an index of depressive illness which, despite its short duration, still confers risk. More information about the measures of depressive symptoms is needed to understand this association. In a study of 5007 men and 2886 women from the National Health and Nutrition Examination Survey (NHANES) who were free of coronary heart disease at baseline, depression on the Center for Epidemiologic Studies depression scale predicted incident coronary heart disease in both men and women, but coronary heart disease mortality only in men controlling for confounding factors.[22]

The nature of depressive symptoms involved was explored in the Normative Aging Study, a community study of 2280 men, which used three self report measures of depression: the MMPI-2D scale measuring feelings of depression, pessimism, and hopelessness; the MMPI Dep content scale measuring depressive thoughts; and the Symptom Checklist 90 (SCL-90) depression subscale.[10] The strongest prospective associations were for the Dep content scale with angina pectoris and total coronary heart disease, suggesting cognitive aspects of depression may be important.

More light is thrown on what may underlie depressive symptoms may be, by the NHANES follow-up study, which examined the predictive power of a single item hopelessness scale and a four item depression subscale from the General Well-Being Schedule on risk of coronary heart disease in 2832 persons from a random population sample.[23] Moderate or severe hopelessness was associated with increased risk of non-fatal and fatal coronary heart disease even after adjusting for age, sex, race, education, marital status, smoking, total cholesterol concentration, systolic blood pressure, body mass index, number of alcoholic drinks consumed per week, and physical activity. Moreover, there seemed to be a dose–response relationship with increasing risk of coronary heart disease for moderate and severe hopelessness. As these results could be explained by undetected physical illness at baseline, the analyses were adjusted for self reported health at baseline, which had no substantial effect on estimates of risk. Although this suggests that hopelessness may be central to the relationship of depression to coronary heart disease, hopelessness is by no means independent of depression, because the hopelessness item correlated moderately with the depressed affect scale (0.58). On the other hand, hopelessness is not always present in depression.[24] Hopelessness may indicate fairly severe depression and may also reflect a persistent attitude to life, which may endure after clinical depression has remitted. There is scope for further exploration of these associations.

Depression, coronary heart disease and mortality in older people

Many studies have identified depression as a risk factor for mortality. Murphy *et al.* found that depression, but not anxiety, measured by a standardised instrument in the Canadian Stirling County study, was predictive of increased mortality risk, controlling for the effects of age, sex, and physical illness at baseline.[25] In the Health and Lifestyle Survey, psychiatric "caseness" on the General Health Questionnaire measuring less severe morbidity was also associated with increased mortality risk.[26] Is the effect of depression on physical health specific to coronary heart disease? This does not seem to be the case, as depressive symptoms predict mortality from both non-cardiac and cardiac causes.[19,26] However, the effect is more consistent for cardiac than non-cardiac causes of death.

The association between depression and all cause mortality has been found more consistently in younger rather than older people. This might mean that there is selective attrition of younger adults who are more vulnerable to this influence, and those who live to a greater age are survivors less vulnerable to the cardiac effects of depression. Thomas *et al.* found no association between depression measured with the Center for Epidemiologic Studies depression scale and mortality in a community based survey of people over 65 years.[27] On the other hand, Fuhrer *et al.* did find an association between depressive symptoms measured by the Center for Epidemiologic Studies depression scale and mortality in a population sample of French adults aged over 65 years.[28] This association was confined to men and to women aged 65–74 years only.

Questionnaire measures of depression have not always been associated with increased coronary risk or mortality in older populations.[27,29] However, depressive symptoms measured on the Center for Epidemiologic Studies depression scale predicted both coronary heart disease (hazard ratio 1.15) and all cause mortality (hazard ratio 1.15) in a prospective cohort study of community dwelling elderly Americans in the Cardiovascular Health Study, adjusting for age, race, sex, education, diabetes, hypertension, smoking, total cholesterol, triglyceride level, congestive heart failure, and physical inactivity.[30] Moreover, increase in depression scores measured by the Center for Epidemiologic Studies depression scale was associated with a 25% increase in the risk of new myocardial infarction and death per each 5 unit increase in depressive symptoms in a clinical trial population (the SHEEP trial) aged 60 years and older (mean age 72).[29] It is not totally convincing from the methodology of this study that the increase in depression score was independent of decline in physical health, although functioning scores and depression were relatively independent and the Activities of Daily Living scale was included as a covariate in the multivariate analyses. As the authors point out, it may be that premonitory signs and symptoms of coronary events could have led to increased depressive symptom scores. This sample was not typical of elderly populations, the participants being generally in better health. In contrast, the New Haven sample of the Established Populations for the Epidemiologic Studies of the Elderly (EPESE) project was representative of the general elderly population.[31] Among 2391 participants aged 65 to 99 years, a linear association was found between depression, measured by the Center for Epidemiologic Studies depression scale, and coronary heart disease mortality and total incident coronary heart disease events, including non-fatal myocardial infarction and coronary heart disease death. However, this was only found in women, and was markedly attenuated after adjustment for physical functioning. The authors interpret these findings as suggesting that the association between depression and coronary risk in elderly women may be explained by the association between impairment of physical functioning and depression. Impairment of physical functioning, possibly resulting from non-cardiac chronic disease, may be a confounding factor in the depression–coronary heart disease relationship. In this case, impairment of physical functioning could be a cause of depression and a risk factor for coronary heart disease. Similarly, Fredman *et al.* found an association between depression and mortality in a community sample of women over 65 years old confined to those suffering from physical illness and functional limitations.[32] In this case it is not clear whether depression is an independent risk factor for mortality or is merely an indicator of the severity of physical illness.

However, stratified analyses in the EPESE project support the original hypothesis: in women without physical functioning impairment a clear association was found between depression and coronary heart disease mortality, similar to that found in younger populations, which was not present in those with impaired physical functioning.[31] There is clearly more work to be done here. Might physical functioning be an early indicator of preclinical coronary disease, or other physical illness carrying increased risk of coronary heart disease? Is depression conferring an independent increased risk of coronary heart disease morbidity and mortality in these elderly populations with impaired functioning, or is depression just an indicator of the degree of physical functioning impairment—a consequence of the physical functioning impairment without independent risk attached?

In the EPESE study the authors also queried whether the effect of depressive symptoms was a continuous effect or whether there was a threshold effect—implying that only severe levels of depressive illness might be associated with coronary heart disease risk. This is especially relevant for two reasons. First, because it may suggest a potential mechanism for the association: severe depressive illnesses are often associated with failure of adrenocortical suppression and high levels of circulating cortisol, potentially leading to metabolic disturbance and coronary heart disease. Second, there are quite different public health and therapeutic implications depending on the type of depression involved. Analyses in women suggested that the continuous model had a better fit than the threshold model. This does not satisfactorily settle the question, because it assumes that high scorers on the Center for Epidemiologic Studies depression scale are equivalent to those with moderate to severe depressive illnesses. This may not be the case, as there are qualitative as well as quantitative differences between mild and severe depression not always picked up by self report rating scales. Also, there may not be a linear relationship between score and clinical severity for scales such as the Center for Epidemiologic Studies depression scale, as has been shown for a similar scale, the General Health Questionnaire.[33] Results from the Amsterdam Study of the Elderly suggest that severe psychotic depression measured by the Geriatric Mental State AGECAT was predictive of all cause mortality at 6 year follow up in both men and women, adjusting for demographic variables, physical illness, and cognitive decline. In support of an effect on mortality related to severity of depression, a higher risk of mortality for neurotic, milder, depression was confined to men.[34]

Apart from severity of depression, duration may influence mortality risk: elderly people depressed on two occasions 5 years apart in a Finnish community study had nearly twice the risk of mortality of those who were not depressed on either occasion.[35] Those who were depressed on the first occasion, but not on the second, did not have an increased mortality risk compared with those depressed on neither occasion, implying that depression present on two occasions—and likely to have persisted across the interval—was associated with higher mortality risk. However, in an American cohort study of community residents aged 65 years or more, the risk for cardiovascular mortality and new cardiovascular disease events was only found in newly depressed persons and not among those who had also been depressed 3 and 6 years previously.[36] The authors argue that physiological disturbances associated with depression are more likely to be triggered by acute illness than by chronic illness where some adaptation has occurred, although they presented no evidence to support this. Chronic depression was associated with increased overall mortality risk, but this became non-significant after adjustment for confounding factors, largely physical disability. These inconsistencies between duration of depression and mortality risk are puzzling, but if physical disability is a consequence of depression and a mediating factor between depression and mortality, it may be misleading to adjust for it. Further research on the more immediate physical consequences of depression may help to elucidate these pathways.

In summary, there may be several pathways between depression and coronary heart disease, and these may be different in younger and older people. In younger people the association between depressive symptoms (as well as clinical depressive illness) and coronary heart disease, and the long latent period between depression and increased coronary risk, suggest that the increased pathophysiological risk operates over a long period. It may be that the experience of depression sets the level of physiological responsivity to stressors which is maintained after the depressive episode remits. Such chronic physiological hyperreactivity could lead to metabolic disturbance contributing to atherosclerosis. (An alternative is that the measures of depression in these studies are inadequate to capture severity of clinical illness, which is important in determining degree of risk.)

In older age groups, the association between depression and coronary heart disease morbidity and mortality is less consistent, particularly by sex. One crucial issue yet to be resolved is whether depression in older age groups is a consequence of early unrecognised coronary heart disease, or of atherosclerotic processes elsewhere (such as in the brain), or a consequence of other physical illnesses—all of which might predict later coronary heart disease rather than depression itself. Decline in physical functioning may lead to depression. Alternatively, depression may be a mediating step on the pathway between early physical ill health and coronary heart disease. Conversely, it is possible that depression may be the primary phenomenon, leading to decline in physical functioning which is, in turn, a risk factor for increased coronary risk. Only prospective studies with multiple waves of data collection can answer these questions.

Vital exhaustion, depression, and coronary heart disease

Vital exhaustion indicates a state of fatigue, which is often present in the weeks prior to myocardial infarction. Carney suggests that insomnia in the weeks prior to myocardial infarction may indicate depressive illness.[12] "Waking up exhausted" doubled the risk of myocardial infarction in a prospective study of male volunteers in Rotterdam, and this effect remained after adjustment for problems in falling or staying asleep.[37,38] Although waking up exhausted might be a symptomatic index of subclinical coronary heart disease, this symptom was not more common in those with electrocardiographic abnormalities. Proximity in time to the myocardial infarction greatly increased the risk, which would be in keeping with exhaustion being an indirect indicator of pathophysiological change. However, there is some evidence that the predictive power of vital exhaustion for new cardiac events in patients following percutaneous transluminal coronary angioplasty is independent of the severity of coronary disease.[39,40] An alternative explanation is that vital exhaustion is the culmination of prolonged exposure to stressors and may reflect decreased activity of the hypothalamic–pituitary–adrenal axis.[41] Additionally, vital exhaustion could be a consequence of a separate unrecognised physical illness, which is independently associated with increased coronary risk.

However, waking up exhausted may also indicate depression. Although the clinical presentation of vital exhaustion overlaps with depressive symptoms, the two conditions are not coterminous. Individuals with depression may be overtired, but not all those with vital exhaustion are depressed. Symptoms of depression such as depressed mood, guilt, and loss of self worth are absent in vital exhaustion.[42] The time course of vital exhaustion suggests that this is either a phenomenon of primarily cardiac origin in which the intense fatigue is the result of a failing heart, or related to nervous system changes due to cardiac insufficiency, or may be the outcome of exposure to chronic stressors resulting in exhaustion rather than depression.

Mechanisms for the association of depression and coronary heart disease and mortality

Depression and mortality

The most obvious mechanisms for the association of depression and mortality are that depressed people may take less exercise, are less likely to eat a healthy diet, and are more likely to smoke, which may incur increased risk to health. In addition, it may be that depressed persons generally take less care and expose themselves more to dangerous situations, thereby increasing their mortality risk through accidents. Depressed people are also at greater risk of committing suicide. However, the increased risk of mortality associated with depression does not seem to be confined to suicides and accidents. There is evidence that depression confers increased risk particularly for death from cardiovascular disease.

Depression and coronary heart disease

If the evidence for the association between depression and coronary heart disease is accepted, what might the possible mechanism of effect be? There are a number of potential pathways (see Figure 7.1).

Behaviours affecting health

Depression may be associated with the adoption of unhealthy behaviours such as smoking, eating fatty foods, drinking alcohol excessively, or lack of exercise.[43] Amount smoked is associated with depression in some populations but not in others.[19] Difficulties in quitting smoking have also been associated with depression.[44] The predictive effect of depressive illness on coronary heart disease appears stronger in some studies of smokers,[15] but in most reported studies adjustment of the association between depressive symptoms or depressive illness and coronary heart disease by smoking has little effect on diminishing the risk. In a more detailed analysis of this question, Anda *et al.* found a strong interaction between hopelessness, smoking, and risk of fatal coronary heart disease.[45] This did not explain the association between hopelessness and coronary heart disease because there was still an increased coronary risk associated with hopelessness in non-smokers, but the risk of coronary heart disease increased in those with depressed affect who were also smokers.

Hostility

The experience of depression may be an indicator of personality characteristics, such as hostility, or the outcome of the interaction between personality characteristics and external circumstances, which relate to higher coronary heart disease risk through chronic physiological hyperreactivity in stressful occupational or domestic contexts.[46] This is further described by Redford Williams in Chapter 6. One intriguing possibility is that expression of high levels of hostility associated with hypomanic mood elevation is an indicator of a *forme fruste* of bipolar disorder, thus linking hostility, depression, and coronary risk.[47]

Psychosocial factors

Depression may be an outcome of exposure to adverse social circumstances and social isolation, which are risk factors for both depression and coronary heart disease.[48] In addition, depression may be the intermediate outcome of exposure to situations of low perceived control both at work and at home.[49] Low control is a powerful explanation for the higher incidence of coronary heart disease associated with lower socioeconomic status.[50]

Direct effects of depression

Depression may act independently of these associated factors and may of itself induce biochemical and physiological changes. These include sympathoadrenal hyperactivity, hypothalamic–pituitary–adrenal axis hyperactivity, diminished heart rate variability, ventricular instability, and myocardial ischaemia in relation to mental stress and alterations in platelet receptors.[46] Sympathoadrenal hyperactivity with raised plasma levels of norepinephrine (noradrenaline) seems to represent a state marker of depression.[51] Sympathoadrenal stimulation modifies the function of circulating platelets and lipids, and inhibits vascular eicosanoid synthesis.[52] Heart rate variability is decreased in depressed patients compared with non-depressed groups,[53] which may reflect decreased parasympathetic tone, predisposing to ventricular arrhythmias.

Vascular depression

Finally, a further mechanism has been postulated to explain the link between depression and coronary heart disease. Could the same vascular pathology that is affecting the heart also be affecting the brain? Thus depression might be the outcome of cerebrovascular lesions. A syndrome of "vascular depression" has been described in highly selected clinical samples; more likely to have onset after 60 years, less likely to have a family history of depression, more likely to be non-psychotic,[54] also having more cognitive impairment, more retardation, less agitation, less guilt, and less insight.[55] This vascular depression has been associated with lesions in the subcortical grey matter, deep white matter and periventricular grey matter. These studies suggest that lesions in the striato–pallido–thalamo–cortical pathways may be responsible for depression. In this situation, the association between depression and subsequent coronary heart disease would be artefactual. A more holistic picture is provided by the Cardiovascular Health Study, a population-based, cross-sectional study of elderly people living in the community.[56] Non-basal ganglia lesions identified on magnetic resonance imaging, rather than basal ganglia lesions, were associated with depression measured with the Center for Epidemiologic Studies depression scale, adjusting for age, sex, history of stroke, and transient ischaemic attack. However, this association was abolished after adjustment for cognitive and physical function. Thus there could be two explanations: either depression is a reaction to increasing disability, or brain lesions that create high levels of disability are also selectively associated with depressive symptoms.

These explanations for the association of depression and coronary heart disease depend on the cerebrovascular lesions probably predating coronary heart disease by some years. Although this seems a plausible explanation in the elderly and could account for the association of relatively mild depressive symptoms and coronary heart disease, it does not seem to explain the association of depression in younger age groups and later coronary heart disease. The cerebrovascular lesions seem to be the result of small vessel disease rather than atherosclerosis, which makes their relevance to the pathological processes involved in coronary heart disease less complementary. The mechanisms may be different in younger samples.

Anxiety and coronary heart disease

The most consistent evidence indicating a specific association between affective disorders and coronary heart disease comes from a group of studies examining the relationship between anxiety and cardiac outcomes, particularly sudden death (Table 7.2). In the first of these studies, the Northwick Park study of 1457 men in the United Kingdom, high levels of phobic anxiety measured by the Crown–Crisp index were associated with a relative risk for fatal coronary heart disease of 3.77 (95% confidence interval 1.64–8.64).[57] In further work, the Crown–Crisp index was used again in 33 999 men aged between 40 and 75 years from the US Health Professionals follow up study.[58] Among men without coronary heart disease at baseline, a dose–response relationship was found between phobic anxiety and fatal coronary heart disease (relative risk 2.5, 95% CI 1.00–5.96). Further analysis revealed that this association was due to an excess risk of sudden death. These findings persisted after adjustment for smoking, alcohol use, and a broad range of cardiovascular risk factors, and in a sample including baseline cases of coronary heart disease. On the other

Table 7.2 Prospective studies of the association between anxiety and coronary heart disease.

Study	Total sample	Age at entry (yr)/sample	Anxiety measure	CHD measure	Follow up (yr)	Number of non-fatal and fatal events	Adjustments*	Relative risk (95% CI)	Summary
Haines et al. (1987)[57]	3500	40–64 Occupational groups	Crown–Crisp Index	Non-fatal/ fatal IHD	6	57 NF IHD 56 F IHD		NF 1·26 (0·62–2·54) F 3·77 (1·64–8·64)	Phobic anxiety associated with CHD
Kawachi et al. (1994)[58]	51 529	40–75 Health professionals	Crown–Crisp Index	Non-fatal/ fatal IHD	2	128 NF 140 F	Age SMK CHOL HYP DIAB FH BMI ALC PA	NF 0·89 (0·45–1·79) F 2·45 (1·00–5·96)	An association between phobic anxiety and fatal CHD
Kawachi et al. (1994)[60]	2280	21–80 Community sample	Five-item anxiety scale from Cornell Medical Index	Non-fatal/ fatal IHD	32	137 NF 131 F	Age BMI SBP DBP CHOL ALC SMK FH	NF 0·71 (0·24–2·09) F 1·94 (0·70–5·41)	An association between anxiety and CHD
Kubzansky et al. (1997)[61]	2280	21–80 Community sample	Worry scale	Non-fatal/ fatal CHD	20	113 NF 86 F	Age DIAB CHOL BMI FH ALC SMK SBP DBP	NF 2·41 (1·40–4·13) F 0·81 (0·45–1·44)	Worrying increases the risk of CHD

*Adjustments: SMK, smoking; ALC, alcohol; PA, physical activity; MS, marital status; SBP, DBP, systolic, diastolic blood pressure; BMI, body mass index; CHOL, cholesterol; HYP, hypertension; DIAB, diabetes; ANG, angina FH, family history.
CHD, coronary heart disease; CI, confidence interval; F, fatal; IHD, ischaemic heart disease; NF, non-fatal.

hand, no association was found between phobic anxiety and either non-fatal myocardial infarction or total coronary heart disease.

One explanation for these results might be that this excess mortality could be a consequence of the drugs prescribed to treat phobic anxiety, as a British case–control study in a general practice setting found increased risk for myocardial infarction among women using benzodiazepines, tricyclic antidepressants, and barbiturates,[59] although it is difficult to separate the risk associated with the drugs from the risk attached to underlying anxiety. Nevertheless, examination of the mortality risk in the subgroup who were drug free in the Health Professionals follow up study showed similar magnitudes of effect, making the explanation of drug side effects less likely.

Two questions arose out of this research—how generalisable might this effect be from the findings in a group of male professionals, and is this effect found only with phobic anxiety or might it occur with other anxiety disorders? Kawachi examined the association between other anxiety disorders and mortality using the Normative Aging Study cohort, involving a community sample of 2271 men, aged 21 to 80 years in 1961.[60] A five item anxiety scale was extracted from the Cornell Medical Index. This correlates moderately with the Crown–Crisp index but contains four items more indicative of generalised anxiety disorder: "Are you considered a nervous person?" "Are you constantly keyed up and jittery?" "Do you often become suddenly scared for no good reason?" "Do you often break out in a cold sweat?"

In a nested case–control analysis, the age adjusted odds ratio for fatal coronary heart disease was elevated (OR = 3.20, 95% CI 1.27–8.09) among men who scored 2 or more on the anxiety symptoms scale compared with those who scored 0. There were no increases in either the age adjusted odds ratios or in multivariate analyses for non-fatal myocardial infarction, non-fatal coronary heart disease, or total coronary heart disease in relation to raised anxiety. As high levels of anxiety have been related to smoking, these analyses were adjusted for smoking, body mass index, systolic and diastolic blood pressure, cholesterol level, family history of heart disease, and alcohol intake. After adjustment for these factors, the multivariate odds ratio for fatal coronary heart disease became non-significant (OR = 1.94, 95% CI 0.7–5.41, for two or more symptoms). Men who scored 1 on the anxiety scale compared with men who scored 0 had elevated odds ratios for sudden cardiac death (OR = 2.96, 95% CI 1.02–8.55). The odds ratios for sudden cardiac death were even larger for men who scored 2 or higher on the anxiety scale (OR = 4.46, 95% CI 0.92–21.6). Risk was not elevated for non-sudden causes of cardiac death.

Further analyses in the Normative Aging Study have examined an additional dimension of anxiety—chronic worrying—as a risk factor for coronary heart disease.[61] Unlike the other anxiety measures already discussed, worrying might be considered as generally not indicative of psychopathology. Five domains of worries were identified: social conditions (for example, economic recession), health, finances, self definition, and ageing. Moderate levels of worry about social conditions were related to elevated age adjusted risks for myocardial infarction (RR = 1.70, 95% CI 1.01–2.86), while for high levels of worry the relative risk was 2.54 (95% CI 1.49–4.31). This risk was not modified by adjustment for potential confounding factors. No association was found with angina pectoris or sudden cardiac death. Financial and health worries showed moderate associations with angina pectoris, the former also with total coronary heart disease. Health worries were also associated with sudden cardiac death (RR = 2.19, 95% CI 1.01–4.76), but the numbers were small and this was not found for the other types of worries. Self definition and ageing worries were not associated with heart disease. Overall worries did demonstrate associations with total coronary heart disease: for a 1 point increase the age adjusted relative risk was 1.40 (95% CI 1.07–1.83). This was not changed substantially after accounting for multiple risk factors. For a 1 point increase in the chronic worrying scale, the age adjusted relative risk for angina pectoris was 1.52 (95% CI 1.02–2.29).

Mechanisms for the effects of anxiety on coronary heart disease risk

The findings relating anxiety and sudden cardiac death are specific. The lack of an association between phobic anxiety and non-fatal coronary heart disease outcomes suggests that a different mechanism is involved from that implicated in the association between depression and coronary heart disease. It seems likely that sudden cardiac death may be the result of ventricular arrhythmias. Hyperventilation associated with anxiety disorders and panic attacks may lead to coronary artery spasm and heightened susceptibility to arrhythmias. Furthermore, intense psychological states burdening daily life are a risk factor for fatal arrhythmias, which may also be triggered by psychological events.[62]

A further pathophysiological pathway relates to reduced heart rate variability (see Chapter 14). Chronically anxious patients have low heart rate variability with decreased capacity for heart rate change in response to stress.[63] Diminished heart rate variability has been identified as a potent risk factor for sudden cardiac death in patients recovering from myocardial infarction and apparently normal subjects.[64,65]

The results relating worrying and coronary heart disease are less consistent with the anxiety findings and may represent a different mechanism. Intense worrying may imply two situations. The first is exposure to adverse environmental conditions and material circumstances, possibly over a prolonged period; this is similar to the increased risk of coronary heart disease in people of low socioeconomic status. It is possible that the effect of prolonged exposure to adverse circumstances on coronary heart disease risk is mediated partly through heightened levels of worrying. Second, worrying implies a perception of lack of control over situations. Lack of control, particularly in the workplace, has been identified as an important psychosocial risk factor for coronary heart disease.[66]

Depression following coronary heart disease

Rates of depression

Many studies have focused on depression following myocardial infarction. As the latter is a severe life event implying considerable threat to life and everyday functioning it is not surprising that it is associated with depression. Between 15% and 20% of survivors of myocardial infarction suffer from major depressive illness.[67,68] Ladwig et al. found that of 552 male survivors assessed 3 weeks after myocardial infarction, 14.5% had severe depression, 22.3% moderate depression, and 63.2% were without depression.[69] In 283 postmyocardial infarction patients Schleifer et al. found 18% suffering from major depression and 27% from minor depression.[68] Rates of major depression measured using a standardised diagnostic interview (Diagnostic Interview Schedule) and applying DSM–III–R criteria yielded similar rates: 16% major depression.[70] Interestingly, the presence of depression was not associated with the severity of the cardiac illness but was associated with the presence of other illnesses.[68]

Course of depression following myocardial infarction

Depressive illness can follow a recurrent course and, for a small proportion of cases, may remain persistent. The same patterns are seen following myocardial infarction, with 25% of patients having persistent psychopathology a year later.[71,72] The course of depression following myocardial infarction has been surveyed by Lesperance et al.[73] Of 222 patients with acute myocardial infarction assessed with the Diagnostic Interview Schedule at 1 week, 6 months, and 12 months, 16% had depression at first assessment and 32% during either initial hospitalisation or during the year after discharge. Of those not depressed at baseline, 21% became depressed during follow up. A prior history of depression was present in 28% of patients, which increased the risk of depression following infarction.

Only 12% of patients were seen by a psychiatrist during the follow up period. Most patients who might have benefited from treatment were not seen by a psychiatrist: only 35% who had major depression during admission and only 39% of those who became depressed during the subsequent year's follow up were referred. This is especially important because of the prognostic implications of depression following myocardial infarction.

Prognostic implications of depression

Depression in the early period following myocardial infarction has prognostic implications.[69] Patients with severe depression, compared with patients with moderate or low levels of depression, have higher levels of angina pectoris subsequently, continuing levels of emotional instability, lower levels of return to work, and higher maintenance of smoking. More than that, patients with high levels of depression or anxiety following myocardial infarction are more likely to die of cardiac causes over the subsequent 5 years than other patients.[7] In a follow up study of 222 acute myocardial infarction patients assessed using the Diagnostic Interview Schedule 7 days after myocardial infarction, 16% had major depression.[70] At 6 month follow up 12 patients had died: 17% of the initially depressed patients and 3% of the initially non-depressed patients. The hazard ratio for depression was 5.74 (95% CI 4.61–6.87, $p = 0.0006$) for mortality at 6 months follow up. After adjustment for other independent predictors related to severity of cardiac damage and cardiac function (Killip class, previous myocardial infarction, left ventricular ejection fraction) the hazard ratio decreased but remained strong at 3.44 (95% CI 2.25–4.63). Despite this increased mortality risk, depressed patients did not have more severe coronary heart disease than non-depressed patients at baseline 7 days after myocardial infarction. Further follow up of this cohort showed that major depression failed to predict mortality after 6 months, but the Beck Depression Inventory continued to predict survival in the later phases of follow up.[74] This could have resulted from selective attrition, with the vulnerable depressed patients dying earlier. This issue has been largely answered by a large follow up study of men and women assessed with the Zung Depression Scale at the time of diagnostic coronary angiography— those with significant coronary artery disease were followed up for a median of 15.2 years in which period there were 488 cardiac deaths.[75] During follow up 51.4% of the moderately severely depressed patients died, compared with 42.4% of the mildly depressed and 35.5% of the non-depressed subjects on the Zung scale. The mortality rate in the severely depressed patients was not much greater than that in the mildly depressed patients. Moreover, analyses using survival curves suggested that the higher mortality risk for depressed patients persisted into the later stages of follow up, against the hypothesis of early selective mortality for the majority of depressed patients.

Mechanism of increased mortality risk for depression following myocardial infarction

Several explanations have been put forward for the mortality risk associated with depression following myocardial infarction. The first is that depressed patients are less likely to adhere to treatment and less likely to adhere to healthy behaviours than patients who are not depressed. Certainly, there is evidence that depressed patients are more likely to continue smoking after myocardial infarction, but this seems unlikely to be a sufficient reason for the increased mortality risk. Depression may lead to decreased heart rate variability, with a greater risk of fatal arrhythmias in a heart already sensitised by myocardial infarction. Frasure-Smith *et al.* found premature ventricular contractions predicted mortality over 18 months in patients with depression following myocardial infarction.[74] The association between depression and cardiac events in those with existing coronary heart disease may be mediated through myocardial ischaemia predisposing to ventricular instability.[76] Alternatively, depression has been associated with possible heightened susceptibility to platelet activation and changes in platelet aggregatability, the latter mediated through changes in serotonin levels, leading to a greater risk of thrombosis.[51] If the mortality risk of depression is maintained over longer periods it may be that depression is also involved in longer term processes, for instance, altering neuroendocrine function or fostering the development of atherosclerosis.

Conclusion

The associations between depression and both the aetiology and the prognosis of coronary heart disease are convincing. Depressive symptoms as much as depressive caseness seem to be influential in predicting coronary heart disease, although it is unclear what the effect of duration of depression is upon risk. On balance, pre-existing ill health does not seem to explain the association between depression and coronary heart disease in younger people, but this may be the case in some older people. In older people, vascular depression resulting from silent cerebral infarction may be an indicator of vascular pathology in the heart. However, there is much about these associations that needs to be better specified. It is not yet clear what the underlying mechanisms of these effects might be and there is scope for much further research in this area. This might include better diagnosis of depressive illness, more emphasis on assessing the effects of duration of depression, better adjustment for baseline coronary heart disease in prospective aetiological studies, and more exploration of intervening factors and the links between cerebrovascular and cardiac pathology.

The studies on phobic anxiety present a clearer picture with risk of sudden death probably related to heightened susceptibility to arrhythmias. Following myocardial infarction, depression is unequivocally a risk factor for poorer prognosis, and susceptibility to premature ventricular contractions may be the crucial intervening risk factor. These associations have clinical therapeutic implications as depressive symptoms, depressive illness, and anxiety states can be treated by psychological and pharmacological methods, potentially leading to reductions in the morbidity and mortality associated with coronary heart disease.[77] Progress will depend on a greater understanding of the pathophysiological and biochemical links between depression and coronary heart disease, and more precise identification of the aspects of depression that confer risk and of the population groups most at risk.

Acknowledgements

We would like to acknowledge with grateful thanks the assistance of Farhat Rasul.

120

References

1 Lewis T. Report upon soldiers retired as cases of 'disordered action of the heart' (DAH) or 'valvular diseases of the heart' (VDH). *MRC Special Report Series 8*. 1917.

2 Wood P. Da Costa's syndrome (or effort syndrome). *BMJ* 1941;**i**:767–72,805–11,845–51.

3 Crisp AH, Queenan M, D'Souza MF. Myocardial infarction and the emotional climate. *Lancet* 1984;**i**:616–19.

4 Skerrit PW. Anxiety and the heart—a historical review. *Psychol Med* 1983;**13**:17–25.

5 Mayou R, Foster A, Williamson B. Psychosocial adjustment in patients one year after myocardial infarction. *J Psychosom Res* 1978;**22**:447–53.

6 Lloyd GG, Cawley RH. Distress or illness: a study of psychological symptoms after myocardial infarction. *Br J Psychiatry* 1983;**142**:120–5.

7 Frasure Smith N. In-hospital symptoms of psychological stress as predictors of long-term outcome after acute myocardial infarction in men. *Am J Cardiol* 1991;**67**:121–7.

8 Booth-Kewley S, Friedman HS. Psychological predictors of heart disease: a quantitative review. *Psychol Bull* 1987;**101**:343–62.

9 Appels A. The year before myocardial infarction. In: Dembroski TM, Schmidt TM, Blumchen G, eds. *Biobehavioural Bases of Coronary Heart Disease*. Karger: Basel, 1983.

10 Sesso HD, Kawachi I, Vokonas PS. Depression and the risk of coronary heart disease in the Normative Aging Study. *Am J Cardiol* 1998;**82**:851–6.

11 Bianchi G, Fergusson D, Walshe J. Psychiatric antecedents of myocardial infarction. *Med J Aust* 1978;**1**:297–301.

12 Carney RM, Freedland KE, Jaffe AS. Insomnia and depression prior to myocardial infarction. *Psychosom Med* 1990;**52**:603–9.

13 Stansfeld SA, Sharp DS, Gallacher JEJ, Yarnell JWG. A population survey of ischaemic heart disease and minor psychiatric disorder in men. *Psychol Med* 1992;**22**:939–49.

14 Aromaa A, Raitasalo R, Reunanen A *et al*. Depression and cardiovascular diseases. *Acta Psychiatr Scand* 1994;**377**:77–82.

15 Ford DE, Mead LA. Depression is a risk factor for coronary artery disease in men: the precursors study. *Arch Intern Med* 1998;**158**:1422–6.

16 Chang PP, Ford DE, Mead LA, Cooper-Patrick L, Klag MJ. Insomnia in young men and subsequent depression: the Precursors study. *Am J Epidemiol* 1997;**146**:1–10.

17 Hippisley-Cox J, Fielding K, Pringle M. Depression as a risk factor for ischaemic heart disease in men: population based case-control study. *BMJ* 1998;**316**:1714–18.

18 Checkley S. The neuroendocrinology of depression and chronic stress. *Br Med Bull* 1996; **52**:597–617.

19 Barefoot JC, Schroll M. Symptoms of depression, acute myocardial infarction, and total mortality in a community sample. *Circulation* 1996;**93**:1976–80.

20 Costa PT, Fleg JL, McCrae RR, Lakatta EG. Neuroticism, coronary artery disease and chest pain complaints: cross-sectional and longitudinal findings. *Exp Aging Res* 1982;**8**:37–44.

21 Costa P. Influence of the normal personality dimension of neuroticism on chest pain symptoms and coronary artery disease. *Am J Cardiol* 1987;**60**:20–26J.

22 Ferketich AK, Schwartzbaum JA, Frid DJ, Moeschberger ML. Depression as an antecedent to heart disease among women and men in the NHANES I study. *Arch Intern Med* 2000; **160**:1261–8.

23 Everson SA, Goldberg DE, Kaplan GA *et al*. Hopelessness and risk of mortality and incidence of myocardial infarction and cancer. *Psychosom Med* 1996;**58**:113–21.

24 Greene SM. The relationship between depression and hopelessness: Implications for current theories of depression. *Br J Psychiatry* 1989;**154**:650–9.

25 Murphy JM, Monson RR, Olivier DC, Sobol AM, Leighton AH. Affective disorders and mortality. A general population study. *Arch Gen Psychiatry* 1987;**44**:473–80.

26 Huppert FA, Whittington JE. Symptoms of psychological distress predict 7-year mortality. *Psychol Med* 1995;**25**:1073–86.

27 Thomas C, Kelman HR, Kennedy GJ, Ahn C, Yang CY. Depressive Symptoms and Mortality in Elderly Persons. *J Gerontol* 1992;**47**:580–7.

28 Fuhrer R, Dufouil C, Antonucci TC, Shipley MJ, Helmer C, Dartigues JF. Psychological disorder and mortality in French older adults: do social relations modify the association? *Am J Epidemiol* 1999;**149**:116–26.

29 Wassertheil-Smoller S, Applegate MD, Berge K *et al*. Change in depression as a precursor of cardiovascular events. *Arch Intern Med* 1996;**156**:553–61.

30 Ariyo AA, Haan M, Tangen CM *et al*. Depressive symptoms and risks of coronary heart disease and mortality in elderly Americans. *Circulation* 2000;**102**:1773–9.

31 Mendes-de-Leon CF, Krumholz HM. Depression and risk of coronary heart disease in elderly men and women: New Haven EPESE, 1982–1991. Established Populations for the Epidemiologic Studies of the Elderly. *Arch Intern Med* 1998;**158**:2341–8.

32 Fredman L, Schoenbach VJ, Kaplan BH *et al.* The association between depressive symptoms and mortality among older participants in the Epidemiologic Catchment Area–Piedmont Health Survey. *J Gerontol* 1989;**44**:S149–56.

33 Duncan-Jones P. Validity and uses of the GHQ. *Br J Psychiatry* 1979;**135**:382.

34 Schoevers RA, Geerlings MI, Beekman ATF *et al.* Association of depression and gender with mortality in old age. *Br J Psychiatry* 2000;**177**:336–42.

35 Pulska T, Pahkala K, Laippala P, Kivela SL. Follow up study of longstanding depression as predictor of mortality in elderly people living in the community. *BMJ* 1999;**318**:432–33.

36 Penninx BWJH, Guralnik JM, Mendes-de-Leon CF *et al.* Cardiovascular events and mortality in newly and chronically depressed persons >70 years of age. *Am J Cardiol* 1998; **81**:988–94.

37 Appels A, Schouten E. Waking up exhausted as risk indicator of myocardial infarction. *Am J Cardiol* 1991;**68**:395–8.

38 Appels A, Otten F. Exhaustion as precursor of cardiac death. *Br J Clin Psychol* 1992;**31**:351–6.

39 Kop WJ, Appels AP, Mendes-de-Leon CF, de-Swart HB, Bar FW. Vital exhaustion predicts new cardiac events after successful coronary angioplasty. *Psychosom Med* 1994;**56**:281–7.

40 Kop WJ, Appels AP, Mendes-de-Leon CF, Bar FW. The relationship between severity of coronary artery disease and vital exhaustion. *J Psychosom Res* 1996;**40**:397–405.

41 Appels A. Exhausted subjects, exhausted systems. *Acta Physiol Scand* suppl. 1997; **640**:153–4.

42 Van Diest R, Appels A. Vital exhaustion and depression: a conceptual study. *J Psychosom Res* 1991;**35**:535–44.

43 Ruuskanen JM, Ruoppila I. Physical activity and psychological well-being among people aged 65–84 years. *Age Aging* 1995;**24**:292–6.

44 Anda RF, Williamson DF, Escobedo LG, Mast EE, Giovino GA, Remington PL. Depression and the dynamics of smoking: a national perspective. *JAMA* 1990; **264**:1541–5.

45 Anda R, Williamson D, Jones D *et al.* Depressed affect, hopelessness and the risk of ischemic heart disease in a cohort of US adults. *Epidemiology* 1993;**4**:285–95.

46 King KB. Psychologic and social aspects of cardiovascular disease. *Ann Behav Med* 1997; **19**:264–70.

47 Barrick CB. Sad, glad, or mad hearts? Epidemiological evidence for a causal relationship between mood disorders and coronary artery disease. *J Affective Disord* 1999; **53**:193–201.

48 Kawachi I, Willett WC, Colditz GA, Stampfer MJ, Speizer FE. A prospective study of coffee drinking and suicide in women. *Arch Intern Med* 1996;**156**:521–5.

49 Stansfeld SA, Fuhrer R, Shipley MJ, Marmot MG. Work characteristics predict psychiatric disorder: prospective results from the Whitehall II study. *Occup Environ Med* 1999; **56**:302–7.

50 Marmot M, Bosma H, Hemingway H, Brunner EJ, Stansfeld SA. Contribution of job control and other risk factors to social variations in coronary heart disease incidence. *Lancet* 1997; **350**:235–9.

51 Musselman DL, Evans DL, Nemeroff CB. The relationship of depression to cardiovascular disease. *Arch Gen Psychiatry* 1998;**55**:580–92.

52 Anfossi G, Trovati M. Role of catecholamines in platelet function: pathophysiological and clinical significance. *Eur J Clin Invest* 1996;**26**:353–70.

53 Miyawaki E, Salzman C. Autonomic nervous system tests in psychiatry: implications and potential uses of heart rate variability. *Integr Psychiatry* 1991;**7**:21–8.

54 Krishnan KRR, Hays JC, Blazer DG. MRI-defined vascular depression. *Am J Psychiatry* 1997;**154**:497–501.

55 Alexopoulos GS, Meyers BS, Young RC, Kakuma T, Silversweig D, Charlson M. Clinically defined vascular depression. *Am J Psychiatry* 1997;**154**:562–5.

56 Salo R, Bryan RN, Fried LP. Neuroanatomic and functional correlates of depressed mood. The Cardiovascular Health Study. *Am J Epidemiol* 1999;**150**:919–29.

57 Haines AP, Imeson JD, Meade TW. Phobic anxiety and ischaemic heart disease. *BMJ* 1987;**295**:297–9.

58 Kawachi I, Colditz GA, Ascherio A *et al.* Prospective study of phobic anxiety and risk of coronary heart disease in men. *Circulation* 1994;**89**:1992–7.

59 Thorogood M, Cowen P, Mann J, Murphy M, Vessey M. Fatal myocardial infarction and use of psychotropic drugs in young women. *Lancet* 1992;**340**:1067–8.

60 Kawachi I, Sparrow D, Vokonas PS, Weiss ST. Symptoms of anxiety and risk of coronary heart disease. The normative aging study. *Circulation* 1994;**90**:2225–9.

61 Kubzansky LD, Kawachi I, Spiro A, Weiss ST, Vokonas PS, Sparrow D. Is worrying bad for your heart? A prospective study of worry and coronary heart disease in the normative aging study. *Circulation* 1997;**95**:818–24.

62 Lown B, DeSilva R, Reich P, Murawski BJ. Psychophysiologic factors in sudden cardiac death. *Am J Psychol* 1980;**137**:1325–35.

63 Yeragani VK, Balon R, Pohl R *et al.* Decreased R-R variance in panic disorder patients. *Acta Psychiatr Scand* 1990;**81**:554–9.

64 Kleiger RE, Miller JP, Bigger JT, Moss AJ. Decreased heart rate variability and its association with mortality after myocardial infarction. *Am J Cardiol* 1987;**59**:256–62.

65 Fei L, Anderson MH, Katrisis D *et al.* Decreased heart rate variability in survivors of sudden cardiac death not associated with coronary artery disease. *Br Heart J* 1994;**71**:16–21.

66 Bosma H, Marmot MG, Hemingway H, Nicholson A, Brunner EJ, Stansfeld S. Low job control and risk of coronary heart disease in the Whitehall II (prospective cohort) study. *BMJ* 1997;**314**:558–65.

67 Carney RM, Rich MW, Tevelde A, Saini J, Clark K, Jaffe AS. Major depressive disorder in coronary artery disease. *Am J Cardiol* 1987;**60**:1273–5.

68 Schleifer SJ, Macari-Hinson MM, Coyle DA *et al.* The nature and course of depression following myocardial infarction. *Arch Intern Med* 1989;**149**:1785–9.

69 Ladwig KH, Roll G, Breithardt G, Budde T, Borggrefe M. Post-infarction depression and incomplete recovery 6 months after acute myocardial infarction. *Lancet* 1994;**343**:20–3.

70 Frasure-Smith N, Lesperance F, Talajic M. Depression following myocardial infarction. Impact on 6 month survival. *JAMA* 1993;**270**:1819–25.

71 Doehrman SR. Psychosocial aspects of recovery from coronary heart disease: A review. *Soc Sci Med* 1977;**11**:199–218.

72 Mayou R. Prediction of emotional and social outcome after a heart attack. *J Psychosom Res* 1984;**28**:17–25.

73 Lesperance F, Frasure-Smith N. Negative emotions and coronary heart disease: getting to the heart of the matter. *Lancet* 1996;**347**:414–15.

74 Frasure-Smith N, Lesperance F, Talajic M. Depression and 18-month prognosis after myocardial infarction. *Circulation* 1995;**91**:999–1005.

75 Barefoot JC, Helms MJ, Mark DB *et al.* Depression and long-term mortality risk in patients with coronary artery disease. *Am J Cardiol* 1996;**78**:613–17.

76 Jiang W, Babyak M, Krantz DS *et al.* Mental stress-induced myocardial ischemia and cardiac events. *JAMA* 1996;**21**:1651–56.

77 Januzzi JL, Stern TA, Pasternak RC, De Sanctis RW. The influence of anxiety and depression on outcomes of patients with coronary artery disease. *Arch Intern Med* 2000;**160**:1913–21.

8: Impact of stress on diet: processes and implications

JANE WARDLE AND E LEIGH GIBSON

Stress may affect health not only through its direct biological effects, but also through changes in behaviours which themselves have an impact on health.[1,2] Clearly, one such health behaviour is eating, and in particular food choice: that is, stress may influence health through adverse changes in diet.[3]

From the point of view of cardiovascular disease risk, there is scientific consensus that diet is a major factor, and specific recommendations have been published.[4,5]

- The contribution of fat to total energy intake should not exceed 35%.
- Saturated fat intake should be no more than one third of total fat intake.
- Cholesterol intake should be less than 300 mg per day.
- Consumption of sources of monounsaturated fats (for example, olive oil) and ω-3 polyunsaturated fats (for example, fish) should be increased to substitute for cholesterogenic saturated fats.
- Intake of carbohydrate should provide at least 50% of total dietary energy.
- Fruit and vegetable consumption should reach a minimum of five servings per day.
- Salt intake should be reduced.
- Alcohol intake should be moderate (1–3 units per day).

It is believed that these changes would lower the risk of cardiovascular disease by stabilising or lessening atherosclerotic plaques, as well as reducing hypertension and thrombosis (see Chapters 11 and 12). In addition, cardiovascular disease risk increases with increasing adiposity,[6,7] so dietary changes that help to lower body weight or maintain body mass index within 20–25 kg/m^2, and reduce obesity related insulin resistance and hyperlipidaemia, would also be beneficial.

Stress could increase the risk of cardiovascular disease by inducing changes in diet that are opposite to the above recommendations. In addition, it is likely that the physiological sequelae of stress will promote or exacerbate cardiovascular disease to a greater extent in the presence of a diet that raises risk factors such as hypercholesterolaemia and hypertension.[8]

Influences on quality of diet

It needs to be recognised at the outset that diet, mediated behaviourally by food choice, is under the influence of a complex array of factors. Foods can be chosen not just for a liked flavour, but also because of cost, availability, convenience, perceived health promoting features, and social, cultural, religious, or psychological considerations.[9] Furthermore, dietary habits and preferences are modified through a lifetime of learning about the consequences of eating,[10] and through reacting to the influence of parents, family, and friends,[11] as well as persuasion from the food industry. Also, it is probable that eating habits may be adapted, and new foods sought, through an intrinsic motivation to explore, albeit cautiously, our nutritional environment.[12]

If stress affects diet, it may do so by interacting with any of these influences on food choice. An obvious non-appetitive influence would be a change in the time available to procure and prepare food: thus, stressed workers pressed for time may simply select the most convenient food available, probably with a reduction in dietary quality as a result. In addition, appetitive effects of stress may alter the choice as well as the amount eaten of particular foods. This could occur through cognitive mechanisms, such as beliefs about how filling a food may be, its appropriateness as a snack item, or a wish to eat a small but healthy meal. Alternatively, physiological processes, reinforced by learning, could bias food consumption in favour of particular sensory or nutritional properties that satisfy the demands of homeostasis or other functional needs and limitations.

Effects of stress on eating behaviour

The dominant and longstanding physiological concept is that stress will inhibit appetite and food intake, through a combination of suppression of upper gastrointestinal motility and stimulation of energy substrate mobilisation, although research continues into the underlying mechanisms and impact of different stressors.[13-15]

Acute stress activates the sympathetic branch of the autonomic nervous system (sympathetic nervous system), as in the classic "fight or flight" defensive response,[16] shunting blood from gut to muscles, and suppressing digestive processes.[17] Release of epinephrine (adrenaline) from the adrenal medulla, and norepinephrine (noradrenaline) from the sympathetic nervous system, stimulates glycogenolysis in the liver and lipolysis in adipose tissue, so increasing the glucose and free fatty acid supply to the muscles and other tissues. It also needs to be recognised that other sequelae of autonomic activation, such as a dry mouth and feelings of excitement, could discourage eating independently of energy status. Despite these apparently appetite suppressant consequences, there is considerable evidence for an increase in eating and/or a change in diet evoked by some stressors.

Studying the effects of stress on human eating behaviour presents obvious ethical and methodological difficulties: in controlled experimental settings the severity of the stress is constrained, while in naturalistic studies the nature of the stressor is often poorly controlled, and measurement of food intake is fraught with difficulty. Not surprisingly, this phenomenon has been studied to a greater extent in laboratory animals.

Stress and eating in laboratory animals

To eat or not to eat?

Animal research offers the opportunity to examine the general, physiologically mediated effect of stress on food intake, while maintaining close control over relevant variables.[18,19] Nevertheless, to date animal research has produced inconsistent results. Many of the studies were designed to model a depressed state, and involved quite severe stressors such as physical restraint (immobilisation) or cold water swims, over which the animal has no control. These sorts of stressor typically suppressed eating (considered to be a validation of the depression model).[20] Another common depression model, the chronic mild stress model, which generally results in reduced food intake (hypophagia), employs a series of milder stressors: for example, lighting and housing changes, noise, cage cleaning, and handling, applied chronically over many weeks.[21] In most animal models of depression, effects on food intake are typically assessed *after* (for example, 24 hours after) the chronic stress has been applied: moreover, other behaviours, such as exploration of novel environments, are often suppressed.[22]

Studies using more acute and arguably milder stressors, such as tail pinching, noise, and low intensity electric shocks, often found an increase in food intake (hyperphagia). One interpretation is that these acute and perhaps less physically engaging, stressors cause a general activation which energises behaviours favoured by the current environment: for instance, tail pinching has been shown to elicit gnawing of wooden blocks, not just eating.[23] Robbins and Fray argued that rats *learn* to eat during the general activation caused by the tail pinch.[19] Others have offered ecological explanations: an increase in eating rate, but smaller meals, with increased vigilance, induced by noise or novel environments, has been proposed to be an adaptive response to threat or stress, permitting refuelling while minimising predation risk.[24,25]

Studies using stressors for which the intensity can be systematically varied, principally electric shock, have generally found that hyperphagia is induced at low intensities, but that hypophagia can be seen at high intensities.[19] Hypophagia induced by stress may be partly due to enhanced activation of competing behaviours such as those aimed at escape or avoidance of the stressor. Alternatively, or additionally, severe stressors such as surgery may trigger overriding physiological processes which act to suppress appetite (see below).[26]

Changing food preferences

Of more importance in relation to cardiovascular disease is the question of whether selection or avoidance of particular foods is altered by stress. Few studies have addressed this issue in animals. However, a longstanding and consistent finding is that stress increases finickiness in rats: the classic example is the suppression of intake caused by stress in rats given diets adulterated by the bitter taste of quinine.[24,27]

This might reflect the same enhanced reactivity to salient stimuli underlying hyperphagia induced by stress, but with hypophagia induced by the innately aversive nature of the stimulus. Neophobia may be an important component,[24] but perhaps only to the extent that novelty increases the aversive strength of the stimulus. This finicky characteristic of ingestive responses to stress suggests a role for particular neural pathways in mediating the effect (see below).

In contrast to the reactions to bitterness, effects of stress on responses to sweetness are inconsistent. Irrespective of whether the stressor consists of repeated electric shocks or chronic mild stress, findings on intake of sweetened food or solutions include no effect of stress,[28–30] decreased intake,[21] or increased intake.[31] Nevertheless, a finding that chronically stressed rats show increased acceptance of diets with high levels of sucrose (30–40%)[29] compares well with a report that people with depression rate concentrated sucrose solutions as more pleasant than do controls.[32]

The impact of having a variety of foods to choose from has been studied in relation to hypophagia following immobilisation stress.[33] However, variety (three foods similar in macronutrient composition) merely enhanced intake to the same extent in stressed and unstressed rats. Indeed, it is well established that dietary variety enhances food intake in rats previously maintained on (unpalatable) laboratory chow.[34] This could be akin to the overeating stimulated by palatable foods in bored human beings.[35,36] It is not clear what cognitive or emotional routes link boredom to eating in humans, but one possibility is the intrusion of anxiogenic or depressing thoughts.

It needs to be recognised that variation in results abounds, and interpretation is hampered by differences in methodology such as strength and length of the stress, the feeding regimen, and the delay between stressor and ingestion test.[18] Prior dietary experience is a little studied but critical variable, because rats, as much as people, will need to learn about the relative benefits of dietary regimens. Indeed, it has recently been shown that experience with an energy dense diet protects rats against the cachectic effects of inescapable stress.[37]

The implications of any appetitive response to an isolated acute stressor for human cardiovascular health may well be rather different from the impact of repeated chronic stress; nevertheless, the relationship between the two forms of stress and their effects on diet, food choice, and cardiovascular disease risk can be addressed by animal studies, and remains an important area of future research.

Stress and human eating behaviour

Human research on stress and food intake has come from several research traditions. Naturalistic studies usually investigate community samples and attempt to gather information on food intake at high and low stress periods of life. The focus in these studies, as in most of the animal research, has been on the general effect of stress on eating over the short or medium term.[18] Laboratory studies typically administer a stressful procedure in parallel with an eating task, then covertly assess food intake. The emphasis therefore is on the acute effects of the stress. Most of the laboratory studies have looked at individual differences, examining stress-related eating in relation either to weight or dietary restraint (the conscious tendency to restrict intake).

Naturalistic studies

There are a variety of naturally occurring, but predictable, stressful circumstances that can provide an experimental context in which to study the effect of stress on variations in diet. School or university examinations have been used as the stressor in several studies, and periods of high work stress in others. Food intake is recorded either in a diary record kept by the study participants, or with a 24 hour recall procedure. The food records are then analysed to obtain estimates of intake of energy and nutrients. Biological measures such as weight or blood lipids have been included in some studies to provide another indicator of dietary change.

McCann *et al.* examined the effects of variation in workload on food intake and serum lipids in a small group of female office workers.[38] The workers reported a higher energy intake, and a higher percentage of energy ingested as fat, in two periods of high workload compared with the normal work period.

Using academic examinations as the stressor, Michaud *et al.* also found higher energy intake from 24 hour food records for the day of the examination compared with a month later, among high school students aged 15–19 years.[39] Increased academic workload and negative affect were associated with a less healthy diet in a study of health behaviours among university students,[40] while in another study, positive affect during examination periods was associated with improved diet.[41]

One problem with these studies is that there were no non-stressed control groups to disconfound high and low stress periods from sequential changes in the environment unrelated to stress. This makes it difficult to rule out the possibility that the dietary changes associated with periods of high stress were the result of different foods being available at the school or workplace (for example, pizza being brought to the office during the high workload period), rather than the individual's choices in the low and high stress periods. In a study of examination stress which included a control group, we found no overall nutritional difference between students taking examinations and others for whom there were no examinations scheduled at that time.[42] O'Donnell *et al.*[43] also failed to find significant differences in the diets of medical students between 3 months and 1 week prior to exams, or compared with a non-student control group. Their sample may have been too small (13 students) to detect dietary differences, but even so, plasma lipoprotein and catecholamine concentrations were raised during the stressful pre-examination week: stress is well known to produce unfavourable changes in blood lipids independently of diet (see Chapter 12).[8] In another study in which time sequence was not a confounding factor, high work load in department store workers was associated with greater intakes of fat, sugar, and total energy, but only in people who habitually restrained their food intake.[8,44] Restrained eating has also been found to differentiate appetitive responses to stress in laboratory studies (see below).

In addition, a number of prospective survey studies have reported a positive association between weight gain and negative life events.[45–48] However, a consistent finding was that such weight gain was temporary in women, though not in men.[45,47,48] Foreyt et al. found that greater weight fluctuation, in 468 normal weight and obese adults, was associated with higher reported stress over 1 year, regardless of initial body weight.[49] Lowe and Fisher analysed mood ratings prior to eating, over 13 days, and found that overweight women ate more snacks during negative than positive moods.[50] Similarly, when nurses and teachers completed diaries of their diet and stress levels, intake of high fat "fast foods" was found to be greater during high stress periods compared with low stress periods.[3]

Thus, from naturalistic studies in the non-clinical population, there is no support for the hypothesis that stress induces hypophagia, and weak support for stress resulting in at least a temporary increase in energy intake and deterioration in healthiness of the diet. This has some resonance with the popular concept of "comfort eating" and its association with eating disorders, albeit there is little evidence that the eating is indeed comforting. Thus, Rand and Stunkard found that obese psychotherapy patients (total $n=84$) were much more likely to report eating during negative emotional periods than normal weight patients (total $n=63$) (71% v 8%).[51] In contrast, 20% of normal weight patients, but none of the obese patients, reported actually losing weight during periods of stress. Such data are, of course, susceptible to the influence of expectations and memory bias.

There has been a small number of self report investigations of stress effects on eating in non-eating-disordered populations, which reveal a bidirectional effect. In one study, middleaged men and women kept daily stress diaries over several weeks and at the same time recorded whether, on that day, they had eaten more, the same, or less than usual.[52] The pattern of results showed that most individuals were consistent in their reactions to stress, with some consistently eating more on higher stress days, and others consistently eating less. Among these consistent responders ($n=80$), the hypophagic response predominated (72% v 28%).

Willenbring et al. administered an eating habits questionnaire to 80 men and women and found that the great majority (92%) reported changes in eating habits with stress; responses were fairly equally distributed between eating more (44% of sample) and eating less (48%), the former preferring energy-dense foods.[53] Weinstein *et al.* found that approximately half of a student sample reported that they "ate more than usual" or "binged" under stress, with the hyperphagic response being more common in restrained eaters.[54] Data were combined for the "ate less than usual" and "no change" response categories, so it was not possible to identify the reported frequency of stress hypophagia.

Comparable results were found in a questionnaire survey of 212 students, in which 42% reported eating more and 38% reported eating less under stress, with reported hyperphagia being twice as likely in dieters than in non-dieters.[55] Oliver and Wardle also asked about perceived changes in intake of a number of specific foods or food categories.[55] This revealed an interesting pattern of effects of stress, which was partly independent of whether eating increased or decreased overall: that is, sweets and chocolate were reported to be eaten more under stress by both hyperphagic and hypophagic students; conversely, fruit and vegetables, and meat and fish, were reportedly eaten less under stress by both groups (Figure 8.1).

One caveat is that reported changes in diet from all the above naturalistic and self report studies need to be interpreted cautiously. Dietary data are notoriously difficult to collect accurately: methods are either crude and limited, or invasive and hard to comply with, as well as subject to systematic misreporting. These shortcomings no doubt contribute to some of the variability in results. Although laboratory studies provide more objective measures of food intake, they are limited by eating context and choice of foods available. This restricts the generalisability of effects on food intake in such studies.

Laboratory studies

Most laboratory studies have been based on the idea that the "biologically natural" response to stress is hypophagia, but that individuals who are overweight, or exert strong cognitive control over their eating (highly "restrained" eaters), are unresponsive to their internal signals.[56,57] Participants (mainly female) are therefore characterised according to these features and are expected to respond differently to stress.

Laboratory stress studies have used a range of stressors, including unpleasant films, false heart rate feedback, task failure, and threat of public speaking. In the typical design, participants are exposed either to the stressor or to a control procedure, and food intake is assessed covertly, often disguised as a "taste test" in which participants are asked to taste and rate some flavours of a palatable food such as ice cream.[18]

Earlier studies grouped subjects by body weight, and in general found that stress increased eating in overweight subjects, whereas subjects of normal weight either were unaffected or ate less.[58,59] However, the stress manipulations did not always affect eating.[60] The majority of studies have followed the design used by Herman and Polivy, who grouped participants by their level of dietary restraint, and found that women who cognitively attempt to restrain their intake show no response to stress, whereas those

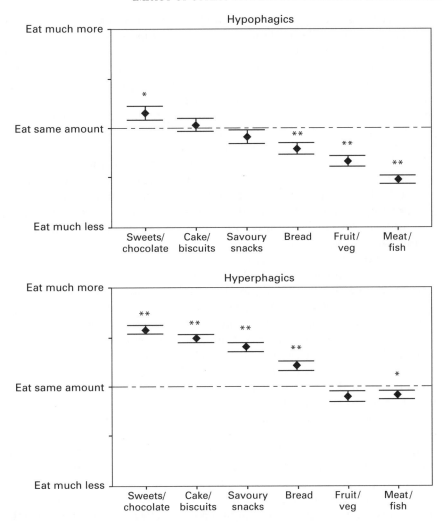

Figure 8.1   Self rated tendency to change the amount eaten of six food categories when stressed (212 students); adapted from Oliver and Wardle, 1999.[55] Upper panel: students who reported eating less when stressed (hypophagics; 38% of sample). Lower panel: students who reported eating more when stressed (hyperphagics; 42% of sample). Irrespective of these general effects on food intake, stress is perceived to increase intake of sweets and chocolates, but to reduce consumption of fruit and vegetables, and meat and fish. Data are expressed as mean $\pm$ SE; asterisks indicate statistically significant perceived changes in intake when stressed.

who are unrestrained reduce their intake under stress.[56] Mitchell and Epstein replicated this finding.[61] However, several groups reported hyperphagia induced by stress in restrainers but not in unrestrained subjects.[62–66]

Heatherton *et al.* have suggested that these different findings may in part reflect whether the stressor is simply fear inducing or ego threatening, the

131

former suppressing appetite in normal unrestrained eaters but not in restrained eaters, while the latter might actually increase eating in highly restrained women.[67] Interactions between restraint and stress have also been demonstrated by defining stress on the basis of subjects' self reports of emotional state after stressful tasks.[68–70] Some support was found for the induction by stress of hyperphagia in restrained eaters and hypophagia in unrestrained eaters. However, attempts to consider the additional impact of perceived hunger are hard to interpret,[68,70] since appetitive state confounds both physiological and psychological reactions to stress.

Bellisle *et al.* compared the mid-day meal intake on the day before a surgical operation with intake at a comparable time of day a few weeks later in 12 middleaged men, and found no difference either in energy intake or dietary composition.[71] However, the men showed a considerable variation, ranging from one man eating 125% more on the day before surgery, to another who ate 53% less.

That study was a rare example of testing the effects of stress on consumption of mixed food meals in humans. Others have addressed the issue of whether stress affected intake of foods differing in taste qualities (sweet, salty, and bland).[72] Men, but not women, ate less when stressed, with no significant effects of taste quality. These sex differences may have reflected differences in dietary restraint, but this was not measured. The ecological validity of these findings may also be limited by the fact that the foods were snack foods presented incidentally to the main task of viewing a film (used for the stress induction), and the amount of food eaten by the participants was very small.[72]

We also tested the effect of stress on intake of foods from sweet, salty, and bland taste categories, and in addition, high fat and low fat foods within those sensory groups.[73] Analysing effects by taste category may be important because stress has been shown to affect taste perception.[32,74] Threat of public speaking was used as the stressor, and the food was presented as a buffet style meal during preparation of the speech task. Dietary restraint and emotional eating tendencies were assessed as possible explanatory variables. Increases in blood pressure and changes in mood confirmed the effectiveness of the stressor. Stress did not alter overall intake, nor intake of the six food categories. However, stressed emotional eaters ate more sweet foods high in fat, and a more energy dense meal, than unstressed emotional eaters or non-emotional eaters in either condition. This suggests that food choice is affected by stress in susceptible individuals, and in a manner that may increase risk of cardiovascular disease.

Physiological and neural processes

Gastric emptying, gastric acid secretion, and upper gut transit time are delayed by acute stress,[15,75] so that nutrient absorption into the portal circulation is also delayed. These effects are likely to delay or decrease subsequent food intake.[76,77] This would seem to be an adaptive response to stress, diverting resources away from food intake and digestion towards processes allowing more active coping with the stressor.[24,78] At the same time, energy needs are met by mobilisation of stored fuels.

It should be noted that it is the neurohormonal responses to changes in fuel supply, metabolism, and storage that govern appetite at the physiological level, not simply plasma levels of glucose, lactate, or fatty acids.[79–82] The primary organ responsible for monitoring fluctuations in energy balance is the liver,[13] although neural signals of nutrient delivery to the upper gut are also essential for integrating substrate supply with normal control of appetite.[83] Hepatic carbohydrate and fat oxidation drive production of adenosine triphosphate (ATP), which provides a metabolic stimulus of energy flux signalled to the brain via vagal afferent sensory neurones.[13] Thus, mobilisation of stored fuels might be expected to reduce food intake, via increased hepatic ATP production, as would energy from food eaten. Energy supply from these two sources should offset each other in achieving energy balance, until factors affecting availability of one or other fuel supply disrupted the equilibrium: stress would be one such factor.[13]

Neurohormonal pathways

A critical neurohormonal system mediating the effects of stress on energy flux and appetite is the hypothalamic–pituitary–adrenal (HPA) axis. It is now well established that corticotrophin releasing hormone release is essential for the suppression of food intake by severe stressors such as immobilisation.[84] Thus, corticotrophin releasing hormone antagonists prevent stress induced hypophagia, while exogenous corticotrophin releasing hormone, administered for example into brain ventricles, reduces food intake.[85] Also, eating induced by tail pinch in rats is blocked by corticotrophin releasing hormone injection, and enhanced by corticotrophin releasing hormone antagonism.[86] It is probable that the involvement of corticotrophin releasing hormone in eating behaviour depends on the presence of either stress or nutrient deficiency: for instance, the enhanced preference for a novel food in rats deficient in protein is disrupted by corticotrophin releasing hormone administration.[87] This suggests a crucial role for the HPA axis in linking stress or deficiency induced redistribution of nutrient supply with changes in eating behaviour. The clinical observation that exogenous glucocorticoids stimulate appetite[88] has been replicated in rats:[89] the effect depends on stimulation of type II glucocorticoid receptors in the paraventricular nucleus of the hypothalamus,[89] and by inhibition of corticotrophin releasing hormone release.[90] However, it should be noted that corticotrophin releasing hormone is known to be released at a number of brain sites, and may influence behaviour, including appetite, independently of pituitary–adrenal activation.[91–93]

The involvement of the HPA axis in mediating the influence of stress on eating behaviour seems especially important for several reasons.

- Glucocorticoid hormones substantially affect energy substrate mobilisation and metabolism, increasing lipolysis, proteolysis, and gluconeogenesis, while protecting hepatic glycogen stores.[94]
- The circadian rhythm of HPA axis responsivity, and of corticotrophin and corticosterone, is dependent on patterns of food ingestion.[95,96]
- Normal meals, of at least 10% protein as energy, activate the HPA axis and release of cortisol in humans.[97,98]
- Food deprivation suppresses the HPA axis response to stress, especially during low levels of basal activity.[95,99]

Furthermore, most animal models of obesity, genetic or otherwise, depend on an intact HPA axis.[100] Indeed, the classic animal model of obesity resulting from lesions of the hypothalamic ventromedial nucleus includes elevated corticosterone levels, basal hyperinsulinaemia and insulin resistance, as well as hyperphagia. Also, akin to effects of stress on food selection in rats, animals with ventromedial nucleus lesions are characteristically finicky, being intolerant of quinine but voracious devourers of highly palatable diets, such as oily foods.[101,102]

Similarly, it has been proposed that disruption of HPA axis function may underlie at least some human obesity, in particular increased visceral adiposity,[103,104] which is strongly linked to raised risk of cardiovascular disease.[105] Indeed, visceral adiposity appears to be most associated with dysfunction of the HPA axis in obese patients suffering from anxiety and depression.[106] The eating disorders, bulimia and anorexia nervosa, are also associated with hypercortisolaemia and disrupted HPA axis activity even in the absence of undernutrition.[107,108] Nevertheless, the role of the HPA axis in human eating behaviour, both normal and abnormal, remains poorly understood.

Another hormone that may be involved in integrating HPA axis activity and food intake is the adipocyte hormone, leptin.[109,110] Leptin is synthesised in adipose tissue, and plasma levels correlate strongly with fat mass in humans,[111] with consistently higher levels in women than men independently of body composition.[112] In genetic rodent models, obesity has been shown to be associated either with the absence of leptin (ob/ob mice) or its receptor (db/db mice; fa/fa rats).[113,114] Glucocorticoids given to humans cause gradual and sustained increases in plasma leptin,[115] and leptin stimulates corticotrophin releasing hormone synthesis.[110] However, plasma leptin is not sensitive to acute food intake in humans,[116] and is not obviously related to depression.[117] Therefore, as yet a specific or critical role for leptin in mediating effects of stress on appetite has not been clearly demonstrated.

Involvement of specific neurotransmitter systems

In the nature of physiological and neurohormonal interactions with behaviour, the systems involved with stress and eating are diverse and complex. Numerous transmitters and hormones have been implicated in this area. Well established examples include norepinephrine (noradrenaline) and neuropeptide Y, both powerful stimulants of food intake when administered near the hypothalamic paraventricular nucleus of the hypothalamus in rats,[118,119] with intake of diets rich in carbohydrate preferentially enhanced.[120,121] Moreover, this hyperphagic effect of both neurochemicals depends on corticosterone release mediated by corticotrophin,[122,123] implying their possible involvement in stress and appetite. There is evidence that enhanced activity of noradrenergic projections to the dorsomedial hypothalamus induced by arousal or stress could facilitate overeating of foods rich in carbohydrate.[124]

Corticosterone enhances, while insulin inhibits, neuropeptide Y release in rats,[125] suggesting a homeostatic pathway encouraging restoration of depleted fuel stores following stress. Interestingly, neuropeptide Y is overexpressed in the brains of obese rodents deficient in leptin,[126] whereas in normal rodents, chronic neuropeptide Y infusion elevates leptin expression.[127] The HPA axis may mediate this link, since neuropeptide Y enhances corticotrophin and corticosterone release.[128] On balance, the evidence suggests that neuropeptide Y mediates initiation of eating provoked by disturbance of nutritional homeostasis,[129,130] which may be the result of stress, or a stressor in itself. An intriguing possibility is that commercial development of neuropeptide Y antagonists for obesity treatment might especially benefit individuals susceptible to stress induced eating.[131]

Two other neurotransmitter systems in particular—serotonin and the opioids—merit closer attention, given the strength of the evidence for their roles in appetite, food preference, and body weight regulation in animals and humans, as well as interactions with the HPA axis and responses to stress.

Serotonin

Serotonin (5-hydroxytryptamine, 5-HT) has a lengthy history of being implicated in control of appetite, food choice, depression, anxiety, stress, and the HPA axis.[132–135] The pattern of influence of 5-HT on these outcomes is complex and by no means fully integrated; nevertheless, with increasing knowledge of 5-HT receptor subtypes and associated specificity of function, recent evidence allows some potentially useful inferences to be made.

Inhibition of 5-HT release, as produced by stimulation of 5-HT somatodentritic 5-HT_{1A} autoreceptors, elicits hyperphagia.[136] More detailed analyses of this behaviour in rats show that there are marked similarities to eating induced by stress: that is, arousal allows a dominant behaviour in the current context, such as gnawing a wooden block, or eating, to be enhanced,[23] so that increased eating can occur, despite the incentive value of the food being reduced.[19,137] Conversely, there is growing evidence for the importance of the 5-HT_{2C} receptor subtype in mediating suppression of appetite, in both rodents and human beings.[138–141]

Can any predictions be made about the impact of stress on food choice or intake, from knowledge of the effect of stress on changes in 5-HT function? One problem is that the nature of the changes may vary with the extent of the stress. Thus, animal studies show that acute stressors such as handling, injection, and exposure to novel environments, are associated with increases in brain 5-HT release.[142] Conversely, chronic stress appears to be associated with lowered brain levels of 5-HT.[133] Interpretation of this area is complicated by evidence suggesting that different 5-HT pathways and terminal fields, as well as receptor subtypes, may have differing and even opposing roles. However, in general, deficient 5-HT function would seem likely to impair coping with stressful events.[133,134,143]

An explanation for the differential serotoninergic consequences of acute and chronic stress may be found in the role of the HPA axis. Increased 5-HT activity in acute stress activates this axis, thus increasing secretion of cortisol (or corticosterone).[135,144] However, chronically raised cortisol release during sustained stress seems to have a profound impact on 5-HT function: 5-HT synthesis is reduced, in part by diversion of its precursor amino acid, tryptophan, into other metabolic pathways, while 5-HT_{1A} receptor sensitivity is reduced and 5-HT_2 receptor sensitivity may be increased.[144–146] These receptor changes are the opposite of those found in response to acute stress. In addition, reduction of hippocampal 5-HT is associated with attenuation of feedback inhibition of the HPA axis by cortisol, which would then maintain the hypercortisolaemia. An inability to recover from these effects is thought to underlie chronic depressed and anxious states in some patients.[135,144]

Clearly, one might expect different effects depending on the temporal nature of the stress. Many data are compatible with an expectation of a reduction in appetite, or increased satiety, during acute stress, perhaps mediated in particular by increased 5-HT_{2C} receptor activation. In contrast, chronic stress may lead to 5-HT dysfunction and receptor changes, which, while not generally increasing appetite, may provide conditions in which a habit of consuming highly salient or reinforcing foods is easily acquired and maintained.[137] This is therefore one way in which stress may influence food choice, via effects on 5-HT function, rather than simply overall intake.

Tryptophan, 5-HT function, macronutrient intake, and dietary "self medication"

Synthesis of 5-HT depends on dietary availability of the precursor essential amino acid, tryptophan, owing to a lack of saturation of the rate limiting enzyme, tryptophan hydroxylase.[147] An important complication is that tryptophan competes with several other amino acids for the same transport system from blood to brain. If the protein content of a meal is sufficiently low, such as 5% (or less) total energy as protein, then relatively few amino acids will be absorbed from the food in the gut, whereas insulin (enhanced by high carbohydrate content) will stimulate tissue uptake of competing amino acids. Thus the plasma ratio of tryptophan to those amino acids will rise, favouring more tryptophan entry to the brain.[148–150] Not surprisingly, such effects also depend on the interval since, and nutrient content of, the last meal.[151] Importantly, there is evidence that dietary availability of tryptophan can influence brain function in humans; that is, feeding a tryptophan free diet (so presumably reducing 5-HT function)[152] can induce depression in previously recovered depressive people or in those with a genetic predisposition to depression.[144,153]

By way of comparison, dieting in women can lead both to reduced plasma levels of tryptophan,[141,154] and to increased 5-HT_{2C} receptor responsiveness after 3 weeks, implying a functional deficit of 5-HT in certain pathways.[140] Such a consequence could undermine adherence to weight loss regimens. However, these findings need to be interpreted with caution, given that fasting, exercise, and stress can all increase uptake of tryptophan into the brain, through greater amounts of free fatty acids competing with tryptophan for binding to albumin in plasma.[155,156] Moreover, prolonged fasting (often associated with dulled appetite) leads to downregulation of 5-HT uptake sites, so increasing 5-HT availability at neuronal synapses.[157] Also, meals of pure carbohydrate, fat, and protein can alter hypothalamic 5-HT release preabsorptively.[158] Nevertheless, in a study of dieting women, high carbohydrate intake was associated with relatively improved mood and a raised plasma ratio of tryptophan to competing amino acids.[159]

It has been proposed that states associated with reduced 5-HT activity, such as depression, lead to preferential selection of carbohydrate over protein by "carbohydrate cravers", in an attempt to "self medicate" or correct their 5-HT levels.[160] The evidence for this idea has been heavily criticised.[161,162] Nevertheless, a recent study provides some support for this model in susceptible individuals: Markus *et al.* found that neurotic ("stress prone") subjects were protected from depressed mood and from raised cortisol levels otherwise induced by a psychological stressor task, by eating a carbohydrate rich, protein poor breakfast and lunch, but not by a carbohydrate poor, protein rich diet.[163] In stable subjects, mood was depressed and cortisol level increased equally after either diet. This result was interpreted as improved coping following a diet-induced increase in tryptophan supply to serotonin synthesis,[163] although differential stimulation of the hypothalamic–pituitary–adrenal axis might also be involved.[98] The implication is that neurotic or stress-prone individuals may be particularly sensitive to dietary effects on brain pathways influencing mood and stress coping. These (mainly female) subjects may well have similar personality characteristics to those who overeat under stress.[164] To learn to "self medicate" through eating in this fashion would probably require ingestion of foods especially low in protein in isolation,[151] such as might be achieved by snacking on sweet and fatty foods while hungry. It has also been suggested that increased insulin secretion in stressed people would exaggerate the effect of carbohydrate rich, protein poor meals on 5-HT function.[165]

Opioids

Endogenous opioids are released during stress, and are known to be central to adaptive effects such as increased analgesia.[166] There is also abundant evidence for their involvement in motivational and reward processes in eating behaviour.[167–169] In humans, opiate antagonists appear able to reduce food intake without appreciably affecting hunger in several,[170,171] but not all,[172] studies, although drug-induced nausea can confound results.[170] The implication that more selective motivational effects than simply hunger are responsible is supported by evidence that opiate receptor blockade selectively reduces intake of the most palatable foods offered,[173,174] and the initial rise in appetite stimulated by eating palatable food is prevented by opiate antagonism.[175] Furthermore, pleasantness ratings, but not sweetness intensity, of sugar and fat mixtures were reduced by the opiate antagonist naloxone,[176] as was intake of such foods by binge eaters.[177]

Perhaps the best evidence for opioid involvement in an interaction between stress and eating is provided by Blass *et al.*[178] They demonstrated, in animals and human infants, that the ingestion of sweet and fatty foods (including milk) alleviates crying and other behavioural signs of stress. This stress reduction effect was blocked by opioid antagonists. The conclusion that adults select sweet, fatty foods for opioid mediated relief of stress is tempting, but remains speculative. Also, such behaviour would need to be explained in the context of stress itself enhancing endogenous opioid release. Nevertheless, it may well be relevant that κ-opioid agonists, which elicit eating in satiated animals,[167] block the inhibition of gastric motility induced by stress and mediated by corticotrophin releasing hormone.[179] The interaction of opioids, stress, and appetite remains a fertile area for research.

Psychological and social processes

Obesity, individual differences, and eating induced by stress

The clinical interest in the effects of stress on eating stemmed from the psychosomatic theory of obesity, which suggested that for the obese, eating met emotional rather than nutritional needs, and that the tendency towards emotional eating explained why they had become obese in the first place.[180] Eating was supposed to provide reassurance, and hence stress was predicted to trigger higher than usual food intake—"emotional" or "comfort eating". There is no doubt that many obese people report that they eat more under stress,[51] but these clinical reports need to be examined in controlled studies, both to establish their validity and to see if stress related eating is specific to obesity.[35,181] Without adequate longitudinal data in this area, the possibility that emotional eating is a consequence of obesity and chronic dieting, rather than its cause, cannot be excluded.

The balance of findings suggests that obesity may be an indicator of a higher risk of hyperphagia—or at least a lower likelihood of hypophagia—induced by stress. However, it remains unclear to what extent this is a result of associated chronic attempts to restrain eating, rather than some other facet of obesity.

The other side of the psychosomatic theory was that eating would have an anxiolytic effect, but this has received less support.[19] Many obese people admit that any solace they derive from eating is transient and rapidly followed by shame and regret at not having shown more self control.

In laboratory studies there has been no evidence that eating is successful in reducing emotional arousal. These observations have largely discredited the basic idea of the psychosomatic theory, namely that obesity represents a disorder of emotional reactions.

However, there is still interest in the idea that the obese (and chronic dieters) have a reduced sensitivity to internal satiety cues,[182,183] and the fact that they do not show stress hypophagia may be a consequence of this lack of internal responsiveness. Chronic attempts to restrain intake could lead to overreliance on cognitive or external influences on eating, so that dietary restraint might be the mediating factor in the obese, and indeed in normal weight, but highly restrained, emotional eaters. Thus, although restrained eaters seem capable of detecting large energy differences in foods, the relative control of eating by internal and external factors may be imbalanced:[184,185] this might lead to overemphasis on sensory, psychosocial, and emotional cues in eating contexts, which could contribute to unhealthy eating and obesity even in childhood.[186,187] The eventual relief of hunger (perhaps by particular foods) in restrained eaters, in a context of sociocognitive turmoil, might rapidly reinforce a "self medicating" habit of emotional eating.

Few naturalistic studies of effects of stress on diet have looked at individual differences, but those that have done so indicate that there are important differences that need to be considered.[44] In surveys asking respondents about how stress affects their eating, dieters are more likely to report stress hyperphagia, and non-dieters to report stress hypophagia.[53-55]

In a laboratory study, incidental snacking during recovery from a stressful task was greatest in subjects showing the least signs of physiological arousal during the task, but this relationship was attenuated among highly cognitively restrained subjects.[69] This supports the idea that eating may be controlled in part independently of physiological state in restrained eaters: normally dominant cognitive strategies for restraint in such individuals may be overridden by other imperatives during stress.

A potential cause of confusion in this area is that dietary restraint, as measured in most studies by the Restraint Scale,[188] includes the tendency for eating to be disinhibited by emotional states.[189] When separate scales were used to measure restraint and emotional eating, the latter was the better predictor of stress eating.[73] Thus, our finding of increased intake of sweet, fatty foods by emotional eaters during stress may underlie previous reports that dietary restraint or female sex predicts eating induced by stress. However, these factors are correlated, and all of them may contribute to release of eating under stress.

Type of stressor

Another explanation for variability in the results is the different kinds of stressors used. The animal literature suggests that physical, more prolonged, and uncontrollable stressors might be more likely to elicit hypophagia, whereas brief, arousing and/or psychosocial stressors might elicit hyperphagia. In human experiences, the stress of surgery for a hernia, which was used in one study, is qualitatively and quantitatively different from the stress of an examination or a period of long working hours used in others, and they could well have a different effect on food intake. Furthermore, it is obviously difficult to study effects of severe stressors for ethical reasons, and grief or family life stress cannot be accurately modelled, only surveyed.

One laboratory study reported differential effects of ego threatening versus fear inducing stressors,[67] although self esteem alone has not been found to be a reliable predictor of eating behaviour. At present, though, there are too few human studies to make any systematic analyses of the differential effects of different types of stressor.

Collateral effects of stress

In the real world, there will frequently be other consequences of stress beyond the emotional and physiological domain, which may often not be under the control of the stressed individual. For instance, stress at work may include increased time pressure and demands on attention and priorities.

These changes could reduce the range of food available no matter what the person actually felt like eating. Such factors may also affect choice in favour of foods that could be rapidly procured and eaten, i.e. from a pragmatic rather than a sensory perspective.

Stress might also be associated with changes in life circumstances, including economic difficulties, novel environments, or loss of family members who had been responsible for providing and cooking the food. All of these could alter a person's diet, irrespective of body weight or attitude to eating.

Conclusion

At first sight there appear to be numerous confusing findings and lack of consensus in this area, but on reflection an overall picture can be seen, and some predictions made (Figure 8.2).

The first indisputable point is that any effect of stress on diet will depend on the nature of the stressor: intensity, duration, and physical or psychological domain will all be important. From the perspective of this book, psychosocial stress, especially in the workplace, is likely to be of most interest. There is a modest amount of evidence for stress at work increasing the amount eaten, particularly of fatty and sweet foods.

In addition, the weight of evidence suggests that an identical stressor can lead to different effects in different people, i.e. hypophagia or hyperphagia, or at least a change in diet in some but not others. Therefore, any model of effects of stress on diet and eating must take individual susceptibility into account. Inherited predispositions, perhaps underpinned by genetic differences in neurochemistry, are probably interacting with experience to produce acquired stress coping strategies.

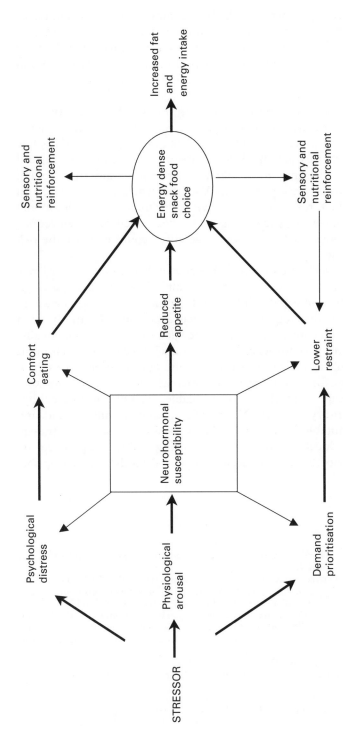

Figure 8.2 Proposed diverse pathways by which stress may lead to a final common effect of eating energy dense snack foods, particularly in susceptible individuals. Stress may thus result in a relative increase in dietary fat intake, and hence cardiovascular disease risk, independently of general effects on appetite.

From a neurochemical viewpoint, the best coping strategies would result in increased activity of relevant serotonergic and opioid mediated pathways. It has been pointed out that both selective carbohydrate consumption (or protein avoidance) and prolonged food restriction can independently result in increased serotonin function, so that either strategy may potentially alleviate stress and deterioration in mood.[190]

During stress, a combination of physiological necessity and neurochemical reinforcement would therefore seem likely to encourage the eating of smaller—but more frequent—amounts of energy dense, fatty, low protein foods. To what extent this leads to disordered eating may depend on the particular experience and cognitive strategies (and thus coping ability) that an individual brings to bear. Also, the demands of appetite and cognition may conflict, resulting in negative rather than positive emotional consequences. In any event, such a change in diet, which may well reduce the intake of antioxidant rich fruits and vegetables, could increase the risk of cardiovascular disease.

It is no unhappy accident that the majority of snack and convenience foods are rich in fat, and often in sugar or salt. Those characteristics go hand in hand with innate palatability, and rapidly learned sensory and nutritional reward, which together drive their acceptance by the hurried consumer. It seems that stress can exaggerate such motives physiologically, neurochemically, and psychosocially. Unfortunately from a research point of view, it is difficult to disentangle the separate contributions of each of these domains to the final common path of increases in unhealthy snacking induced by stress, especially when most available snacks share (unhealthy) nutritional and sensory profiles. Nevertheless, even dominant snacking habits are not immutable.[191] In the future, a possible therapeutic strategy could involve re-education to modify snacking habits, supported by appropriate pharmacotherapy, or even "functional foods", in susceptible individuals.

References

1 Adler N, Matthews K. Health psychology: why do some people get sick and some stay well? *Ann Rev Psychol* 1994;45:229–59.
2 Steptoe A. The links between stress and illness. *J Psychosom Res* 1991;35:633–44.
3 Steptoe A, Lipsey Z, Wardle J. Stress, hassles and variations in alcohol consumption, food choice and physical exercise: a diary study, *Br J Health Psychol* 1998;3:51–63.
4 Department of Health. *Nutritional aspects of cardiovascular disease*. London: HMSO, 1994.
5 Wood D, Durrington P, Poulter N, McInnes G, Rees A, Wray R. Joint British recommendations on prevention of coronary heart disease in clinical practice. *Heart* 1998;80(suppl. 2):S1–29.
6 Garrow J. Importance of obesity. *BMJ* 1991;303:704–6.
7 Willett WC, Dietz WH, Colditz GA. Guidelines for healthy weight. *N Engl J Med* 1999;341:427–34.
8 Brindley DN, McCann BS, Niaura R, Stoney CM, Suarez EC. Stress and lipoprotein metabolism: modulators and mechanisms. *Metabolism* 1993;42(suppl. 1):3–15.
9 Shepherd R. Overview of factors influencing food choice. *BNF Nutr Bull* 1990; 15(suppl. 1):12–30.

10 Booth DA. *Psychology of Nutrition*. London: Taylor & Francis, 1994.

11 Wardle J. Parental influences on children's diets. *Proc Nutr Soc* 1995;**54**:747–58.

12 Day JEL, Kyriazakis I, Rogers PJ. Food choice and intake: towards a unifying framework of learning and feeding motivation. *Nutr Res Rev* 1998;**11**:25–43.

13 Friedman MI. Control of energy intake by energy metabolism. *Am J Clin Nutr* 1995;**62**:1096s–100s.

14 Hagstrom Toft E, Arner P *et al*. Adrenergic regulation of human adipose tissue metabolism in situ during mental stress. *J Clin Endocrinol Metab* 1993;**76**:392–8.

15 O'Brien JD, Thompson DG, Burnham WR, Holly J, Walker E. Action of centrally mediated autonomic stimulation on human upper gastrointestinal transit: a comparative study of two stimuli. *Gut* 1987;**28**:960–9.

16 Cannon WB. *Bodily changes in pain, hunger, fear and rage, 2nd ed*. New York: Appleton, 1915.

17 Gue M, Bueno L. Brain-gut interaction. *Semin Neurol* 1996;**16**: 235–43.

18 Greeno CG, Wing RR. Stress-induced eating. *Psychol Bull* 1994;**115**:444–64.

19 Robbins TW, Fray PJ. Stress-induced eating: fact, fiction or misunderstanding? *Appetite* 1980;**1**:103–33.

20 Stunkard AJ, Fernstrom MH, Price A, Frank E, Kupfer DJ. Direction of weight change in recurrent depression. Consistency across episodes. *Arch Gen Psychiatry* 1990;**47**:857–60.

21 Willner P. Validity, reliability and utility of the chronic mild stress model of depression: a 10-year review and evaluation. *Psychopharmacol* 1997;**134**:319–29.

22 Curzon G. 5-Hydroxytryptamine and corticosterone in an animal model of depression. *Prog Neuropsychopharmacol Biol Psychiatry* 1989;**13**:305–10.

23 Fletcher PJ. 8-OH-DPAT elicits gnawing, and eating of solid but not liquid foods. *Psychopharmacol* 1987;**92**:192–5.

24 Job RFS, Barnes BW. Stress and consumption: Inescapable shock, neophobia, and quinine finickiness in rats. *Behav Neurosci* 1995;**109**:106–16.

25 Krebs H, Macht M, Weyers P, Weijers HG, Janke W. Effects of stressful noise on eating and non-eating behavior in rats. *Appetite* 1996;**26**:193–202.

26 Varma M, Chai JK, Meguid MM, Gleason JR, Yang ZJ. Effect of operative stress on food intake and feeding pattern in female rats. *Nutrition* 1999;**15**:365–72.

27 Dess NK, Minor TR, Brewer J. Suppression of feeding and body weight by inescapable shock: Modulation by quinine adulteration, stress reinstatement, and controllability. *Physiol Behav* 1989;**45**:975–83.

28 Kant GJ, Bauman RA. Effects of chronic stress and time of day on preference for sucrose. *Physiol Behav* 1993;**54**:499–502.

29 Sampson D, Muscat R, Phillips G, Willner P. Decreased reactivity to sweetness following chronic exposure to mild unpredictable stress or acute administration of pimozide. *Neurosci Biobehav Rev* 1992;**16**:519–24.

30 Strongman KT, Coles MGH, Remington RE, Wookey PE. The effect of shock duration and intensity on the ingestion of food varying in palatability. *Q J Exp Psychol* 1970;**22**:521–5.

31 Dess NK. Divergent responses to saccharin vs. sucrose availability after stress in rats. *Physiol Behav* 1992;**52**:115–25.

32 Amsterdam JD, Settle RG, Doty RL, Abelman E, Winokur A. Taste and smell perception in depression. *Biol Psychiatry* 1987;**22**:1481–5.

33 Zylan KD, Brown SD. Effect of stress and food variety on food intake in male and female rats. *Physiol Behav* 1996;**59**:165–9.

34 Rolls BJ, Van Duijvenvoorde PM, Rowe EA. Variety in the diet enhances intake in a meal and contributes to the development of obesity in the rat. *Physiol Behav* 1983;**31**:21–7.

35 Ganley RM. Emotion and eating in obesity: A review of the literature. *Int J Eat Disord* 1989;**8**:343–61.

36 Rolls BJ, Rowe EA, Rolls ET, Kingston B, Megson A, Gunary R. Variety in a meal enhances food intake in man. *Physiol Behav* 1981;**26**:215–21.

37 Dess NK, Choe S, Minor TR. The interaction of diet and stress in rats: high-energy food and sucrose treatment. *J Exp Psychol Anim Behav Process* 1998;**24**:60–71.

38 McCann BS, Warnick GR, Knopp RH. Changes in plasma lipids and dietary intake accompanying shifts in perceived workload and stress. *Psychosom Med* 1990;**52**:97–108.

39 Michaud C, Kahn JP, Musse N, Burlet C, Nicolas JP, MeJean L. Relationships between a critical life event and eating behaviour in high-school students. *Stress Med* 1990;**6**:57–64.

40   Weidner G, Kohlmann CW, Dotzauer E, Burns LR. The effects of academic stress on health behaviors in young adults. *Anxiety Stress Coping Int J* 1996;**9**:123–33.
41   Griffin KW, Friend R, Eitel P, Lobel M. Effects of environmental demands, stress, and mood on health practices. *J Behav Med* 1993;**16**:643–61.
42   Pollard TM, Steptoe A, Canaan L, Davies GJ, Wardle J. The effects of academic examination stress on eating behaviour and blood lipid levels. *Int J Behav Med* 1995;**2**:299–320.
43   O'Donnell L, O'Meara N, Owens D, Johnson A, Collins P. Plasma catecholamines and lipoproteins in chronic psychological stress. *J R Soc Med* 1987;**80**:339–42.
44   Wardle J, Steptoe A, Oliver G, Lipsey Z. Stress, dietary restraint and food intake. *J Psychosom Res* 2000;**48**:195–202.
45   Deurenberg P, Hautvast JG. Prevalence of overweight and obesity in The Netherlands in relation to sociodemographic variables, lifestyle and eating behavior: starting points for the prevention and treatment of obesity. *Bibl Nutr Dieta* 1989;**44**:8–21.
46   Gerace TA, George VA. Predictors of weight increases over 7 years in fire fighters and paramedics. *Prev Med* 1996;**25**:593–600.
47   Rookus MA, Burema J, Frijters JER. Changes in body mass index in young adults in relation to number of life events experienced. *Int J Obes* 1988;**12**:29–39.
48   Van Strien T, Rookus MA, Bergers GP, Frijters JE, Defares PB. Life events, emotional eating and change in body mass index. *Int J Obes* 1986;**10**:29–35.
49   Foreyt JP, Brunner RL, Goodrick GK, Cutter G, Brownell KD, St Jeor ST. Psychological correlates of weight fluctuation. *Int J Eat Disord* 1995;**17**:263–75.
50   Lowe MR, Fisher EB. Emotional reactivity, emotional eating and obesity: a naturalistic study. *J Behav Med* 1983;**6**:135–48.
51   Rand C, Stunkard AJ. Obesity and psychoanalysis. *Am J Psychiatry* 1978;**135**:547–51.
52   Stone A, Brownell KD. The stress-eating paradox: multiple daily measurements in adult males and females. *Psychol Health* 1994;**9**:425–36.
53   Willenbring ML, Levine AS, Morley JE. Stress-induced eating and food preference in humans: a pilot study. *Int J Eat Disord* 1986;**5**:855–64.
54   Weinstein SE, Shide DJ, Rolls BJ. Changes in food intake in response to stress in men and women: psychological factors. *Appetite* 1997;**28**:7–18.
55   Oliver G, Wardle J. Perceived effects of stress on food choice. *Physiol Behav* 1999;**66**:511–15.
56   Herman CP, Polivy J. Anxiety, restraint and eating behavior. *J Abnorm Psychol* 1975;**84**:666–72.
57   Schachter S, Goldman R, Gordon A. Effects of fear, food deprivation, and obesity on eating. *J Pers Soc Psychol* 1968;**10**:91–7.
58   McKenna RJ. Some effects of anxiety level and food cues on the eating behavior of obese and normal subjects: a comparison of the Schachterian and Psychosomatic conceptions. *J Pers Soc Psychol* 1972;**22**:311–19.
59   Pine CJ. Anxiety and eating behavior in obese and nonobese American Indians and White Americans. *J Pers Soc Psychol* 1985;**49**:774–80.
60   Abramson EE, Wunderlich RA. Anxiety, fear, and eating: a test of the psychosomatic concept of obesity. *J Abnorm Psychol* 1972;**79**:317–21.
61   Mitchell SL, Epstein LH. Changes in taste and satiety in dietary-restrained women following stress. *Physiol Behav* 1996;**60**:495–9.
62   Baucom DH, Aiken PA. Effect of depressed mood on eating among obese and non-obese dieting and non-dieting persons. *J Pers Soc Psychol* 1981;**41**:577–85.
63   Cools J, Schotte DE, McNally RJ. Emotional arousal and overeating in restrained eaters. *J Abnorm Psychol* 1992;**101**:348–51.
64   Frost RO, Goolkasian GA, Ely RJ, Blanchard FA. Depression, restraint, and eating behavior. *Behav Res Ther* 1982;**20**:113–21.
65   Polivy J, Herman CP, McFarlane T. Effects of anxiety on eating: does palatability moderate distress-induced overeating in dieters? *J Abnorm Psychol* 1994;**103**:505–10.
66   Schotte DE, Cools J, McNally RJ. Film-induced negative affect triggers overeating in restrained eaters. *J Abnorm Psychol* 1990;**99**:317–20.
67   Heatherton TF, Herman CP, Polivy J. Effects of physical threat and ego threat on eating behaviour. *J Pers Soc Psychol* 1991;**60**:138–43.
68   Herman CP, Polivy J, Lank CN, Heatherton TF. Anxiety, hunger and eating behaviour. *J Abnorm Psychol* 1987;**96**:264–9.
69   Rutledge T, Linden W. To eat or not to eat: affective and physiological mechanisms in the stress-eating relationship. *J Behav Med* 1998;**21**:221–40.

70   Steere J, Cooper PJ. The effects on eating of dietary restraint, anxiety, and hunger. *Int J Eat Disord* 1993;**13**:211–9.

71   Bellisle F, Louis-Sylvestre J, Linet N *et al*. Anxiety and food intake in men. *Psychosom Med* 1990;**52**:452–7.

72   Grunberg NE, Straub RO. The role of gender and taste class in the effects of stress on eating. *Health Psychol* 1992;**11**:97–100.

73   Oliver G, Wardle J, Gibson EL. Stress and food choice: a laboratory study. *Psychosom Med* 2001; (**in press**).

74   Dess NK, Edelheit D. The bitter with the sweet: the taste/stress/temperament nexus. *Biol Psychol* 1998;**48**:103–19.

75   Blair EH, Wing RR, Wald A. The effect of laboratory stressors on glycemic control and gastrointestinal transit time. *Psychosom Med* 1991;**53**:133–43.

76   Hunt JN. A possible relation between the regulation of gastric emptying and food intake. *Am J Physiol* 1980;**239**:1–4.

77   McHugh PR, Moran TH. Calories and gastric emptying: a regulatory capacity with implications for feeding. *Am J Physiol* 1979;**236**:R254–60.

78   Dess NK. Ingestion and emotional health. *Hum Nature* 1991;**2**:235–69.

79   Lavin JH, Wittert G, Sun WM, Horowitz M, Morley JE, Read NW. Appetite regulation by carbohydrate: role of blood glucose and gastrointestinal hormones. *Am J Physiol* 1996;**271**:E209–14.

80   Mellinkoff SM, Frankland M, Boyle D, Greipel M. Relation between serum amino acid concentration and fluctuations in appetite. *Am J Physiol* 1956;**8**:535–8.

81   Tordoff MG, Friedman MI. Hepatic portal glucose infusions decrease food intake and increase food preference. *Am J Physiol* 1986;**251**:192–6.

82   Warwick ZS, Hall WG, Pappas TN, Schiffman SS. Taste and smell sensations enhance the satiating effect of both a high-carbohydrate and a high-fat meal in humans. *Physiol Behav* 1993;**53**:553–63.

83   Lavin JH, Read NW. The effect on hunger and satiety of slowing the absorption of glucose: relationship with gastric emptying and postprandial blood glucose and insulin responses. *Appetite* 1995;**25**:89–96.

84   York DA. Central regulation of appetite and autonomic activity by CRH, glucocorticoids and stress. *Prog Neuroendocrinimmunol* 1992;**5**:153–65.

85   Krahn DD, Gosnell BA, Grace M, Levine AS. CRF antagonist partially reverses CRF- and stress-induced effects on feeding. *Brain Res Bull* 1986;**17**:285–9.

86   Heinrichs SC, Cole BJ, Pich EM, Menzaghi F, Koob GF, Hauger RL. Endogenous corticotropin-releasing factor modulates feeding induced by neuropeptide Y or a tail-pinch stressor. *Peptides* 1992;**13**:879–84.

87   Heinrichs SC, Koob GF. Corticotropin-releasing factor modulates dietary preference in nutritionally and physically stressed rats. *Psychopharmacol* 1992;**109**:177–84.

88   Baxter JD, Forsham PH. Tissue effects of glucocorticoids. *Am J Med* 1972;**53**:573–89.

89   Tempel DL, Leibowitz SF. Adrenal steroid receptors: interactions with brain neuropeptide systems in relation to nutrient intake and metabolism. *J Neuroendocrinol* 1994;**6**:479–501.

90   Dallman MF, Strack AM, Akana SF *et al*. Feast and famine: critical role of glucocorticoids with insulin in daily energy flow. *Front Neuroendocrinol* 1993;**14**:303–47.

91   Dunn AJ, Berridge CW. Physiological and behavioral responses to corticotropin-releasing factor administration: is CRF a mediator of anxiety or stress responses? *Brain Res Rev* 1990;**15**:71–100.

92   Merali Z, McIntosh J, Kent P, Michaud D, Anisman H. Aversive and appetitive events evoke the release of corticotropin-releasing hormone and bombesin-like peptides at the central nucleus of the amygdala. *J Neurosci* 1998;**18**:4758–66.

93   Rothwell NJ. Central effects of CRF on metabolism and energy balance. *Neurosci Biobehav Rev* 1990;**14**:263–71.

94   McMahon M, Gerich J, Rizza R. Effects of glucocorticoids on carbohydrate metabolism. *Diabetes Metab Rev* 1988;**4**:17–30.

95   Akana SF, Strack AM, Hanson ES, Dallman MF. Regulation of activity in the hypothalamo-pituitary-adrenal axis is integral to a larger hypothalamic system that determines caloric flow. *Endocrinol* 1994;**135**:1125–34.

96   Dallman MF, Akana SF, Bradbury ES *et al*. Diurnal rhythms in adrenocortical function are primarily determined by feeding and calories. In: Nakagawa H, Oomura Y, Nagai K, eds. *New functional aspects of the suprachiasmatic nucleus of the hypothalamus*. London: John Libbey, 1993.

97 Follenius M, Brandenberger G, Hietter B, Simeoni M, Reinhardt B. Diurnal cortisol peaks and their relationships to meals. *J Clin Endocrinol Metab* 1982;**55**:757–61.

98 Gibson EL, Checkley S, Papadopoulos A, Poon L, Daley S, Wardle J. Increased salivary cortisol reliably induced by a protein-rich midday meal. *Psychosom Med* 1999;**61**:214–24.

99 Kirschbaum C, Bono EG, Rohleder N *et al*. Effects of fasting and glucose load on free cortisol responses to stress and nicotine. *J Clin Endocrinol Metab* 1997;**82**:1101–5.

100 Bray GA. Food intake, sympathetic activity, and adrenal steroids. *Brain Res Bull* 1993;**32**:537–41.

101 Ferguson NB, Keesey RE. Effect of a quinine-adulterated diet upon body weight maintenance in male rats with ventromedial hypothalamic lesions. *J Comp Physiol Psychol* 1975;**89**:478–88.

102 Sclafani A, Aravich PF, Landman M. Vagotomy blocks hypothalamic hyperphagia in rats on a chow diet and sucrose solution, but not on a palatable mixed diet. *J Comp Physiol Psychol* 1981;**95**:720–34.

103 Bjorntorp P. Metabolic implications of body fat distribution. *Diabetes Care* 1991;**14**:1132–43.

104 Dallman MF, Akana SF, Strack AM, Hanson ES, Sebastian RJ. The neural network that regulates energy balance is responsive to glucocorticoids and insulin and also regulates HPA axis responsivity at a site proximal to CRF neurons. *Ann NY Acad Sci* 1995;**771**:730–42.

105 Seidell JC. Regional obesity and health. *Int J Obes* 1992;**16**:S31–4.

106 Rosmond R, Bjorntorp P. Endocrine and metabolic aberrations in men with abdominal obesity in relation to anxio-depressive infirmity. *Metabolism* 1998;**47**:1187–93.

107 Mortola JF, Rasmussen DD, Yen SSC. Alterations of the adrenocorticotrophin-cortisol axis in normal weight bulimic women: evidence for a central mechanism. *J Clin Endocrinol Metab* 1989;**68**:517–22.

108 Ward A, Brown N, Lightman S, Campbell IC, Treasure J. Neuroendocrine, appetitive and behavioural responses to d-fenfluramine in women recovered from anorexia nervosa. *Br J Psychiatry* 1998;**172**:351–8.

109 Licinio J, Mantzoros C, Negrao AB *et al*. Human leptin levels are pulsatile and inversely related to pituitary-adrenal function. *Nature Med* 1997;**3**:575–9.

110 Uehara Y, Shimizu H, Ohtani K, Sato N, Mori M. Hypothalamic corticotropin-releasing hormone is a mediator of the anorexigenic effect of leptin. *Diabetes* 1998;**47**:890–3.

111 Klein S, Coppack SW, Mohamed Ali V, Landt M. Adipose tissue leptin production and plasma leptin kinetics in humans. *Diabetes* 1996;**45**:984–7.

112 Rosenbaum M, Nicolson M, Hirsch J *et al*. Effects of gender, body composition, and menopause on plasma concentrations of leptin. *J Clin Endocrinol Metab* 1996;**81**:3424–7.

113 Pelleymounter MA, Cullen MJ, Baker MB *et al*. Effects of the obese gene product on body weight regulation in ob/ob mice. *Science* 1995;**269**:540–3.

114 Campfield LA, Smith FJ, Guisez Y, Devos R, Burn P. Recombinant mouse OB protein: evidence for a peripheral signal linking adiposity and central neural networks. *Science* 1995;**269**:546–9.

115 Newcomer JW, Selke G, Melson AK, Gross J, Vogler GP, Dagogo JS. Dose-dependent cortisol-induced increases in plasma leptin concentration in healthy humans. *Arch Gen Psychiatry* 1998;**55**:995–1000.

116 Korbonits M, Trainer PJ, Little JA *et al*. Leptin levels do not change acutely with food administration in normal or obese subjects, but are negatively correlated with pituitary-adrenal activity. *Clin Endocrinol Oxf* 1997;**46**:751–7.

117 Deuschle M, Blum WF, Englaro P *et al*. Plasma leptin in depressed patients and healthy controls. *Horm Metab Res* 1996;**28**:714–7.

118 Clark JT, Kalra PS, Crowley WR, Kalra SP. Neuropeptide Y and human pancreatic polypeptide stimulate feeding behavior in rats. *Endocrinol* 1984;**115**:427–9.

119 Leibowitz SF. Paraventricular nucleus: a primary site mediating adrenergic stimulation of feeding and drinking. *Pharmacol Biochem Behav* 1978;**8**:163–75.

120 Jhanwar Uniyal M, Beck B, Jhanwar YS, Burlet C, Leibowitz SF. Neuropeptide Y projection from arcuate nucleus to parvocellular division of paraventricular nucleus: specific relation to the ingestion of carbohydrate. *Brain Res* 1993;**631**:97–106.

121 Leibowitz SF, Weiss GF, Yee F, Tretter JB. Noradrenergic innervation of the paraventricular nucleus: specific role in control of carbohydrate ingestion. *Brain Res Bull* 1985;**14**:561–7.

122 Hanson ES, Dallman MF. Neuropeptide Y (NPY) may integrate responses of hypothalamic feeding systems and the hypothalamo-pituitary-adrenal axis. *J Neuroendocrinol* 1995;**7**:273–9.

146

123 Leibowitz SF. Hypothalamic paraventricular nucleus: interaction between α_2-noradrenergic system and circulating hormones and nutrients in relation to energy balance. *Neurosci Biobehav Rev* 1988;**12**:101–9.

124 Booth DA, Gibson EL, Toase AM, Freeman RPJ. Small objects of desire: the recognition of appropriate foods and drinks and its neural mechanisms. In: Legg CR, Booth DA, eds. *Appetite: neural and behavioural bases*. Oxford: Oxford University Press, 1994.

125 Strack AM, Sebastian RJ, Schwartz MW, Dallman MF. Glucocorticoids and insulin: reciprocal signals for energy balance. *Am J Physiol* 1995;**268**:R142–9.

126 Jang M, Romsos DR. Neuropeptide Y and corticotropin-releasing hormone concentrations within specific hypothalamic regions of lean but not ob/ob mice respond to food-deprivation and refeeding. *J Nutr* 1998;**128**:2520–5.

127 Schwartz MW, Baskin DG, Bukowski TR *et al*. Specificity of leptin action on elevated blood glucose levels and hypothalamic neuropeptide Y gene expression in ob/ob mice. *Diabetes* 1996;**45**:531–5.

128 Miell JP, Englaro P, Blum WF. Dexamethasone induces an acute and sustained rise in circulating leptin levels in normal human subjects. *Horm Metab Res* 1996;**28**:704–7.

129 White BD, He B, Dean RG, Martin RJ. Low protein diets increase neuropeptide Y gene expression in the basomedial hypothalamus of rats. *J Nutr* 1994;**124**:1152–60.

130 Woods SC, Figlewicz DP, Madden L, Porte D, Sipols AJ, Seeley RJ. NPY and food intake: discrepancies in the model. *Regul Pept* 1998;**75–6**:403–8.

131 Curzon G, Gibson EL. Pharmacological treatment of obesity. In: Watson SJ, ed. *Psychopharmacology: the fourth generation of progress*. Baltimore: Lippincott, Williams & Wilkins, 1998. URL: http://www.acnp.org/citations/GN 401/000156.

132 Blundell JE. Serotonin and appetite. *Neuropharmacol* 1984;**23**:1537–51.

133 Cowen PJ. The serotonin hypothesis: necessary but not sufficient. In: Feighner JP, Boyer WF, eds. *Selective serotonin re-uptake inhibitors: advances in basic research and clinical practice*. London: John Wiley, 1996.

134 Deakin JFW, Graeff FG. 5-HT and mechanisms of defence. *J Psychopharmacol* 1991;**5**:305–15.

135 Dinan TG. Glucocorticoids and the genesis of depressive illness. A psychobiological model. *Br J Psychiatry* 1994;**164**:365–71.

136 Hutson PH, Dourish CT, Curzon G. Neurochemical and behavioural evidence for mediation of the hyperphagic action of 8-OH-DPAT by 5-HT cell body autoreceptors. *Eur J Pharmacol* 1986;**129**:347–52.

137 Balleine BW, Fletcher N, Dickinson A. Effect of the 5-HT$_{1A}$ agonist 8-OH-DPAT on instrumental performance in rats. *Psychopharmacol* 1996;**125**:79–88.

138 Curzon G, Gibson EL, Oluyomi AO. Appetite suppression by commonly used drugs depends on 5-HT receptors but not on 5-HT availability. *Trends Pharmacol Sci* 1997;**18**:21–5.

139 Tecott LH, Sun LM, Akana SF *et al*. Eating disorder and epilepsy in mice lacking 5-HT$_{2C}$ serotonin receptors. *Nature* 1995;**374**:542–6.

140 Cowen PJ, Clifford EM, Walsh AE, Williams C, Fairburn CG. Moderate dieting causes 5-HT$_{2C}$ receptor supersensitivity. *Psychol Med* 1996;**26**:1155–9.

141 Walsh AES, Oldman AD, Franklin M, Fairburn CG, Cowen PJ. Dieting decreases plasma tryptophan and increases the prolactin response to d-fenfluramine in women but not men. *J Affect Disord* 1995;**33**:89–97.

142 Marsden CA. The neuropharmacology of serotonin in the central nervous system. In: Feighner JP, Boyer WF, eds. *Selective serotonin re-uptake inhibitors: advances in basic research and clinical practice*. London: John Wiley, 1996.

143 Spoont MR. Modulatory role of serotonin in neural information processing: implications for human psychopathology. *Psychol Bull* 1992;**112**:330–50.

144 Van Praag HM. Faulty cortisol/serotonin interplay. Psychopathological and biological characterisation of a new, hypothetical depression subtype (SeCA depression). *Psychiatry Res* 1996;**65**:143–57.

145 Chaouloff F. Physiopharmacological interactions between stress hormones and central serotonergic systems. *Brain Res Rev* 1993;**18**:1–32.

146 Porter RJ, McAllister Williams RH, Lunn BS, Young AH. 5-Hydroxytryptamine receptor function in humans is reduced by acute administration of hydrocortisone. *Psychopharmacol* 1998;**139**:243–50.

147 Fernstrom JD. Role of precursor availability in control of monoamine biosynthesis in brain. *Physiol Rev* 1983;**63**:484–546.

147

148 Fernstrom JD, Wurtman RJ. Brain serotonin content: physiological regulation by plasma neutral amino acids. *Science* 1972;**178**:414–16.

149 Teff KL, Young SN, Blundell JE. The effect of protein or carbohydrate breakfasts on subsequent plasma amino acid levels, satiety and nutrient selection in normal males. *Pharmacol Biochem Behav* 1989;**34**:829–37.

150 Yokogoshi H, Wurtman RJ. Meal composition and plasma amino acid ratios: effect of various proteins or carbohydrates, and of various protein concentrations. *Metabolism* 1986;**35**:837–42.

151 Fernstrom MH, Fernstrom JD. Brain tryptophan concentrations and serotonin synthesis remain responsive to food consumption after the ingestion of sequential meals. *Am J Clin Nutr* 1995;**61**:312–9.

152 Stancampiano R, Melis F, Sarais L, Cocco S, Cugusi C, Fadda F. Acute administration of a tryptophan-free amino acid mixture decreases 5-HT release in rat hippocampus in vivo. *Am J Physiol* 1997;**272**:R991–4.

153 Heninger GR, Delgado PL, Charney DS. The revised monoamine theory of depression: a modulatory role for monoamines, based on new findings from monoamine depletion experiments in humans. *Pharmacopsychiatry* 1996;**29**:2–11.

154 Anderson IM, Parry Billings M, Newsholme EA, Fairburn CG, Cowen PJ. Dieting reduces plasma tryptophan and alters brain 5-HT function in women. *Psychol Med* 1990;**20**:785–91.

155 Chaouloff F. Effects of acute physical exercise on central serotonergic systems. *Med Sci Sports Exerc* 1997;**29**:58–62.

156 Curzon G, Joseph MH, Knott PJ. Effects of immobilisation and food deprivation on rat brain tryptophan metabolism. *J Neurochem* 1972;**19**:1967–74.

157 Zhou D, Huether G, Wiltfang J, Hajak G, Ruther E. Serotonin transporters in the rat frontal cortex: lack of circadian rhythmicity but down-regulation by food restriction. *J Neurochem* 1996;**67**:656–61.

158 Rouch C, Nicolaidis S, Orosco M. Determination, using microdialysis, of hypothalamic serotonin variations in response to different macronutrients. *Physiol Behav* 1999;**64**:653–7.

159 Schweiger U, Laessle RG, Pirke KM. Macronutrient intake and mood during weight-reducing diets. *Ann NY Acad Sci* 1987;**499**:335–7.

160 Wurtman RJ, Wurtman JJ. Brain serotonin, carbohydrate-craving, obesity and depression. *Obes Res* 1995;**3**(suppl. 4):477s–80s.

161 Booth DA. Central dietary feedback onto nutrient selection—not even a scientific hypothesis. *Appetite* 1987;**8**:195–201.

162 Thibault L, Booth DA. Macronutrient-specific dietary selection in rodents and its neural bases. *Neurosci Biobehav Rev* 1999;**23**:457–528.

163 Markus CR, Panhuysen G, Tuiten A, Koppeschaar H, Fekkes D, Peters ML. Does carbohydrate-rich, protein-poor food prevent a deterioration of mood and cognitive performance of stress-prone subjects when subjected to a stressful task? *Appetite* 1998;**31**:49–65.

164 Van Strien T, Frijters JER, Bergers GPA, Defares PB. Dutch Eating Behaviour Questionnaire for assessment of restrained, emotional and external eating behaviour. *Int J Eat Disord* 1986;**5**:295–315.

165 Tuiten A, Panhuysen G, Koppeschaar H *et al*. Stress, serotonergic function, and mood in users of oral contraceptives. *Psychoneuroendocrinol* 1995;**20**:323–34.

166 Grossman A. Opioids and stress in man. *J Endocrinol* 1988;**119**:337–81.

167 Cooper SJ, Jackson A, Kirkham TC, Turkish S. Endorphins, opiates and food intake. In: Rodgers RJ, Cooper SJ, eds. *Endorphins, opiates and behavioural processes*. Chichester: John Wiley, 1988.

168 Doyle TG, Berridge KC, Gosnell BA. Morphine enhances hedonic taste palatability in rats. *Pharmacol Biochem Behav* 1993;**46**:745–9.

169 Mercer ME, Holder MD. Food cravings, endogenous opioid peptides, and food intake: a review. *Appetite* 1997;**29**:325–52.

170 Spiegel TA, Stunkard AJ, Shrager EE, O'Brien CP, Morrison MF, Stellar E. Effect of naltrexone on food intake, hunger, and satiety in obese men. *Physiol Behav* 1987;**40**:135–41.

171 Trenchard E, Silverstone T. Naloxone reduces the food intake of normal human volunteers. *Appetite* 1983;**4**:43–50.

172 Wolkowitz OM, Doran AR, Cohen MR, Cohen RM, Wise TN, Pickar D. Single-dose naloxone acutely reduces eating in obese humans: behavioral and biochemical effects. *Biol Psychiatry* 1988;**24**:483–7.

148

173 Yeomans MR, Wright P, Macleod HA, Critchley JA. Effects of nalmefene on feeding in humans. Dissociation of hunger and palatability. *Psychopharmacol* 1990;**100**:426–32.

174 Yeomans MR, Wright P. Lower pleasantness of palatable foods in nalmefene-treated human volunteers. *Appetite* 1991;**16**:249–59.

175 Yeomans MR, Gray RW. Effects of naltrexone on food intake and changes in subjective appetite during eating: evidence for opioid involvement in the appetizer effect. *Physiol Behav* 1997;**62**:15–21.

176 Drewnowski A, Krahn DD, Demitrack MA, Nairn K, Gosnell BA. Taste responses and preferences for sweet high-fat foods: evidence for opioid involvement. *Physiol Behav* 1992;**51**:371–9.

177 Drewnowski A, Krahn DD, Demitrack MA, Nairn K, Gosnell BA. Naloxone, an opiate blocker, reduces the consumption of sweet high-fat foods in obese and lean female binge eaters. *Am J Clin Nutr* 1995;**61**:1206–12.

178 Blass EM, Shide DJ, Weller A. Stress-reducing effects of ingesting milk, sugars, and fats. A developmental perspective. *Ann NY Acad Sci* 1989;**575**:292–305.

179 Gue M, Honde C, Pascaud X, Junien JL, Alvinerie M, Bueno L. CNS blockade of acoustic stress-induced gastric motor inhibition by kappa-opiate agonists in dogs. *Am J Physiol* 1988;**254**:G802–7.

180 Bruch H. *Eating disorders: anorexia, obesity and the person within.* London: Routledge & Kegan Paul, 1974.

181 Allison DB, Heshka S. Emotion and eating in obesity? A critical analysis. *Int J Eat Disord* 1993;**13**:289–95.

182 Craighead LW, Allen HN. Appetite awareness training: A cognitive behavioral intervention for binge eating. *Cogn Behav Pract* 1995;**2**:249–70.

183 Rodin J. Current status of the internal/external hypothesis for obesity: What went wrong? *Am Psychol* 1981;**36**:361–72.

184 Heatherton TF, Polivy J, Herman CP. Restraint and internal responsiveness: Effects of placebo manipulations of hunger state on eating. *J Abnorm Psychol* 1989;**98**:89–92.

185 Ogden J, Wardle J. Cognitive restraint and sensitivity to cues for hunger and satiety. *Physiol Behav* 1990;**47**:477–81.

186 Birch LL, McPhee L, Shoba BC, Steinberg L, Krehbiel R. "Clean up your plate": Effects of child feeding practices on the conditioning of meal size. *Learning Motiv* 1987;**18**:301–17.

187 Braet C, Van Strien T. Assessment of emotional, externally induced and restrained eating behaviour in nine to twelve-year-old obese and non-obese children. *Behav Res Ther* 1997;**35**:863–73.

188 Herman CP, Polivy J. Restrained eating. In: Stunkard AJ, ed. *Obesity.* Philadelphia: Saunders, 1980.

189 Van Strien T. On the relationship between dieting and "obese" and bulimic eating patterns. *Int J Eat Disord* 1996;**19**:83–92.

190 Huether G, Schmidt S, Ruther E. Nutritional effects on central serotonergic activity: a hypothesis on the unconscious self-manipulation of mood by food intake and dietary selection. *Nutr Neurosci* 1998;**1**:3–7.

191 Gibson EL, Desmond E. Chocolate craving and hunger state: implications for the acquisition and expression of appetite and food choice. *Appetite* 1999;**32**:219–40.

9: Smoking and stress

MARTIN JARVIS

The relationship between smoking and stress has long been recognised as puzzling. Nicotine is a stimulant drug. It increases heart rate, desynchronises the electroencephalographic trace, produces a pattern of autonomic arousal,[1] and is a psychomotor stimulant.[2] Human subjects given nicotine intravenously and double blind reliably identified it as a stimulant and frequently confused it with amphetamine or cocaine.[3] Sedative or anxiolytic effects of nicotine are hard to detect in non-smokers.[4,5] Despite these observations, which would suggest that nicotine should act as a pharmacological stressor, smokers frequently report that they want to smoke most when stressed and that smoking calms them down. Even adolescent smokers as young as 15 identify the calming effect of smoking as its most important subjective effect.[6] The mismatch between physiological and subjective effects of smoking has become known as the nicotine paradox,[7] and numerous attempts have been made to provide an explanation for it.[8-10]

Understanding how nicotine might reduce stress is important in considering smoking's role in relation to heart disease. Cigarette smoking has a number of known biological mechanisms through which it increases the risk of cardiovascular disease. It promotes thrombosis, produces endothelial and oxidant damage, acutely increases catecholamine release, leads to increased myocardial work, higher fibrinogen levels, and so on.[11] Not surprisingly, rates of myocardial infarction are greatly elevated in smokers in comparison with non-smokers, especially in younger age groups where other causes of cardiovascular disease are less prominent. At ages 30–49 rates of myocardial infarction in smokers are about five times those in non-smokers.[12] If this were all that there were to say about smoking in the context of heart disease, there would no room for anything other than outright condemnation. However, if smoking genuinely helps people manage stress, and if stress is itself a contributor to risk of heart disease, a more nuanced approach may be needed. It may be unhelpful simply to condemn smoking without understanding its role in people's lives.[13] If, for example, smoking by disadvantaged women is a means by which they cope with the challenge of caregiving in isolation and poverty, then simple preaching is unlikely to have much effect.[14] In this chapter, I briefly review the links between smoking, stress, and disadvantage, and outline attempts to explain the paradox.

Patterns of smoking prevalence and indicators of stress

Smoking is intimately linked to a variety of indicators of disadvantage throughout the life span. Children who are destined later to become smokers have been reported to show higher levels of neuroticism,[15] and to exhibit attention deficit disorder (Beresford, in preparation) and conduct disorder.[16] Among adults, patterns of smoking prevalence closely follow the contours of disadvantage.[17,18] There is a marked gradient in smoking by indicators of deprivation such as social class, housing tenure, car ownership, unemployment, and educational level, such that prevalence rises from about 15% in professional owner occupiers to 70% or more in the most disadvantaged groups. In addition to this, other indicators of stressful living circumstances, such as being a lone parent or being divorced or separated, independently predict higher prevalence (Table 9.1). It has been suggested that so strong are these relationships, that any measurable indicator of disadvantage—whether personal, material, or cultural—is likely to bear an

Table 9.1 Predictors of current cigarette smoking among men and women in the UK: General Household Survey 1988–1996. Reproduced from Jarvis and Wardle.[18]

	Men		Women		All	
	OR	95% CI	OR	95% CI	OR	95% CI
Social class						
I	1·00		1·00		1·00	
II	1·37	1·20–1·56	1·47	1·29–1·68	1·41	1·28–1·54
III NM	1·18	1·04–1·35	1·46	1·28–1·66	1·31	1·20–1·44
III M	1·65	1·45–1·88	1·86	1·63–2·12	1·74	1·59–1·90
IV	1·58	1·38–1·82	1·74	1·52–1·99	1·63	1·49–1·80
V	1·59	1·35–1·88	1·88	1·60–2·21	1·71	1·52–1·91
Rented tenure	1·88	1·78–1·99	1·85	1·75–1·95	1·87	1·80–1·95
No car	1·43	1·33–1·53	1·33	1·25–1·41	1·38	1·32–1·45
Unemployed	1·59	1·46–1·74	1·43	1·28–1·58	1·53	1·44–1·64
Crowding	1·25	1·15–1·35	1·10	1·01–1·19	1·17	1·10–1·23
Education						
Degree level	1·00		1·00		1·00	
Higher < degree	1·51	1·34–1·71	1·84	1·58–2·12	1·63	1·48–1·79
A level	1·62	1·44–1·82	1·62	1·40–1·87	1·61	1·47–1·76
O level	1·95	1·74–2·18	2·02	1·78–2·30	1·94	1·78–2·10
CSE grade	2·03	1·79–2·39	2·50	2·18–2·86	2·22	2·07–2·43
No qualification	2·49	2·23–2·78	3·10	2·72–3·53	2·73	2·52–2·97
Lone parent	0·90	0·73–1·10	1·49	1·36–1·64	1·33	1·22–1·44
Divorced or separated	1·73	1·56–1·92	1·38	1·26–1·51	1·53	1·43–1·64

CI, confidence interval; CSE, Certificate of Secondary Education; M, manual; NM, non-manual; OR, odds ratio.

151

independent predictive relationship to cigarette smoking.[18] The closeness of smoking's relationship to social disadvantage, which is in itself a marker for stress, suggests that cigarette smoking is intimately linked to the experience and management of stress, whether through self medication to enable coping or through other pathways.

Association of smoking with psychiatric morbidity

Social disadvantage leading to stressful circumstances translates at the individual level into impaired psychological wellbeing. Concepts of adverse mood states, stress, and neurotic symptoms are not well differentiated in surveys of minor psychiatric morbidity in the general population. Instruments such as the General Health Questionnaire,[19] the Malaise Inventory,[20] and the Perceived Stress Scale,[21] have a considerable degree of overlap in tapping a fairly non-specific dimension of minor psychiatric morbidity. The Clinical Interview Schedule – Revised (CIS-R) is designed as a survey instrument, assessing 14 different areas of neurotic symptomatology.[22] Scores for the individual symptoms are summed to derive an overall judgement of the presence or absence of significant current psychiatric morbidity ("caseness"), and also to diagnose particular neurotic disorders. The CIS-R has been employed in a large and representative survey of the general population in Great Britain to assess the prevalence of psychiatric morbidity and its relationship to socioeconomic circumstances, drug and alcohol dependence, and cigarette smoking.[23]

Here data from the survey are used to assess the relationship of cigarette smoking status (and the degree of dependence within smokers) to particular symptoms and diagnoses and to the prevalence of psychiatric caseness. Time to first cigarette of the day (measured in six categories ranging from less than 5 minutes to 2 hours or more) is used as an indicator of dependence in smokers.[24] Odds ratios for psychiatric morbidity associated with cigarette smoking status were calculated from logistic regression models which adjusted for sex, age, socioeconomic deprivation, alcohol consumption, and drug dependence. The scale used to measure socioeconomic deprivation incorporated information on occupational class, housing tenure, employment status, and access to a car.

As shown in Figure 9.1, odds for scoring as a current case of neurotic psychiatric disorder were slightly but significantly raised in ex-smokers by comparison with never-smokers (odds ratio 1.30, 95% confidence interval 1.10–1.53). Smokers in general were at increased risk of scoring as a current case, and there was a trend to higher odds with shorter time to first cigarette of the day. Among smokers who lit up within 5 minutes of waking, the odds of caseness were 3.21 (95% CI 2.51–4.11) by comparison with never-smokers. Odds of caseness were also raised among people from more disadvantaged socioeconomic circumstances, but the associations with smoking were independent of this, and there was no significant interaction between cigarette smoking and deprivation.

152

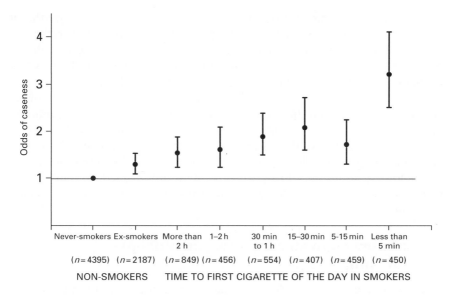

Figure 9.1   Current psychiatric disorder by smoking habit: the OPCS psychiatric morbidity survey. Odds adjusted for age, sex, deprivation, alcohol consumption, and drug dependence. Plots show odds ratios and 95% confidence intervals.

On a symptom by symptom basis, ex-smokers did not in general differ from never-smokers. One exception to this was that ex-smokers complained significantly more of somatic symptoms. Smokers had raised scores on all symptoms, and except for compulsions, there was a dose–response trend with time to first cigarette. Associations were particularly marked for the symptoms of depression, worry, anxiety, fatigue, panic, and irritability. Similarly, for most neurotic diagnoses, especially the three most common ones, there was a trend to increased prevalence with increased dependence on smoking. Compared with never-smokers, prevalence in the most dependent smokers who lit up within 5 minutes of waking was 15.3% (61/398) versus 6.2% (284/4552) for mixed anxiety and depression, 13.3% (53/399) versus 3.1% (143/4552) for generalised anxiety disorder, and 9.3% (37/398) versus 1.4% (65/4552)for depression.

These findings point to a remarkably pervasive association between cigarette smoking and minor psychiatric morbidity, an association that extends to the whole range of symptoms and diagnoses in addition to a measure of overall dysphoria. The associations are similar in men and women and across all levels of socioeconomic deprivation. Similar findings have been reported from surveys in the USA.[25,26] As with all cross-sectional data, interpretation of the associations is problematic. It could be that those who experience the most difficulties and stress in their lives are drawn to cigarette smoking. This could be either because smoking acts as a form of self medication that enables people to cope better, or because giving up smoking is especially difficult for those who encounter psychological and other problems. If smoking is self medication, then it has to be said that it is not very effective (other than perhaps very transiently) in normalising affect, as those who smoke the most also rate their psychological wellbeing as lowest while at steady state blood nicotine levels. Another possibility is that smoking itself may contribute to impaired psychological wellbeing. It is not implausible that there could be causal pathways in both directions: smoking could be both a manifestation and a cause of stress. The greater similarity of ex-smokers to never-smokers than to current smokers might suggest that much of the association is reversible with cessation, unless those who are able to quit successfully are strongly selected for relatively higher psychological wellbeing. Prospective studies are needed to unpick the relationships between smoking cessation, stress, and psychological wellbeing more precisely.

What happens to stress levels when people give up smoking?

The first few days and weeks of smoking abstinence are accompanied by a well delineated withdrawal syndrome, largely attributable to loss of nicotine.[27,28] Prominent symptoms include irritability, difficulty in concentrating, and depression. Withdrawal is acutely stressful, and is thought to be the cause of many quit attempts failing. It might, therefore, be thought that quitting would exacerbate stress, and this seems to be something that many smokers believe. However, in the numerous studies that have followed smokers after quitting there is a consistent finding that successful cessation leads to lowered stress and improved psychological wellbeing. Cohen and Lichtenstein found that perceived stress levels reduced with cessation, but increased again among those who relapsed to smoking.[29] Very similar results were reported by Carey et al., who followed smokers up for 12 months after quitting and found lower perceived stress in those who succeeded.[30] State anxiety has also been found to decline in successful quitters.[31] Finally, psychological wellbeing has been reported to improve 6 months after giving up smoking successfully.[32] Taken together, these studies consistently point to a benefit in terms of improved wellbeing and lowered stress in those smokers who succeed in becoming ex-smokers. Partly this may reflect an increase in self esteem through achievement of a difficult personal goal, but it once again raises the possibility that smoking, far from improving the ability to cope with stress, may itself cause increased stress.

Could the perceived stress management effects of smoking be illusory?

The notion that any effects of smoking in managing stress and mood are more apparent than real has received increasing attention in recent years.[8,33,34] Underlying this view is the fact that nicotine withdrawal has an onset within a few hours of not smoking, certainly with overnight abstinence during sleep, and possibly in embryonic form within 1–2 hours from the last cigarette. Symptoms of nicotine withdrawal include irritability, depression, anxiety, and difficulty in concentrating, as well as cognitive and performance deficits. These symptoms are eliminated by smoking a cigarette. So, the argument goes, dependent smokers become used to experiencing an improvement in mood state and performance when they smoke, because a considerable amount of their smoking behaviour is driven by a need to avert incipient nicotine withdrawal. Smoking is then perceived by the smoker as calming and stress reducing. This it is, but only to the extent of normalising deficits induced by abstinence, rather than in an absolute sense. This view was expressed forcibly by Schachter as long ago as 1978, when he wrote:

It has been widely reported that smoking increases with stress and that smoking is calming. These observations ... appear to support the assertion that nicotine or tar or some component of the act of smoking is anxiety reducing. The experimental facts are peculiarly at variance with this interpretation. Smokers are not more or less calm than a control group of non-smokers. They are, however, considerably calmer than groups of smokers who are prevented from smoking or permitted to smoke only low nicotine cigarettes. This fact can be interpreted as indicating that smoking isn't anxiety reducing, but that not smoking or insufficient nicotine is anxiety increasing.[10]

This model has the merit of reconciling smokers' perceptions of calming effects with the possibility that smoking/nicotine may at the same time be a physiological stressor.

Parrot has conducted a number of studies of moods in smokers over the course of a day which lend further support to this interpretation.[35] In each study, feelings of anxiety or stress were significantly lower after smoking than before smoking. However, while moods improved immediately after smoking, mood impairments occurred between cigarettes. People whose questionnaire responses indicated that they smoked to sedate themselves reported above average stress prior to smoking, rather than below average stress after smoking. Thus stress modulation represented mainly the relief of adverse moods, rather than the attainment of beneficial moods.

Conclusion

It seems unlikely that we have reached a definitive understanding of the enigmatic relationship between cigarette smoking and stress. It may be that a true anxiolytic or sedative property of smoking remains to be discovered. There have been suggestions that nicotine's effects on brain serotonergic pathways may provide such a mechanism, although convincing data are lacking.[36] Equally, it may be that the increased risk of suicide found in smokers and currently regarded as a paradigm of a meaningless epidemiological association will come to be viewed as attributable to stressor effects of nicotine or smoking.[37] What is abundantly clear is that smoking is intimately linked with the experience of adverse mood and stress and that smoking cessation has beneficial effects in improving wellbeing. This observation has the potential for sensitive exploitation to encourage smokers who place a high value on the use of cigarettes for stress reduction to quit and experience life as a non-smoker.

References

1 Benowitz NL. Pharmacologic aspects of cigarette smoking and nicotine addiction. *N Engl J Med* 1988;**319**:1318–30.
2 West RJ, Jarvis MJ. Effects of nicotine on finger tapping rate in non-smokers. *Pharmacol Biochem Behav* 1986;**25**:727–31.
3 Jones HE, Garrett BE, Griffiths RR. Subjective and physiological effects of intravenous nicotine and cocaine in cigarette smoking cocaine abusers. *J Pharmacol Exp Ther* 1999; **288**:188–97.
4 Foulds J, Stapleton JA, Bell N, Swettenham J, Jarvis MJ, Russell MAH. Mood and physiological effects of subcutaneous nicotine in smokers and never-smokers. *Drug Alcohol Depend* 1997;**44**:105–15.
5 Foulds J, Stapleton J, Swettenham J, Bell N, McSorley K, Russell MAH. Cognitive performance effects of subcutaneous nicotine in smokers and never-smokers. *Psychopharmacol* 1996;**127**:31–8.
6 McNeill AD, Jarvis MJ, West R. Subjective effects of cigarette smoking in adolescents. *Psychopharmacol* 1987;**92**:115–17.
7 Gilbert DG. Paradoxical tranquilizing and emotion-reducing effects of nicotine. *Psychol Bull* 1979;**86**:643–61.
8 Parrott A. Does cigarette smoking cause stress? *Am Psychol* 1999;**54**:817–20.
9 Epstein LH, Perkins KA. Smoking, stress, and coronary heart disease. *J Consult Clin Psychol* 1988;**56**:342–9.
10 Schachter S. Pharmacological and psychological determinants of smoking. In: Thornton R, ed. *Smoking Behaviour: Physiological and Psychological Influences*. Edinburgh: Churchill Livingstone, 1978.
11 Benowitz NL, Gourlay SG. Cardiovascular toxicity of nicotine: Implications for nicotine replacement therapy. *J Am Coll Cardiol* 1997;**29**:1422–31.
12 Parish S, Collins R, Peto R *et al*. Cigarette smoking, tar yields, and non-fatal myocardial infarction: 14000 cases and 32000 controls in the United Kingdom. *BMJ* 1995; **311**:471–7.
13 Carroll D, Bennett P, Davey-Smith G. Socio-economic health inequalities: their origins and implications. *Psychol Health* 1993;**8**:295–316.
14 Stewart MJ, Brosky G, Gillis A *et al*. Disadvantaged women and smoking. *Can J Pub Health* 1996;**87**:257–60.
15 Cherry N, Kiernan K. Personality scores and smoking behaviour. A longitudinal study. *Br J Prev Soc Med* 1976;**30**:123–31.
16 Lynskey MT, Fergusson DM. Childhood conduct problems, attention deficit behaviors, and adolescent alcohol, tobacco, and illicit drug use. *J Abnorm Child Psychol* 1995;**23**:281–302.
17 Jarvis MJ. A profile of tobacco smoking. *Addiction* 1994;**89**:1371–6.
18 Jarvis MJ, Wardle J. Social patterning of health behaviours: the case of cigarette smoking. In: Marmot M, Wilkinson R, eds. *Social Determinants of Health*. Oxford: OUP, 1999.
19 Johnstone A, Goldberg D. Psychiatric screening in general practice. A controlled trial. *Lancet* 1976;**i**(7960):605–8.
20 Ferri E, ed. *Life at 33: the fifth follow-up of the National Child Development Study*. London: National Children's Bureau, 1993.
21 Cohen S, Kamarck T, Mermelstein R. A global measure of perceived stress. *J Health Soc Behav* 1983;**24**:385–96.
22 Lewis G, Pelosi A, Araya R, Dunn G. Measuring psychiatric disorder in the community: a standardised assessment for use by lay interviewers. *Psychol Med* 1992;**22**:465–86.
23 Meltzer H, Gill B, Pettigrew M, Hinds K. The prevalence of psychiatric morbidity among adults living in private households. *OPCS Surveys of Psychiatric Morbidity in Great Britain, Report 1*. London: HMSO, 1995.

24 Heatherton TF, Kozlowski LT, Frecker RC, Rickert W, Robinson J. Measuring the heaviness of smoking: Using self-reported time to the first cigarette of the day and number of cigarettes smoked per day. *Br J Addict* 1989;**84**:791–800.

25 Anda RF, Williamson DF, Escobedo LG, Mast EE, Giovino GA, Remington PL. Depression and the dynamics of smoking: A national perspective. *JAMA* 1990;**264**:1541–5.

26 Schoenborn CA, Horm J. Negative moods as correlates of smoking and heavier drinking: Implications for health promotion. *Advance Data from Vital and Health Statistics*. Hyattsville National Center for Health Statistics, 1993.

27 West RJ, Jarvis MJ, Russell MAH *et al*. Effect of nicotine replacement on the cigarette withdrawal syndrome. *Br J Addict* 1984;**79**:215–19.

28 Gross J, Stitzer ML. Nicotine replacement: ten-week effects on tobacco withdrawal symptoms. *Psychopharmacol* 1989;**98**:334–41.

29 Cohen S, Lichtenstein E. Perceived stress, quitting smoking, and smoking relapse. *Health Psychol* 1990;**9**:466–78.

30 Carey MP, Kalra DL, Carey KB, Halperin S, Richards CS. Stress and unaided smoking cessation: a prospective investigation. *J Consult Clin Psychol* 1993;**61**:831–8.

31 West R, Hajek P. What happens to anxiety levels on giving up smoking? *Am J Psychiatry* 1997;**154**:1589–92.

32 Stewart AL, King AC, Killen JD, Ritter PL. Does smoking cessation improve health-related quality of life? *Ann Behav Med* 1995;**17**:331–8.

33 West R. Beneficial effects of nicotine: fact or fiction? *Addiction* 1993;**88**:589–90.

34 Parrott AC. Nebitt's paradox resolved? Stress and arousal modulation during cigarette smoking. *Addiction* 1998;**93**:27–39.

35 Parrott AC. Stress modulation over the day in cigarette smokers. *Addiction* 1995;**90**:233–244.

36 Royal College of Physicians. *Nicotine Addiction in Britain*. London: Royal College of Physicians, 2000.

37 Smith GD, Phillips AN, Neaton JD. Smoking as 'independent' risk factor for suicide: Illustration of an artifact from observational epidemiology? *Lancet* 1992;**340**(8821):709–12.

157

10: Physical activity and stress

KAMALDEEP BHUI

Physical activity is not commonly recognised as having value in the prevention or alleviation of mental disorder. It has been demonstrated to have significant benefits for recovery and rehabilitation from physical ill health. Exercise has been advocated at a population level to reduce the risk of coronary heart disease, hypertension, and obesity, and was most recently popularised in Britain by encouraging people to walk or take part in any activity that made them breathless on a daily basis; such activities included walking the dog or gardening, and using stairs whenever possible. On occasions, leisure activities and exercise may be recommended to individual patients as a general measure to encourage participation in ordinary activities of daily living.[1] The benefit of exercise on the moods of normal non-depressed individuals is unverified.[2] Nonetheless, improvements of cognitive function in the elderly,[3] menopausal symptoms,[4] quality of life of multiple sclerosis patients,[5] chronic obstructive airways disease,[6] eating disorders in women,[7] and chronic fatigue,[8] have all been enthusiastically reported. The rationale for considering physical activity to be a potentially effective intervention in mental disorders, as argued in this and other chapters (Chapters 7, 16), is that coronary heart disease and stress share social risk factors, pathophysiological mediating pathways, and biological predisposition. This chapter briefly summarises the evidence in support of exercise as a preventive intervention in coronary heart disease and as an ingredient in recovery packages after cardiac events or surgery, and reviews the evidence that physical activity is effective in the alleviation of stress and mental disorder. An assumption is that the stress–vulnerability model of mental disorder is valid, and that mental disorders, stress, and coronary heart disease may share risk factors and pathophysiological processes.

Coronary heart disease and psychosocial stress

A psychosocial factor may be defined as a measurement that potentially relates psychological phenomena to the social environment, and to pathophysiological change.[9] Such a definition of the more generally used

158

term "stress" affords the opportunity to investigate the impact of measurable psychosocial factors on health status. This distinction between mind and body reflects the approach of medical researchers and writers, rather than representing the form in which distress manifests in a subjective manner. Thus distressed individuals' response to environmental challenge, although initially adaptive, can culminate in neurophysiological and psychosociobehavioural modification that results in pathophysiological changes of body function as well as psychological distress. Comorbidity of physical and psychiatric disorders has been demonstrated in many epidemiological studies,[10] but the degree of shared aetiology remains the subject of much research activity. It is possible that psychiatric disorders share a common pathophysiology with physical illness; for example, coronary heart disease and gastric ulcers are influenced by psychosocial factors giving rise to a need for holistic biopsychosocial models of disease.[11,12] Cerebrovascular disease can give rise to depression (see Chapter 7). Coronary heart disease is probably the best studied physical illness in which psychosocial factors are known to have a profound impact. It is known that psychological traits (hostility), psychological states (depression and anxiety), psychological interaction with the organisation (job control, demands, and support) and social support have aetiological roles in coronary disease.[9]

The sequence that links coronary heart disease and mental disorder can be conceptualised in several ways. First, depression may precede coronary heart disease and predispose to it. Ford and Mead, in a 37 year follow up of medical students, demonstrated that depression was a risk factor for the onset of coronary heart disease, independent of cardiac events.[13] Depression may also lead to high risk behaviours that include smoking, poor diet, and weight gain. Ziegelstein et al. studied 106 men and 88 women admitted to an inpatient unit following myocardial infarction over an 18 month period.[14] Patients found to have mild to moderate depression, or to have major depression and/or dysthymia, reported lower adherence to a regimen of low fat diet, regular exercise, reducing stress, and recruiting social support 4 months later. Those with major depression and/or dysthymia also showed poorer adherence to the prescribed medication regimen. Thus depression does lead to higher risk behaviour and poorer adherence to pharmacological and psychosocial interventions. Coelho et al. conducted a case–control study that included 153 community resident men with acute myocardial infarction and 156 men randomly selected as controls.[15] Cases of acute infarction demonstrated more type A behaviour, more depressive symptoms, poorer general wellbeing scores, less education, more hypertensive histories, more unfavourable lipid profiles, more type I obesity, more smoking, less exercise, and more non-insulin-dependent diabetes. Type A behaviour and depression persisted as strong associations after adjusting for all other cardiac risk factors. There are, however, almost certainly other social factors that influence the course of coronary heart disease.

For example, rehabilitation after coronary artery bypass grafting is strongly influenced by the presurgical level of employment and poverty.[16] Everson *et al.* reported that middleaged men who showed blood pressure reactivity induced by stress and who reported high job demands experienced the greatest atherosclerotic progression.[11] The social origins of depression and anxiety have been well described. In summary, there is significant evidence that depression can lead to coronary heart disease, and vice versa, with social, environmental and pathophysiological factors having influence over causation and recovery.

Coronary heart disease and exercise

Public health campaigns advocating a daily minimum of physical activity to prevent coronary heart disease are based on evidence showing health advantages.[17-19] Menotti and Seccareccia conducted a study of 99 029 men aged 40–59 and employed on the Italian railroad system.[20] They classified men into three levels of physical activity at work and three levels of job responsibility. Low physical activity and high job responsibility increased the risk of myocardial infarction. Overall, mortality from all causes was not significantly different in different classes of physical activity and job responsibility. This study shows some interaction between physical activity and working environments. There appear to be a complex profile of risk factors contributing to the development of coronary heart disease. A systematic review by Ebrahim and Davey-Smith did not show great benefit from complex risk factor interventions in the primary prevention of coronary heart disease in population samples, but concluded that such interventions should be targeted at high risk hypertensive patients.[21] Jolliffe *et al.* completed a systematic review on exercise-based interventions for rehabilitation from coronary heart disease.[22] They compared the benefits of a comprehensive package of interventions with exercise only interventions. This meta-analysis included 2582 patients in the exercise only group and 5101 in the comprehensive cardiac rehabilitation package. Exercise only intervention reduced all cause and cardiac cause mortality to a slightly greater extent than a comprehensive package, but the difference between the two was not significant. Neither intervention affected non-fatal myocardial infarction occurrence rates. The exercise only intervention did not reduce total cholesterol or low density lipoprotein levels, whereas the comprehensive interventions did so. There is strong evidence that exercise can be beneficial for coronary heart disease patients, and it may mitigate the effects of psychosocial risk factors that are of aetiological significance in coronary heart disease. Psychosocial risk factors are known to be significant in the development of mental disorders, and persistent states of stress may culminate in mental disorder. These findings suggest that exercise may be an effective intervention in stress and stress related mental disorders.

Stress and mental disorders

The distinction between a common mental disorder and common states of suffering is one of intensity rather than quality. Suffering or distress can be caused by interpersonal conflict, poverty, poor housing, unemployment, fear about living in impoverished and crime ridden neighbourhoods, violence, and fears about safety. The individual's resilience to adverse life events and circumstances is determined by the intensity of these events, but also by individual vulnerability dependent upon temperamental or personality factors and genetic factors as well as social support. Some stress, as opposed to distress, is considered helpful in problem solving and improves task performance. Yet if this "healthy" stress becomes persistent or too intense it can compromise problem solving; it may then diminish self esteem and confidence, leading to an inability to escape or modify stressors and resulting in a state of subjective distress. This is further complicated by the term "mental health" being used to describe many aspects of wellbeing: quality of life, relief from social sources of distress, and the alleviation of specific psychiatric disorders. Stress is therefore a multidimensional and inevitable part of daily life. Its detrimental forms warrant individualised approaches as well as public health interventions to minimise the precipitation of mental illness.

The distribution of mental disorders

In 1992 the Royal College of Psychiatrists, in conjunction with the Royal College of General Practitioners, launched a well publicised 'Defeat Depression' campaign.[23] The purpose was not only to reduce the stigma attached to depression and mental illness, but also to educate the public at population level and to encourage people to seek help should they suspect they were suffering from any of the minor psychiatric disorders (anxiety and depressive states). The Office of Population Censuses and Surveys (OPCS) national psychiatric morbidity survey indicated that 18% of the sample scored above the diagnostic cut-off of 12 (indicating the presence of a disorder) on the clinical interview schedule.[24,25] These disorders are relatively common and the public generally do not automatically consider these states to require medication or consultation with general practitioners.[26]

At some time in their lives, 45% of women and 27% of men will suffer from a depressive episode.[27] The majority of patients experience an episodic but recurring illness.[28] In primary care settings, mixed anxiety and depression states have a worse prognosis than depression alone.[29] The argument that minor psychiatric disorders (anxiety and minor depression) can be better prevented by a population preventive strategy seems useful. The population strategy of shifting a risk factor in a favourable direction and its usefulness in the context of developing health policy has been reviewed.[30] Could the benefits of regular exercise include better

161

psychological health? I now turn to the evidence in support of using physical activity and exercise in the management of varieties of stress where these manifest as mental disorders.

Exercise and mental disorders

In 1984 the American National Institute of Mental Health produced a consensus statement,[31] asserting that:

- physical fitness was positively associated with mental health and wellbeing
- exercise has been associated with a reduction in mild to moderate depression
- severe depression requires professional treatment, involving drug and electroconvulsive therapy, and exercise as an adjunctive treatment
- exercise has potential beneficial effects for all ages and both sexes.

Despite this statement, it is unusual to find exercise routinely prescribed for specific conditions, and its use as a population based approach to managing stress is still not widespread. In Britain, the government's report into inequalities in health emphasises exercise as one of ten interventions for a healthier nation. Improved mental health is specifically mentioned as an outcome. Little consideration has, to date, been given to a population strategy to prevent minor psychiatric disorders by considering the use of physical activity.

Reports of the benefits of exercise in combating the harmful effects of stress emerge from the specialities of sports medicine, sports physiology, epidemiology, public health, cardiology, psychiatry, and rehabilitation medicine. Each of these specialities has their specific definitions of mood disorders, exercise packages of interest, and comorbid conditions. Byrne and Byrne reviewed the evidence in favour of exercise becoming a routine intervention.[1] Although many studies reported equivocal results, the conclusions reached were in favour of exercise relieving mood and anxiety states. It was not important whether aerobic or anaerobic activity was involved. The physiological changes in response to increased fitness appears not to be the active "ingredient". Perhaps distraction from life's stresses is a component. Other reported therapeutic components of exercise regimens include a sense of mastery, a capacity for change being acknowledged, a habit that feels positive, symptom relief "even if temporary", and an alteration of conscious awareness. One study indicated a change in self esteem for the better, and greater self awareness.[32]

A number of plausible physiological aetiologies have been advanced to explain the anxiolytic and mood elevating action of physical activity: an alteration of cerebral monoamine neurotransmitters; a reduction in neuromuscular responsiveness (that is, relaxation of muscular tensions); a release of endorphins (this is thought to explain "exerciser's euphoria"); a complex interplay of increased β-endorphins, and an increase in corticotrophin, growth hormone, and prolactin levels.[33] Psychological stress has been associated with increased plasma corticotrophin levels,[34] and anticipated or perceived psychological stress may elicit such changes.[35] Morris *et al.* reported that the cessation of exercise was followed by symptoms of anxiety, insomnia, and an increase in depressive feelings, with a loss of the antidepressive effects of exercise training reflecting a "withdrawal syndrome" and perhaps a true reversibility of the phenomenon.[36] There remains controversy about isolating a single specific mechanism, and the competing hypotheses do not together comprise a consistent explanation. For example, if β-endorphins are responsible, then the opiate antagonist naloxone would be expected to reverse the effects; but naloxone does not influence the antidepressive effects of exercise, and may even produce slight euphoria.[37]

There is consensus that activity does have an effect on anxiety and mood states, with a number of plausible mediating biochemical, physiological, and psychological pathways. Physical activity has, indeed, been reported to be as effective as psychotherapy and superior to an inactive control group in the treatment of mild to moderate depression.[38] More specifically, Veale *et al.* demonstrated that aerobic and low intensity exercise gave better results compared with a control group, where measures of trait anxiety and the results of a psychiatric interview were used as outcomes.[38] Again, there was no correlation with the improved fitness observed following exercise. Berger and Owen examined mood changes in college swimmers who reported less tension, less anxiety, less depression, less anger, and less confusion and bewilderment following exercise.[39] Doyne *et al.* examined the effects of weightlifting, running, or being on a waiting list control over an 8 week period.[40] Weightlifting and running were equally beneficial compared with the control group. Chastain *et al.* advocated a fitness programme for psychiatric inpatients.[41] Sessions three times a week for 6 weeks enhanced patients' self esteem and body image. Yet, although the American consensus statement advocates regular exercise, this does not form part of the routine advice given to psychiatric patients, let alone to populations at risk of psychiatric disorder. This is the case despite widespread knowledge that physical disorders are more common among psychiatric populations,[42] and that physical illness is an important aetiological factor in minor and major psychiatric disorders.

Most of the studies have involved the prescription of certain exercise programmes involving vigorous types of exercise, and have not considered that less intense activity may be beneficial. Indeed, many studies did not enquire after other daily activities such as walking, which may have varied significantly between experimental groups. Few studies used randomly assigned groups, and most used volunteers, reflecting a multitude of potential biases especially where small samples were used. Some studies had single exercise groups and few had comparisons between different types of activity, the exceptions arising where a differential effect for aerobic and anaerobic activity was sought. Peer reviewed published studies contain samples of students or normal non-clinical populations although the potential interventions were targeted mainly at clinical populations. Byrne and Byrne highlight several methodological limitations of studies to date: the exercise programme is poorly described; clinical mood scales used may be insensitive to mood changes in normal populations; and results are limited by a differential selection of subjects, mainly chosen for availability and convenience with little or no concern about their exercise status before inclusion.[1]

Longitudinal and follow up studies are typically absent from the literature and hence it is unclear whether indefinite activity is necessary to maintain the effect. There are few studies examining more specific characteristics about the type of exercise involved or its duration, and none examining the potential for physical activity at a population level as a risk factor. In line with Rose's strategy of preventive medicine,[43] such a population strategy is likely to be of greater benefit than targeting only those who are defined as "cases" by practitioners.

Bhui and Fletcher have completed a nested case–control study using data from the Health and Lifestyle Survey, a large longitudinal survey.[44,45] The General Health Questionnaire, which measures common mood and anxiety states, was the outcome measure. They demonstrated a protective effect for men engaged in at least 92 minutes of exercise a day. Although no such effect was demonstrated in women, women tended to exercise for less time, and were generally younger and from households with lower incomes. Thus one might conclude that physical activity is of benefit only if individuals have adequate income and leisure time. It is possible that the effect of low intensity activity is attributable not to the activity itself but to other associated factors; for example, distraction may be an important component; creative activity may be the critical ingredient in home improvement and gardening. The sample was not sufficiently large to examine the effects of separate activities. Gardening as an activity requires that individuals have access to a garden; home improvement requires that people have a home that they wish to (and financially can) improve. Yet, rather perplexingly, social class appeared not to contribute to the models. Perhaps the most important ingredient at a population level is leisure time. Tkachuk and Martin concluded that exercise was a viable and cost effective treatment for mild to moderate depression, and may be a useful adjunct in more severe forms of disorder.[46] Non-aerobic forms of exercise were as effective as aerobic forms. There was a reduction in disruptive and stereotypical behaviours among those with learning difficulties, and it was helpful in the management of mild to moderate chronic pain. Although exercise was better than placebo in the treatment of panic disorder, it was no better than an antidepressant drug. Regular exercise was also effective in body image disturbance, but the evidence to support an adjunctive role in schizophrenia, conversion disorders, and substance misuse (including nicotine) was lacking.

Future work

This book sets out the impact of stress on coronary heart disease. Although this chapter aims to discuss stress independent of physical illness, there is a growing literature that emphasises the role of exercise in the alleviation of distress associated with cardiac and respiratory conditions. The data are not sufficiently sophisticated to isolate a benefit to mental health independent of improvement in physical health. Some stress accompanying physical illness arises as a direct result of the physical condition, for example, dyspnoea or angina. Other stress might be considered as a neurotic response to actual physical illness, where the distress may be disproportionate to the actual physical disability and associated risks. As far as psychiatric conditions are concerned, one could investigate the effect of exercise on distress associated with having a chronic disabling psychiatric condition, as well as distress associated with the individual response to the condition. It is known that expressed emotion in families may contribute to relapse in chronic mental disorders, and it is known that life events can contribute to the development of depression and precipitate psychotic episodes in the vulnerable.

Future research should aim at developing population based exercise programmes using standardised schedules of physical activity and more specific measures of psychiatric status before and at regular intervals during the programme, to investigate the effect of activity on specific stress disorders. The action of physical activity on wellbeing, and on distress in the psychoses, could also be the focus of future interventions in these groups. Rarely do studies examine or report sex differences,[47] or differential effects based on other population characteristics.[48] The time scales and intensity of interventions as well as the duration of the effect also require better definition. Specific packages should also be evaluated in randomised clinical trials. One possible explanation that requires more detailed evaluation is the effect of leisure. More leisure time or less work time, even if inactive, might be compared to active leisure, and each of these could be compared to better defined physical activities. Exercise is of value in the treatment of physical disorders associated with psychoses, for example, obesity, ischaemic heart disease, and smoking related disorders, as it is in the treatment of physical disorders in the population generally. Thus it has an impact on stress and the development of mental disorders. The next series of research questions must investigate its influence on pathophysiological processes common to physical and mental disorders, with special attention to psychosocial factors and the impact of exercise on psychophysiological states of tension.

References

1 Byrne A, Byrne D. The effect of exercise on depression, anxiety and other mood states: a review *J Psychosom Res* 1993;**6**:565–74.
2 Lennox SS, Bedell JR, Stone AA. The effect of exercise on normal mood. *J Psychosom Res* 1990;**34**:629–36.

3   Williams P, Lord SR. Effects of group exercise on cognitive functioning and mood in older women. *Austr NZ J Public Health* 1997;**21**:45–52.

4   Coope J. Hormonal and non-hormonal interventions for menopausal symptoms. *Maturitas* 1996;**23**:159–68.

5   Petajan JH, Gappmaier E, White AT *et al*. Impact of aerobic training on fitness and quality of life in multiple sclerosis. *Ann Neurol* 1996;**39**:434–41.

6   Weaver TE, Richmond TS, Narsavage GL. An explanatory model of functional status in chronic obstructive pulmonary disease. *Nurs Res* 1997;**46**:26–31.

7   Wurtman JJ. Depression and weight gain: the serotonin connection. Special Issue. Towards a new psychobiology of depression in women. *J Affective Disord* 1993;**29**: 183–92.

8   Fulcher KY, White PD. Randomised controlled trial of graded exercise in patients with chronic fatigue syndrome. *BMJ* 1997;**314**(7095):1674–52.

9   Hemingway H, Marmot M. Psychosocial factors in the aetiology and prognosis of coronary heart disease: systematic review of prospective studies. *BMJ* 1999;**318**:1460–7.

10 Stansfeld SA, Smith GD, Marmot M. Association between physical and psychological morbidity in the Whitehall II Study. *J Psychosom Res* 1993;**37**:227–38.

11 Everson S, Everson SA, Lynch JW *et al*. Interaction of workplace demands and cardiovascular reactivity in progression of carotid atherosclerosis: population based study. *BMJ* 1997;**314**:553.

12 Levenstein S. Stress and peptic ulcer: life beyond helicobacter. *BMJ* 1998;**316**:538–41.

13 Ford DE, Mead LA. Depression is a risk factor for coronary artery disease in men: the precursors study. *Arch Intern Med* 1998;**13**:1422–6.

14 Ziegelstein RC, Fauerbach JA, Stevens SS, Romanelli J, Richter DP. Patients with depression are less likely to follow recommendations to reduce cardiac risk during recovery from myocardial infarction. *Arch Intern Med* 1999;**160**:1818–23.

15 Coelho R, Ramos E, Prata J, Maciel MJ, Barros H. Acute myocardial infarction: psychosocial and cardiovascular risk factors in men. *J Cardiovasc Res* 1999;**6**:157–62.

16 Boulay FM, David PP, Bourassa MG. Strategies for improving the work status of patients after coronary artery bypass surgery. *Circulation* 1982;**66**:III43–9.

17 Wenger NK, Froelicher ES, Smith LK *et al*. Cardiac rehabilitation as secondary prevention. Agency for Health Care Policy and Research and National Heart, Lung, and Blood Institute. *Clinical Practice Guidelines Quick Reference Guide* 1995;**17**:1–23.

18 Rieu M. Role of physical activities in a public health policy. *Bull Acad Natl Med* 1995;**179**:1417–26.

19 King AC, Jeffrey R, Fridinger F *et al*. Environmental and policy approaches to cardiovascular disease prevention through physical activity: issues and opportunities. *Health Educ Q* 1995;**22**:499–511.

20 Menotti A, Seccareccia F. Physical activity at work and job responsibility as risk factors for fatal coronary heart disease and other causes of death. *J Epidemiol Community Health* 1985;**39**:325–9.

21 Ebrahim S, Davey-Smith G. Multiple risk factor interventions for primary prevention of coronary heart disease (Cochrane Review). *Cochrane Library*. Issue 4. Oxford: Update Software, 2000.

22 Jolliffe JA, Rees K, Taylor RS, Thompson D, Oldridge N, Ebrahim S. Exercise based rehabilitation for coronary heart disease (Cochrane Review). *Cochrane Library*. Issue 4. Oxford: Update Software, 2000.

23 Sims A. The scar that is more than skin deep: the stigma of depression. *Br J Gen Pract* 1993;**43**(366):30–1.

24 OPCS. *A National Survey of Psychiatric Morbidity*. London: HMSO, 1995.

25 Lewis G, Pelosi AJ, Araya R, Dunn G. Measuring psychiatric disorder in the community: a standardised assessment for use by lay interviewers. *Psychol Med* 1992;**22**:465–86.

26 Priest RG, Vize C, Roberts A, Roberts M, Tylee A. Lay people's attitudes to treatment of depression: results of opinion poll for Defeat Depression Campaign just before its launch. *BMJ* 1996;**313**(7061):829–30.

27 Rorsman B, Grasbeck A, Hagnell O *et al*. Prospective study of first-incidence depression. The Lundby study, 1957–72. *Br J Psychiatry* 1990;**156**:336–42.

28 Angst J. How predictable is depressive illness? In: Montgomery SA, Rouillon R, eds. *Long Term Treatment of Depression: Perspectives in Psychiatry, vol. 3*. Chichester: John Wiley, 1992.

29 Ormel J, Oldehinkel T, Brilman E, vanden Brink W. Outcome of depression and anxiety in primary care. A three-wave 3 1/2-year study of psychopathology and disability. *Arch Gen Psychiatry* 1993;**50**:759–66.

30 Borst-Eilers E. Perspectives of Epidemiology in Europe. *Int J Epidemiol* 1996;**25**:469.

31 Morgan W, Goldstern S, eds. *Exercise in Mental Health.* Washington: Hemisphere, 1987.

32 Jorgensen C, Jorgensen D. Effects of running on perception of self and others. *J Perception Motor Skills* 1979;**48**:242.

33 Steinberg H, Sykes E. Introduction to a symposium on endorphins and behavioural processes. A review of the literature on endorphins and exercise. *Pharmacol Biochem Behav* 1985;**23**:357–62.

34 Seyle H. *The Stress of Life.* New York: McGraw Hill, 1976.

35 Oltras M. Beta-endorphin and ACTH in plasma: effects of physical and psychological stress. *Life Sci* 1987;**40**:1683–6.

36 Morris M, Steinberg H, Sykes EA, Salmon P. Effects of temporary withdrawal from regular running *J Psychosom Res* 1990;**34**:493–500.

37 Markoff RA, Ryan P, Young T. Endorphins and mood changes in long distance running. *Med Sci Sports Exerc* 1982;**13**:15.

38 Veale D, Le Fevre K, Pantelis C. Aerobic exercise in the adjunctive treatment of depression: a randomised controlled trial. *J R Soc Med* 1992;**85**:541–4.

39 Berger BG, Owen DR. Mood alteration with swimming. Swimmers really do feel better. *Psychosom Med* 1983;**45**:425–33.

40 Doyne, E Ossip-Klein DJ, Bowman ED, Osborn KM, McDougall-Wilson IB, Neimeyer RA. Running versus weightlifting in the treatment of depression *J Consult Clin Psychol* 1987;**55**:738–54.

41 Chastain P, Shapiro GE. Physical fitness programme for patients with psychiatric disorders: a clinical report. *Phys Ther* 1987;**67**:545–8.

42 Honig A, Pop P, Tan ES, Philipsen H, Romme MA. Physical illness in chronic psychiatric patients from a community psychiatric unit. The implications for daily practice [see comments]. *Br J Psychiatry* 1989;**155**:58–64.

43 Rose G. *The strategy of preventive medicine.* Oxford: Oxford Medical 1992.

44 Bhui K, Fletcher A. Common mood and anxiety states: gender effects of the protective effect of physical activity. *Soc Psychiatry Psychiatr Epidemiol* 2000;**35**:28–35.

45 Cox B. *The health and lifestyle survey: seven years on.* Aldershot, Hants. Dartmouth 1993.

46 Tkachuk GA, Martin GL. Exercise therapy for patients with psychiatric disorders: research and clinical implications. *Prof Psychol Res Pract* 1999;**30**:275–2.

47 Raglin JS, Morgan WP, O'Connor PJ. Changes in mood states during training in female and male college swimmers. *Int J Sports Med* 1991;**12**:585–9.

48 Pistacchio T, Weinberg R, Jackson A. The development of a psychobiologic profile of individuals who experience and those who do not experience exercise related mood enhancement. *J Sport Behav* 1989;**12**:151–66.

11: Psychophysiological responsivity in coronary heart disease

ANDREW STEPTOE AND GONNEKE WILLEMSEN

All behavioural states and activities are underpinned by physiological responses, and are dependent on specific patterns of cardiovascular, neuroendocrine, and metabolic adjustment. These physiological responses are adapted to sustain the motoric and metabolic requirements of the individual, ensuring that behaviour and biology are coordinated in states ranging from sleep to vigorous physical activity. However, physiological responses are also elicited by psychological and social factors in a way that might increase risk for serious disease. Psychophysiological stress responses are particularly relevant to coronary heart disease, since there is accumulating evidence that they may be partly responsible for the increases in risk associated with psychosocial factors.

This chapter describes the psychophysiological stress responses that are relevant to heart disease, discusses methods of assessing these responses in humans, and outlines the evidence linking them with heart disease. Psychophysiology in humans is characterised by the measurement of physiological function in relation to behaviour and psychological states, in contrast to the cross-sectional snapshots of physiology recorded in many epidemiological studies. We argue that psychophysiological processes can be reliably measured in clinical and population studies, and that they are involved both in the longterm aetiology of coronary heart disease, and in the triggering of acute cardiac events in patients with established coronary artery disease. These studies provide insight into the mechanisms through which psychosocial influences on coronary heart disease are mediated.

Psychophysiological stress responses

Psychophysiological stress responses involve many systems in the body, not all of which are relevant to cardiovascular disease.[1,2] When healthy humans and other animals are faced with acute challenges or threats, they typically show increases in blood pressure and heart rate. Tasks such as mental arithmetic or visual problem solving elicit increases in systolic and diastolic blood pressure and heart rate of 20–40% in healthy adults, together with vasodilation in skeletal muscle and reduced blood flow to the kidneys and viscera. The high heart rate is the result of sympathetic activation coupled with parasympathetic (vagal) withdrawal, while blood pressure increases because the rise in cardiac output is not matched by reductions in total peripheral resistance. The sensitivity of the cardiac baroreceptor reflex is inhibited, and heart rate variability is reduced. Increases in the concentration of the catecholamines epinephrine (adrenaline) and norepinephrine (noradrenaline) in the venous circulation are inconsistent.[3] However, techniques such as the measurement of radiolabelled norepinephrine spillover from sympathetic nerve terminals indicate that the increase in sympathetic activity during mental stress is particularly prominent in the nerves serving the coronary vessels.[4]

Sympathetic nervous stimulation and catecholamine release are coupled with other neuroendocrine responses, notably activation of the hypothalamic–pituitary–adrenocortical axis. The consequence is the synthesis of corticotrophin, which stimulates production of steroid hormones by the adrenal glands. The most important corticosteroid in the stress response is cortisol. This has a range of actions including stimulation of glucose production by the liver, release of free fatty acids from adipose tissue, the modification of water balance and kidney function, and the promotion of anti-inflammatory responses. Acute psychological stress may also result in increases in the concentration in the blood of total cholesterol, low density lipoprotein (LDL) cholesterol, and apolipoprotein B. These lipid responses are partly due to alterations in plasma volume and changes in haemoconcentration, since a reduction in plasma volume will lead to an apparent increase in concentration of substances in the blood. However, studies indicate that the increases in lipids are genuine responses, probably stimulated by catecholamine and cortisol secretion, and are not merely secondary to plasma volume effects.[5]

Other biological processes stimulated during acute mental stress include factors related to haemostasis and blood clotting. One of the early stages of the clotting process is the adhesion of blood platelets to the lips of a wound. However, platelets are also involved in atherogenesis, since they adhere to the damaged vascular endothelium and release soluble proteins (cytokines) that stimulate the proliferation of monocytes and smooth muscle cells in the vascular wall.[6] Platelet activation rapidly increases during acute stress, probably through the action of catecholamines.[7] The influence of stress on other factors related to coagulation such as fibrinogen is outlined in Chapter 12 by Brunner, while effects on endothelial function are reviewed by Hemingway in Chapter 13.

The pattern of psychophysiological activation outlined here is adaptive under conditions of threat, which call for a vigorous physical response. The stress response ensures that the muscles are well supplied with energy, that clotting mechanisms are stimulated to prevent blood loss from wounds, and that vegetative functions, which are not essential for short-term survival, are suppressed.[8] However, in humans, responses are also elicited in circumstances in which no vigorous activity is required, and chronic stress can lead to sustained activation which becomes maladaptive. For example, disturbances of corticosteroid output can lead to chronic increases in blood cholesterol levels, deposition of fat in abdominal adipose tissue, decalcification of bone, and chronic immunosuppression.[2,9]

There are two general methods of assessing the significance of potentially maladaptive psychophysiological stress responses in heart disease. The first is to evaluate the relationship between physiological responses and cardiovascular risk: do people at greater risk of heart disease (such as people with hypertension, or those experiencing chronic work stress) display different physiological reactions from those at lower risk? The second method is to study the prognostic significance of psychophysiological reactions: are physiologically more responsive individuals at greater risk than those who are less responsive? The evidence related to these two issues is discussed below. First, however, we describe the laboratory and naturalistic methods used to study psychophysiological responses, since these have a bearing on the interpretation of empirical findings.

Laboratory and naturalistic studies

The majority of studies of psychophysiological responsivity have taken place in the laboratory, allowing strict control of the situation and the standardisation of conditions across participants and occasions.[10] The standard laboratory procedure for studying stress reactivity is to record the response of a number of physiological parameters to one or more behavioural challenges. A variety of standardised tasks have been used to elicit stress responsivity, such as mental arithmetic, video games, speech tasks, and cold pressor tasks which involve endurance of a cold stimulus (hand or foot immersion in iced water). To ensure the tasks are provoking a stress response, they are often made more taxing; participants might have to compete for a monetary bonus, perform in front of an audience or video camera, or be punished by loud bursts of noise when they do not reach performance criteria. To quantify stress responses, task-induced changes in physiological parameters are calculated as the difference between the levels during the task period and a baseline period. This baseline period is usually a time of relaxation prior to the task, although sometimes baseline levels are obtained after the task or during a separate session. However, levels measured after a task may reflect recovery from the stressful challenge, and play an independent role in the relation between stress responsivity and disease development.[9] Laboratory studies have consistently shown clear individual differences in the magnitude and even the pattern of physiological responses to behavioural challenges.

The measurement of stress responsivity in the laboratory rests on the assumption that psychophysiological responsivity is an individual characteristic, which expresses itself in a similar manner to a broad range of situations; that is, laboratory stress responsivity reflects responses during everyday life situations. If psychophysiological responsivity plays a part in the longterm development of cardiovascular disease, then we must assume that this results from responses being elicited repeatedly during everyday life for months or even years. The availability of automated ambulatory monitors of blood pressure and heart rate has allowed the assumptions underlying laboratory stress studies to be tested. Many investigators have evaluated the associations between laboratory responses and cardiovascular activity during everyday life, and reviews have concluded that there is evidence for generalisation from the laboratory to real life, supporting the use of laboratory studies of psychophysiological responsivity.[11]

In contrast to the experimental setting of laboratory studies, ambulatory monitoring of physiological parameters such as heart rate and blood pressure allows the direct assessment of the effects of everyday psychosocial influences on physiological functioning. The intricate psychosocial interactions that take place in daily life are impossible to replicate in a laboratory, and might provide important additional information regarding an individual's physiological functioning. This is supported by the fact that blood pressure obtained by ambulatory monitoring predicts cardiovascular events and mortality in hypertensive patients, independently of blood pressure readings obtained in the clinic.[12]

In addition, monitoring during everyday life is important because the classification of an individual as a hyperresponder to laboratory stress in itself does not determine risk of cardiovascular disease; the individual should also experience frequent or prolonged exposure in everyday life to the challenging situations that provoke this hyperresponsivity.[13] Ambulatory monitoring may provide an indication of the individual's exposure to events that elicit stress responses in everyday life.

Most of the studies involving ambulatory monitoring have been restricted to the measurement of heart rate and blood pressure, as only recently has ambulatory monitoring of other physiological variables become possible. Ambulatory monitoring in studies of stress usually takes place on one or more typical working days and possibly also at weekends. The monitor is usually worn from early morning until the end of the day, sometimes even throughout the night, with readings being obtained every 15–30 minutes. Physiological function is influenced by many factors such as posture, physical activity, smoking, and alcohol and caffeine intake. This complicates the analysis of responses to psychosocial experiences. To control for these effects, participants are often asked to keep diaries during the monitoring period to provide a record of their activities. By combining the self report information with the physiological data, the effects of psychosocial factors on physiological functioning can be determined.[11,14]

Stress responses and heart disease risk

Psychophysiological stress responses are associated with biological risk factors such as hypertension, with psychosocial risk factors like work stress, and with behavioural risk factors such as cigarette smoking. The question underlying psychophysiological studies of heart disease is whether associations with risk factors throw light on mediating mechanisms. High stress responsivity has generally been taken to reflect increased cardiovascular risk. There may, however, be circumstances in which heightened risk is associated with a downgrading of responsivity, particularly in neuroendocrine pathways, due to functional adaptation and downregulation of regulatory mechanisms.[9,15]

The area of biological risk that has been studied most extensively is hypertension.[16] A large number of studies have compared the blood pressure responses to mental stress of hypertensive and normotensive individuals, and hypertensive subjects typically show greater systolic and diastolic pressure reactions.[17] Patients with borderline or mild hypertension tend to display enhanced heart rate responsivity as well, indicative of sympathoadrenal involvement. Hypertensive patients may, in addition, display larger reductions in renal blood flow during mental stress, together with greater catecholamine release.

Several investigations have studied associations between cardiovascular stress responsivity and elevated lipid levels. Results have been inconsistent, although some have found heightened stress responsivity among individuals with elevated cholesterol.[18] High blood pressure monitored at work and at home has also been linked with elevated levels of total and LDL cholesterol.[19]

Abdominal obesity is associated with increased vascular resistance during acute mental stress, and with heightened systolic pressure responsivity.[20] Individuals with abdominal obesity may also have disturbances of cortisol regulation both during acute stress testing and over the working day.[21]

Psychophysiological stress responses vary with many of the psychosocial factors discussed elsewhere in this book. Investigations of work stress have typically assessed physiological responses under naturalistic conditions using ambulatory techniques. For example, several studies have examined ambulatory blood pressure at work in relation to job strain as conceptualised in the demand–control model.[22] The general finding is that blood pressure is elevated at work in people who experience job strain. However, results can be difficult to interpret because blood pressure is strongly related to ongoing physical activity. Since high strain jobs often involve a hectic work pace and high levels of physical activity, blood pressure differences may result in part from these factors, rather than physiological stress related processes.

We have recently measured blood pressure over the working day in a sample of people reporting high and low job strain in a single occupation: schoolteaching.[23] Blood pressure at work did not vary with job strain, possibly because the physical demands of work were relatively uniform. Interestingly, a difference emerged after work and in the evening. Figure 11.1 shows the average reductions of blood pressure from the working day (08.30–17.40) to the evening (18.00–22.30). It can be seen that individuals

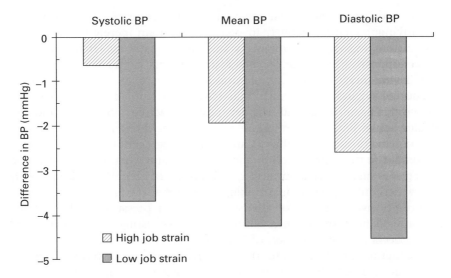

Figure 11.1   Average differences in ambulatory blood pressure (BP) between the working day and evening in schoolteachers experiencing high and low job strain. From Steptoe et al.[23]

experiencing job strain showed less blood pressure reduction in the evening. This sustained activation may reflect a difficulty in unwinding after work, and similar findings have been reported with respect to catecholamine excretion, particularly among women.[24] Different patterns may emerge for cortisol, where job strain appears to stimulate heightened output early in the morning, but not later in the working day.[25]

The associations between work stress and acute physiological responsivity are less consistent. Heightened blood pressure responses to uncontrollable tasks have been observed among individuals categorised as experiencing high job strain according to the demand–control model.[23] In contrast, high levels of effort–reward imbalance were associated with diminished blood pressure, epinephrine (adrenaline), and cortisol responses, in a study of middle managers.[26] The explanation for this discrepancy is unclear, but it may relate to the time of day at which observations were obtained, or the stage of the individual's work career. Siegrist et al. have suggested that work stress may initially stimulate high psychophysiological responses, which are later replaced by attenuated reactions reflecting functional adaptation to excessive stimulation.[26]

The physiological correlates of social support and social networks have been widely studied.[27] Psychophysiological methods have also been used to understand the mechanisms linking social support with reduced heart disease risk. The typical paradigm involves monitoring physiological responses to mental stress tests performed in the presence of a supportive individual, a non-supportive person, or alone. The pattern of results has been variable, but several studies indicate that the presence of a supportive

173

person reduces physiological reactivity.[28] This appears particularly true when the supporter is actively involved, rather than merely being present without making any encouraging statements or gestures. It is likely that social support reduces the perceived stressfulness of the situation, rather than having direct effects on biological function.

The behavioural risk factors that have been studied most extensively are cigarette smoking and regular physical activity. Smoking induces cardiovascular and neuroendocrine responses including increases in blood pressure, heart rate, cortisol level, and platelet aggregation. These responses are similar to those produced by mental stress, and when stress is imposed during smoking, effects appear to be additive.[29] In contrast, measurements not carried out during actual smoking suggest that regular smokers may be hyporesponsive in terms of cortisol and blood pressure.[30] These acute responses depend on the interval between stress testing and smoking, and some effects may be the result of temporary abstinence.

The literature relating acute stress reactivity with regular physical activity is also quite extensive. A number of studies have compared physiological responses to mental stress in relatively active and inactive people, and have shown that regular activity is associated with lower cardiovascular and neuroendocrine responses.[31] However, changes in stress responsivity following aerobic or anaerobic training have generally not been observed.[32] It may be that the duration of exercise training has been insufficient to translate into psychophysiological changes.

We have summarised the relationships between physiological stress responsivity and individual risk factors, but it should be recognised that a pattern of risks will be present in any particular individual. Interactions between risks are only beginning to be investigated. One example is an analysis of our cohort of schoolteachers, examining associations between job strain and abdominal obesity.[33] We found that low job control interacted with abdominal obesity in determining blood pressure at work. Elevated blood pressure was recorded among men with high waist–hip ratios who also reported low job control, but neither factor was significant on its own. It is likely that future studies will explore interactions of this kind more extensively.

Longitudinal studies of heart disease risk

The best possible evidence that psychophysiological responsivity plays a part in the development of coronary heart disease would be provided by longitudinal studies, with high responsivity predicting later morbidity or mortality independently of other established risk factors. Up to now, only three studies have examined the association between responsivity and later coronary heart disease, and the results have been rather inconsistent. A 23 year follow up study of 265 men, aged 47–57 at the time of initial testing, showed exaggerated diastolic blood pressure responses to a cold pressor test to be a risk factor for development of myocardial infarction and death from coronary heart disease.[34] However, in a second prospective study, which followed 905 men aged 19–35 at initial testing for 24–40 years, no association was found between blood pressure responses and the risk of developing coronary heart disease.[35] Similarly, a 9 year follow up of 1493 men, with an average age at entry of 56.8 years, reported that blood pressure reactions to the cold pressor test did not add significantly to the prediction of coronary heart disease.[36]

Considerably more studies have focused on the predictive power of psychophysiological responsivity for hypertension, as a risk factor for the development of coronary heart disease. For studies that have used the cold pressor test to elicit responsivity, results are again inconclusive, since some have found supportive evidence for an association between stress responsivity and the development of hypertension while others have not. There are also other inconsistencies. For instance, in one study blood pressure responses to the cold pressor test were found to be predictive of hypertension, but only for individuals who developed hypertension before 45 years of age,[37] whereas another study found that cold pressor reactivity was only predictive for those who were over 40 at the time of initial testing.[38] The results of studies using mental stressors have generally been more positive. Although negative findings have been reported,[39] the majority of the studies found that responsivity added significantly to the prediction of hypertension (for example, see references 40 and 41). Prospective associations between cardiovascular stress responses and end organ changes such as left ventricular hypertrophy have also been described.[42]

Psychophysiological studies have evaluated the influence of stress responsivity on the development of other markers of coronary heart disease as well. The thickness of the intimal and medial layers of the carotid artery wall can be assessed non-invasively using high resolution ultrasonography, and is an index of early coronary atherosclerosis.[43] Cardiovascular responses to mental stress in the laboratory are associated with greater carotid atherosclerosis cross-sectionally.[44] A recent study of 254 postmenopausal women found that pulse pressure responses induced by mental stress were positively associated with intima and media thickness more than 2 years later.[45] One particularly interesting study showed that stress responsivity interacted with low socioeconomic status in predicting the progression of carotid atherosclerosis.[46] Figure 11.2 summarises the changes in carotid atherosclerosis over 4 years in middleaged men from Finland, classified by socioeconomic status (based on education) and systolic pressure stress responses. The change, adjusted for age and baseline atherosclerosis, was greatest in high stress responders of low social status. This is consistent with the notion that stress responsiveness is particularly relevant to people exposed during their everyday lives to psychosocial adversity.

The overall picture emerging is that there is evidence that psychophysiological responsivity plays a role in the development of coronary heart disease. Although the evidence for a direct relationship between responsivity and hard disease endpoints is weak, it should be noted that the three existing

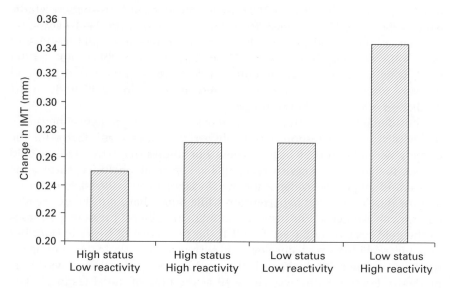

Figure 11.2 Mean increases in the maximum carotid intima–media thickness (IMT) in mm, adjusted for age and baseline intima–media thickness, over a 4 year period in middleaged men. Participants were divided on the basis of education into high and low socioeconomic status groups, and on the basis of systolic blood pressure stress reactions into high and low response groups. From Lynch et al.[46]

studies all used the cold pressor test.[34,35,36] As well as being psychologically stressful, this task is very painful, and there is a strong physiological reflex component to the cardiovascular responses elicited. The more positive findings for mental stressors with hypertension and carotid atherosclerosis as endpoints suggest that the relation between responsivity and coronary heart disease might be more consistent with cognitive and emotionally challenging stimuli. Moreover, blood pressure and heart rate changes only reflect a small part of the stress response, and it may be that the underlying haemodynamic process or the associated neuroendocrine changes are more relevant. Longitudinal studies assessing the stress response more fully by including such variables as cardiac output and vascular resistance might provide strong additional support for the predictive value of psychophysiological tests. In addition, the interactive effects of stress responsivity and other risk factors such as high fat diet, abdominal obesity, or smoking behaviour deserve attention, and might add to our understanding of the relation between psychophysiological responsivity and the development of coronary heart disease.

Stress responses and acute cardiac events

The studies described thus far have been concerned with the role of psychophysiological processes in the longterm aetiology of coronary heart disease. There is now growing interest in the parallel topic of psychophysiological stress in patients with established disease.[47] A variety of imaging techniques such as positron tomography and radionuclide ventriculography have demonstrated that coronary ischaemia is elicited acutely during mental stress testing. For example, Rozanski et al. found that 72% of a series of patients with exercise induced ischaemia showed abnormalities of left ventricular wall motion during tasks such as simulated public speaking.[48] Anger induction is another potent trigger of myocardial ischaemia in the laboratory.[49] An important issue about these responses concerns the underlying haemodynamics. Ischaemia is induced by exertion when metabolic demands on the heart (typically indexed by the product of heart rate and blood pressure) exceed the supply available through narrowed coronary arteries. Interestingly, myocardial ischaemia induced by stress is typically elicited at a lower heart rate and rate–pressure product than the ischaemic threshold, indicating that it does not simply result from raised metabolic demands. Both abnormalities in sympathetic peripheral vasoconstriction and endothelial dysfunction at the sites of coronary vascular damage appear to be involved.[50]

Ischaemic episodes, as defined by changes in the ST segment of the electrocardiogram, occur during ambulatory Holter monitoring in a substantial proportion of cardiac patients. Many of these episodes are clinically silent, in that they occur in the absence of chest pain or other symptoms. The relationship between ischaemia during ambulatory monitoring and emotional state has been evaluated by asking patients to complete diaries of mood and activities, and matching ischaemia with concurrent behaviour and emotional state. Of course, most myocardial ischaemia does not occur during extreme emotional states, since the latter are relatively rare in a typical day. However, if the data are corrected for the time spent in an emotionally disturbed state, then the occurrence of myocardial ischaemia is more likely during periods of negative emotion such as tension or anger. One study showed that the relative risk of myocardial ischaemia was more than doubled in the hour following high levels of tension, frustration, or sadness, after adjusting statistically for physical activity and time of day.[51] The likelihood of myocardial ischaemia during daily life is greater in patients who respond to laboratory and mental stress testing with substantial heart rate and haemodynamic responses,[52] suggesting that a predisposition to heightened psychophysiological reactivity may underlie vulnerability in susceptible individuals.

Evidence for psychophysiological influences on cardiac arrhythmia is rather more mixed. The strongest findings have emerged in animal experiments, which demonstrate that the threshold for ventricular fibrillation is reduced during stress.[53] However, in studies with cardiac patients, associations between emotional arousal and arrhythmia are not always observed,[54] although heightened susceptibility to ventricular arrhythmia has been put forward as a possible mechanism for the association observed between phobic anxiety and mortality (see Chapter 14).

How important is stress induced myocardial ischaemia for the health of patients with coronary heart disease? It should be remembered that transient ischaemia of any origin is only moderately related to the longterm health of patients with stable angina.[55] Evidence for the prognostic significance of responses induced by stress is slight at present, although prospective studies are currently under way. One investigation followed 126 cardiac patients for up to 5 years, during which 28 (22%) experienced at least one cardiac event.[56] The likelihood of cardiac events was significantly higher in those who showed ischaemic responses to mental stress tests at baseline, after controlling for potential confounding factors. Another study followed 79 patients for an average of 3.5 years.[57] Cardiac events occurred in 44% (20/45) of the mental stress responders, and in only 23% (8/34) of non-responders. Unfortunately, most of the cardiac "events" in these studies were angioplasties or coronary artery bypass surgeries, rather than hard events such as myocardial infarction, so the strength of the finding is limited. Nevertheless, we might speculate that stress induced ischaemia underlies the associations between acute myocardial infarction and anger that have been observed in interview studies with survivors.[58,59]

Conclusion

Psychophysiological methods provide information about the influence of psychosocial factors on coronary heart disease that is complementary to pathophysiological research on one hand, and epidemiology on the other. By studying the actual changes in physiological function associated with stress and other behavioural states, we can help to complete the jigsaw concerning mediating mechanisms. Evidence is growing that psychological and social factors affect coronary heart disease risk partly through the mobilisation of physiological processes related to stress. Developments in measurement technology and understanding of molecular pathology will allow psychophysiology to play an increasingly important part in future research on stress and coronary heart disease.

References

1 Hugdahl K. *Psychophysiology*. Cambridge: Harvard University Press, 1996.
2 Weiner H. *Perturbing the Organism: The Biology of Stressful Experience*. Chicago: University of Chicago Press, 1992.
3 Grassi G, Esler M. How to assess sympathetic activity in humans. *J Hypertension* 1999; 17:719–34.
4 Esler M, Jennings G, Lambert G. Measurement of overall and cardiac norepinephrine release into plasma during cognitive challenge. *Psychoneuroendocrinology* 1989;14:477–81.
5 Stoney CM, Bausserman L, Niaura R *et al*. Lipid reactivity to stress. II. Biological and behavioral influences. *Health Psychol* 1999;18:251–61.
6 Ross R. Atherosclerosis—an inflammatory disease. *N Engl J Med* 1999;340:115–26.
7 Patterson SM, Krantz DS, Gottdiener JS *et al*. Prothrombotic effects of environmental stress: changes in platelet function, hematocrit, and total plasma protein. *Psychosom Med* 1995;57:592–9.

8 Steptoe A. Psychophysiological bases of disease. In: Johnston M, Johnston D, eds. *Comprehensive Clinical Psychology Volume 8: Health Psychology*. New York: Elsevier Science, 1998.

9 McEwen BS. Protective and damaging effects of stress mediators. *N Engl J Med* 1998;**338**:171–9.

10 Turner JR. *Cardiovascular reactivity and stress: Patterns of physiological response*. New York: Plenum Press, 1994.

11 Fahrenberg J. Ambulatory assessment: Issues and perspective. In: Fahrenberg J, Myrtek M, eds. *Ambulatory Assessment: Computer-assisted psychological and psychophysiological methods in monitoring and field studies*. Seattle: Hogrefe & Huber, 1996.

12 Perloff D, Sokolow M, Cowan R. The prognostic value of ambulatory blood pressure. *JAMA* 1983;**249**:2792–8.

13 Krantz DS, Manuck SB. Acute psychophysiologic reactivity and risk of cardiovascular disease: A review and methodologic critique. *Psychol Bull* 1984;**96**:435–64.

14 Kamarck TW, Shiffman SM, Smithline L *et al*. The diary of ambulatory behavioral states: a new approach to the assessment of psychosocial influences on ambulatory cardiovascular activity. In: Krantz DS, Baum A, eds. *Technology and Methods in Behavioral Medicine*. Mahwah, NJ: Erlbaum, 1998.

15 Chrousos GP, Gold PW. The concepts of stress and stress system disorders. Overview of physical and behavioral homeostasis. *JAMA* 1992;**267**:1244–52.

16 Steptoe A. Behavior and blood pressure: implications for hypertension. In: Zanchetti A, Mancia G, eds. *Handbook of Hypertension—Pathophysiology of Hypertension*. Amsterdam: Elsevier Science, 1997.

17 Fredrikson M, Matthews KA. Cardiovascular responses to behavioral stress and hypertension: A meta-analytic review. *Ann Behav Med* 1990;**12**:30–9.

18 Fredrikson M, Tuomisto M, Bergman-Losman B. Neuroendocrine and cardiovascular stress reactivity in middle-aged normotensive adults with parental history of cardiovascular disease. *Psychophysiology* 1991;**28**:656–64.

19 Lundberg U, Fredrikson M, Wallin L *et al*. Blood lipids as related to cardiovascular and neuroendocrine functions under different conditions in healthy males and females. *Pharm Biochem Behav* 1989;**33**:381–6.

20 Barnes VA, Treiber FA, Davis H *et al*. Central adiposity and hemodynamic functioning at rest and during stress in adolescents. *Int J Obes* 1998;**22**:1079–83.

21 Rosmond R, Dallman MF, Bjorntorp P. Stress-related cortisol secretion in men: relationships with abdominal obesity and endocrine, metabolic and hemodynamic abnormalities. *J Clin Endocrinol Metab* 1998;**83**:1853–9.

22 Schnall PL, Landsbergis PA, Baker D. Job strain and cardiovascular disease. *Ann Rev Public Health* 1994;**15**:381–411.

23 Steptoe A, Cropley M, Joekes K. Job strain, blood pressure, and responsivity to uncontrollable stress. *J Hypertension* 1999;**17**:193–200.

24 Lundberg U, Frankenhaeuser M. Stress and workload of men and women in high-ranking positions. *J Occup Health Psychol* 1999;**4**:142–51.

25 Steptoe A, Cropley M, Griffith J *et al*. Job strain and anger expression predict early morning elevations in salivary cortisol. *Psychosom Med* 2000;**62**:286–92.

26 Siegrist J, Klein D, Voigt KH. Linking sociological with physiological data: the model of effort-reward imbalance at work. *Acta Physiol Scand* 1997;**161**(suppl. 640):112–16.

27 Uchino BN, Cacioppo JT, Kiecolt-Glaser JK. The relationship between social support and physiological processes: a review with emphasis on underlying mechanisms and implications for health. *Psychol Bull* 1996;**119**:488–531.

28 Lepore SJ. Problems and prospects for the social support–reactivity hypothesis. *Ann Behav Med* 1998;**20**:257–69.

29 Pomerleau OF, Pomerleau CS. Stress, smoking, and the cardiovascular system. *J Subst Abuse* 1989;**1**:331–43.

30 Tsuda A, Steptoe A, West R *et al*. Cigarette smoking and psychophysiological stress responsiveness: effects of recent smoking and temporary abstinence. *Psychopharmacology* 1996; **126**:226–33.

31 Steptoe A, Moses J, Edwards S *et al*. Exercise and responsivity to mental stress: Discrepancies between the subjective and physiological effects of aerobic training. *Int J Sport Psychol* 1993;**24**:110–29.

32 Blumenthal JA, Siegel WC, Appelbaum M. Failure of exercise to reduce blood pressure in patients with mild hypertension. *JAMA* 1991;**266**:2098–104.

33 Steptoe A, Cropley M, Griffith J *et al*. The influence of abdominal obesity and chronic work stress on ambulatory blood pressure in men and women. *Int J Obes* 1999;**23**:1184–91.

34 Keys A, Longstreet H, Blackburn H, Brozek J, Anderson JT, Simonson E. Mortality and coronary heart disease among men studied for 23 years. *Arch Intern Med* 1971; **128**:201–24.

35 Coresh J, Klag MJ, Mead LA, Liang KY, Whelton PK. Vascular reactivity in young adults and cardiovascular disease: A prospective study. *Hypertension* 1992;**19**:II-218–23.

36 Carroll D, Davey Smith G, Willemsen G *et al*. Blood pressure reactions to the cold pressor test and the prediction of ischaemic heart disease: data from the Caerphilly Study. *J Epidemiol Community Health* 1998;**52**:528–9.

37 Menkes MS, Matthews KA, Krantz DS *et al*. Cardiovascular reactivity to the cold pressor test as a predictor of hypertension. *Hypertension* 1989;**14**:524–30.

38 Kasagi F, Akahoshi M, Shimaoka K. Relation between cold pressor test and development of hypertension based on 28-year follow-up. *Hypertension* 1995;**25**:71–6.

39 Carroll D, Davey Smith G, Sheffield D *et al*. Pressor reactivity to psychological stress and prediction of future blood pressure: data from the Whitehall II study. *BMJ* 1995;**310**:771–6.

40 Light K, Dolan C, Davis M *et al*. Cardiovascular responses to an active coping challenge as predictors of blood pressure patterns 10 to 15 years later. *Psychosom Med* 1992;**54**:217–30.

41 Markovitz JH, Raczynski JM, Wallace D *et al*. Cardiovascular reactivity to video game predicts subsequent blood pressure increases in young men: The CARDIA study. *Psychosom Med* 1998;**60**:186–91.

42 Georgiades A, Lemne C, De Faire U *et al*. Stress-induced blood pressure measurements predict left ventricular mass over three years among borderline hypertensive men. *Eur J Clin Invest* 1997;**27**:733–9.

43 O'Leary DH, Polak JF, Kronmal RA *et al*. Carotid-artery intima and media thickness as a risk factor for myocardial infarction and stroke in older adults. Cardiovascular Health Study Collaborative Research Group. *N Engl J Med* 1999;**340**:14–22.

44 Kamarck TW, Everson SA, Kaplan GA *et al*. Exaggerated blood pressure responses during mental stress are associated with enhanced carotid atherosclerosis in middle-aged Finnish men. *Circulation* 1997;**96**:3842–8.

45 Matthews KA, Owens JF, Kuller LH *et al*. Stress-induced pulse pressure change predicts women's carotid atherosclerosis. *Stroke* 1998;**29**:1525–30.

46 Lynch JW, Everson SA, Kaplan GA *et al*. Does low socioeconomic status potentiate the effects of heightened cardiovascular responses to stress on the progression of carotid atherosclerosis? *Am J Public Health* 1998;**88**:389–94.

47 Rozanski A, Blumenthal JA, Kaplan J. Impact of psychological factors on the pathogenesis of cardiovascular disease and implications for therapy. *Circulation* 1999;**99**:2195–217.

48 Rozanski A, Bairey CN, Krantz DS *et al*. Mental stress and the induction of silent myocardial ischemia in patients with coronary artery disease. *N Engl J Med* 1988;**318**:1005–11.

49 Ironson G, Taylor CB, Boltwood M *et al*. Effects of anger on left ventricular ejection fraction in coronary artery disease. *Am J Cardiol* 1992;**70**:281–5.

50 Yeung AC, Vekshtein VI, Krantz DS *et al*. The effect of atherosclerosis on the vasomotor response of coronary arteries to mental stress. *N Engl J Med* 1991;**325**:1551–6.

51 Gullette EC, Blumenthal JA, Babyak M *et al*. Effects of mental stress on myocardial ischemia during daily life. *JAMA* 1997;**277**:1521–6.

52 Stone PH, Krantz DS, McMahon RP *et al*. Relationship among mental stress-induced ischemia and ischemia during daily life and during exercise: the Psychophysiological Investigations of Myocardial Ischemia (PIMI) study. *J Am Coll Cardiol* 1999;**33**:1476–84.

53 Lown B, Verrier RL, Rabinowitz SH. Neural and psychologic mechanisms and the problem of sudden cardiac death. *Am J Cardiol* 1977;**39**:890–902.

54 Follick MJ, Ahern DK, Gorkin L *et al*. Relation of psychosocial and stress reactivity variables to ventricular arrhythmias in the Cardiac Arrhythmia Pilot Study (CAPS). *Am J Cardiol* 1990;**66**:63–7.

55 Mulcahy D, Gunning M, Knight C *et al*. Long-term (5 year) effects of transient (silent) ischaemia on left ventricular systolic function in stable angina. *Eur Heart J* 1998;**19**:1342–7.

56 Jiang W, Babyak M, Krantz DS *et al*. Mental stress-induced myocardial ischemia and cardiac events. *JAMA* 1996;**275**:1651–6.

57 Krantz DS, Santiago HT, Kop WJ *et al*. Prognostic value of mental stress testing in coronary artery disease. *Am J Cardiol* 1999;**84**:1292–7.

58 Mittleman MA, Maclure M, Sherwood JB *et al*. Triggering of acute myocardial infarction onset by episodes of anger. *Circulation* 1995;**92**:1720–5.

59 Moller J, Hallqvist J, Diderichsen F *et al*. Do episodes of anger trigger myocardial infarction? A case-crossover analysis in the Stockholm Heart Epidemiology Program (SHEEP). *Psychosom Med* 1999;**61**:842–9.

12: Stress mechanisms in coronary heart disease

ERIC BRUNNER

There is widespread and increasing concern about the effects of modern life on health. The Labour Force Survey in 1995 found that half a million people in England and Wales believed they were suffering from work related stress, indicating a substantial rise over 5 years. Depression, anxiety, and physical illness are increasingly being attributed to stress, either as a primary cause or as an aggravating factor. Litigation is on the increase. Outside work, unemployment and job insecurity, family problems, and social isolation are considered by many to be further stressors with potentially serious health consequences. Among these consequences there is great public concern that angina, heart attack, and sudden death are in part due to stress. Earlier chapters have addressed key aspects of the evidence, including influences at different life course stages, socially patterned exposures such as smoking and diet, and working conditions. The aim of this chapter is to examine potential mechanisms from a biological and epidemiological perspective.

One policy response has been to fund stress research, and to begin to translate findings into guidance on stress avoidance and reduction in official health messages. The UK Health Education Authority, in a press release in June 1999, told individuals that the usual advice to quit smoking, cut down drinking, eat less fat, and get down to the gym, remains sound. To these familiar messages, the Health Education Authority added stress or psychosocial factors as important considerations in the quest for positive health. The key advice is to take control at work, and to pay more attention to the social and emotional dimensions of working and personal life.

The shift towards a more holistic approach to health promotion can be seen as a response to two contrasting influences. One is the relative weakness of the knowledge–attitudes–behaviour model, with its modest if not disappointing achievements in the field of health related behaviour change.[1] The other influence stems from social epidemiology, or population health, the body of research represented in this book, which places disease causation in a social, psychological, and biological context. An indicator of the shift in policy thinking comes from the World Health Organization (WHO)

181

Europe's Centre for Urban Health, in the form of a booklet published in 1998 which emphasises structural and social, rather than behavioural, factors as important determinants of public health.

This chapter focuses on the biological mechanisms connecting psychosocial stressors to coronary heart disease. In particular, it examines the evidence for a *direct* effect of stress on the disease process, which is to say effects operating independently of conventional risk factors such as smoking and lack of exercise. It is intended that the stress perspective will lead to a deeper understanding of determinants of health at the individual level, and provide insight for those working for broader health gain.

A direct stress effect?

A major question in the field of research into stress and degenerative disease is whether chronic stress exerts its effects directly, or whether it operates indirectly by influencing the pattern of health behaviours such as smoking (Figure 12.1). The pathways are by no means mutually exclusive. A period of high work demands may create competition for time usually devoted to sport. Alternatively, an individual may experience the stress of chronic low control at work, with adverse health consequences, while maintaining a healthy lifestyle.

Attempting to distinguish between the direct and indirect stress pathways is of considerable policy importance, and not a question of mere academic interest. This can readily be appreciated in the case of social differences in health. At risk of caricature, one may contrast biomedical and public health explanations for the inverse social gradient in coronary heart disease. The former tends to emphasise factors such as genetic susceptibility and smoking behaviour, while the latter focuses on wider influences such as material and social deprivation, and stress.

In reality these alternative perspectives are not mutually exclusive, but advocacy of one rather than the other denotes a preference either for individual or for social policy solutions. Our caricature "biomedical

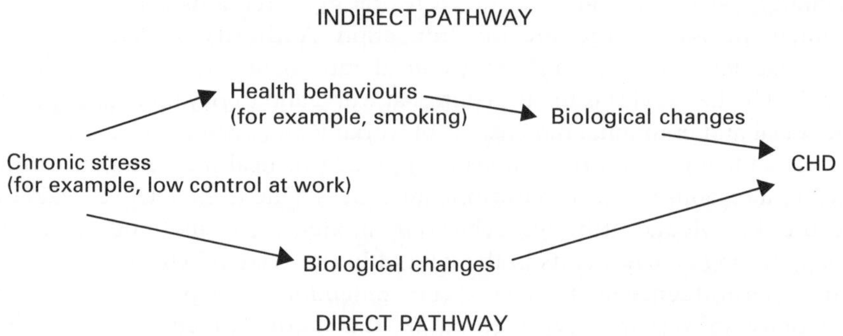

INDIRECT PATHWAY

Figure 12.1 Direct and indirect stress pathways to coronary heart disease (CHD).

explanation" is that more lower status individuals smoke, and they must give up if they do not want to have a heart attack or develop lung cancer. However, individuals do not exist in isolation; rather they interact with family, friends, and neighbours, and are influenced by wider economic and environmental conditions. A public health view, therefore, looks for the explanation of socially patterned disease rates, at least in part at the social level. An individual's smoking habit belongs not only to that individual: it is socially and culturally determined, and, in turn, it shapes the smoking behaviour and tobacco smoke exposure of others around that person.

Returning to the stress model shown in Figure 12.1, we can see in principle that stress may operate to cause coronary heart disease through smoking and other behaviours, or through involuntary, biological mechanisms.

Biological mechanisms

This section first reviews the broad concepts of homeostasis and allostasis in relation to stress and disease, and then presents evidence for the involvement of the autonomic nervous system, the hypothalamic–pituitary–adrenal axis, and other pathways in the stress related development of coronary risk.

The main candidate mechanisms for the link between stress and coronary heart disease involve:

- homeostatic and allostatic changes in response to stress
- neuroendocrine changes and alteration of autonomic functioning
- development of the metabolic syndrome and insulin resistance
- disturbances of coagulation
- inflammatory and immune responses.

Homeostasis and allostasis

The main axes of neuroendocrine response appear to be the sympathoadrenal and hypothalamic–pituitary–adrenal systems. Cannon, Professor of Physiology at Harvard from 1906 to 1942, elucidated the role of the sympathetic branch of the autonomic nervous system and circulating catecholamines in the dynamics of metabolic self regulation. He coined the term "homeostasis" to refer to the feedback mechanisms that maintain constant internal conditions—such as body temperature—in the face of environmental change. Hans Selye, a Czech–Canadian physician, focused on the glucocorticoids, which like catecholamines have widespread effects both centrally and peripherally. He proposed a three stage non-specific stress response: first, the alarm reaction, when the body responds to danger; second, resistance, when the body attempts to restore itself; and third, if the stress continues, exhaustion, with the risk of stress-related disorder.[2] Evidence for the third of these stages is comparatively weak.

The concept of allostasis, the ability to achieve physiological stability through change, extends the idea of homeostasis to include processes leading to disease. The allostatic load hypothesis links the psychosocial environment

183

to physical disease by neuroendocrine mechanisms,[3] particularly those described by Cannon and Selye.[2] Allostatic load, potentially leading to damage induced by stress, is considered relevant in cardiovascular disease, cancer, infection, and cognitive decline, and has been described as a sign of accelerated ageing. The price of adaptation to external and internal stress may be wear and tear on the organism, the result of chronic over- or underactivity of physiological systems to produce allostatic load. For instance, the endocrine system controlling blood glucose may be pushed toward diabetes.

Allostatic load was investigated in a longitudinal study of older Americans,[4] where it was defined by elevations of five established cardiovascular risk factors—systolic and diastolic blood pressure, waist–hip ratio, ratio of total cholesterol to high density lipoprotein (HDL) cholesterol, and HDL cholesterol level—plus raised concentrations of glycated haemoglobin, urinary epinephrine (adrenaline), norepinephrine (noradrenaline) and cortisol, and the adrenal androgen, serum dehydroepiandrosterone sulphate. Subjects with lower baseline allostatic load scores had better physical and mental functioning. Over the follow up period the same group showed less decline in functioning and were less likely to develop cardiovascular disease.

Neuroendocrine pathways

The cardiovascular system is regulated by the autonomic nervous system and by neurohormonal axes regulating the action of catecholamines, insulin, glucagon, growth hormone, and glucocorticoids. Potentially, several neuroendocrine pathways exist by which chronic psychological stress may contribute to cardiovascular disease development through metabolic, haemostatic, and inflammatory changes. The autonomic nervous system and the hypothalamic–pituitary–adrenal axis are, on the basis of physiological and epidemiological evidence as well as the theoretical perspectives outlined above, the most important systems to study.

Rapid release of epinephrine from the adrenal medulla and norepinephrine from sympathetic nerve endings produces cognitive arousal, sensory vigilance, bronchodilation, tachycardia, alteration of organ blood flows, raised blood pressure, haemoconcentration, and energy mobilisation. The precise nature of the activation varies according to the stressor and its duration, but its function is essentially to prepare for or maintain physical exertion. Wide variation between individuals in the size and duration of autonomic responses is attributed to individual differences in psychological coping resources.[5] The size and nature of physiological responses to a given stressor varies between laboratory animals, reflecting differences in prior stress history.[6] This points to the possibility of interactions between immediate and chronic psychosocial adversity, and protective factors such as a high level of control at work and adequate social support.

The autonomic nervous system has long been a target for both stress research and ageing research, although until recently, population based measurement has been impractical. Catecholamines have a halflife of some

2 minutes in the circulation, and so the blood level is volatile. Heart rate and blood pressure readings have therefore often been used as markers of sympathetic activity for reasons of reproducibility and economy (see Chapter 11).[7] Urinary catecholamine output is of interest as a measure of stress responsiveness, because it is a time integrated measure of sympathoadrenal activity. Collection of a 24 hour urine sample is desirable in order to obtain a reliable estimate of output, but it is inconvenient for participants.[8]

The technique of heart rate variability measurement—in particular, power spectral analysis—is proving to be a powerful tool for investigating the balance between sympathetic and parasympathetic activity (see Chapter 14).[9] Total variability is reduced by sympathetic activity and increased by vagal activity. Power spectral density analysis of heart rate variability yields low frequency (0.04–0.15 Hz) and high frequency (0.18–0.4 Hz) components.[10] The low frequency component is increased by mental stress and physical exercise. The high frequency component is abolished by atropine, and therefore appears to index vagal activity. An increase in low frequency and in low frequency/high frequency ratio, and a reduction in total power, indicates sympathetic predominance.

Low heart rate variability has been shown to predict prognosis among those with established coronary heart disease.[11] More recently, a case–cohort study has shown that low variability predicts incident coronary heart disease.[12] Sympathetic predominance has been linked with adverse work characteristics, depression, hostility, and anxiety, and separately with increased risk of sudden death.[13] Depression, also linked with excessive glucocorticoid production,[14] predicts future coronary disease (see Chapter 7).[15] To date, however, there are few population based cohort studies of heart rate variability and its predictive power for coronary heart disease.

Indirect evidence for such an effect comes from the Whitehall II study.[16] The relation between social position and heart rate variability is of great interest within this study, with its emphasis on testing psychosocial explanations for the inverse social gradient in heart disease. Demonstration of a link between low social occupational status and low heart rate variability would add to the psychometric and other evidence that, in a hierarchical society, low status can be viewed as a chronic stressor, with adverse health effects.[16] At the third medical examination of the Whitehall II study, 4000 participants provided a 5 minute electrocardiogram recording after a period of rest in a quiet, darkened room. Preliminary analysis shows that lower heart rate variability, indicating a pattern of sympathetic predominance, is associated with increasing age and lower employment grade. Loss of autonomic function is known to be an important component of the ageing process, but has not been linked previously to lower social position. Analyses of the associations between psychosocial factors, heart rate variability, and markers of subclinical disease will shed light on the nature of stress pathways (see Figure 12.1).

The second and less rapid component of the stress response involves cortisol release from the adrenal cortex. The glucocorticoid cortisol has multiple metabolic and psychological effects. It plays a key role in the maintenance of basal and stress related metabolic homeostasis. Cortisol antagonises the effects of insulin, acting to mobilise energy reserves by raising blood glucose concentration and promoting fatty acid release from adipose tissue. In the physically inactive state these superfluous energy substrates will lead to increased hepatic lipoprotein output. The potent immunosuppressive action of glucocorticoids is well known. Activation of the hypothalamic–pituitary–adrenal (HPA) axis appears to protect the individual from the potentially malign effects of inflammation and infection, and the accompanying host response. For example, leucocytes from patients with sepsis were more sensitive in vitro to the antiproliferative action of dexamethasone than those of controls, using the mitogen stimulated lymphocyte proliferation assay. During recovery, sensitivity declined. Cytokines antagonise the glucocorticoid effect, providing a mechanism by which systemic inhibition of immune response may be accompanied by an appropriate local immune reaction.[17]

There are several feedback loops (Figure 12.2) that regulate the activity of the HPA axis. The control system, involving three hormones—corticotrophin releasing factor, corticotrophin, and cortisol itself—provides three levels of negative feedback to adjust the circulating cortisol level during everyday life and in stress situations. Like the sympathoadrenal system,[18] functioning of the HPA axis appears to be conditioned by psychosocial factors including self esteem,[19,20] chronic unemployment,[21] and low social rank.[22] Prolonged elevations or blunted responses seem to be characteristic of an actual or projected failure to cope with challenge. These patterns of cortisol secretion contrast with an adaptive sharp response and rapid return to a low baseline, and correspond to Selye's proposed non-specific stress mechanism.[2]

Blood cortisol has a halflife of about 1 hour, and there is a marked and pulsatile diurnal pattern with significant day to day variability. The invasive sampling method of venepuncture is being replaced by saliva collections in laboratory or usual life settings.[23,24] Urinary output of adrenal steroids and their metabolites can be measured to obtain integrated measures of secretion. Findings support the expectation that HPA axis function depends on tissue responsiveness as well as on secretion of cortisol. For instance, study participants with a family history of essential hypertension,[25] and those with insulin resistance,[26] show increased tissue sensitivity to glucocorticoids.

Large scale prospective studies of HPA axis function in coronary disease are as yet lacking. The neuroendocrine hypothesis[27,28] proposes that chronic stress drives susceptible individuals towards the metabolic syndrome pattern of abnormalities,[29] consisting of glucose intolerance, insulin resistance, lipoprotein disturbances, reduced fibrinolysis, and often central obesity.[30] According to this model, sensory information prompts cortical and limbic responses, the HPA axis and other neuroendocrine pathways, to push the body into a pathological state. This centrally driven push towards disease development is also part of the concept of allostatic load.[3]

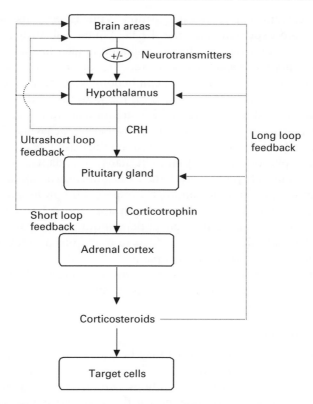

Figure 12.2 The hypothalamic–pituitary–adrenal axis. CRH, corticotrophin releasing hormone. Redrawn from Brown, 1994.[31]

A behavioural explanation for the observed cross-sectional associations among HPA and metabolic syndrome variables is worth considering.[32] In this hypothesis, inappropriate diet and physical inactivity lead to central obesity among those so predisposed. The increased mass of abdominal fat tissue, with its high concentration of glucocorticoid receptors, pulls cortisol out of the circulation and thereby alters feedback to the pituitary and hypothalamus. Here, modified neuroendocrine function is the consequence, and behavioural and constitutional factors are the causes. The push and pull pathways are probably not alternatives; they are likely to be synergistic. Psychosocial and other factors over the life course are related to development of adult risk,[33,34] as is fetal programming (see Chapter 3). Early influence on HPA function in adulthood has now been identified. Lower birthweight was associated with higher morning plasma cortisol level among men 59–70 years old.[35] These related findings give evidence that plasma cortisol levels, in the upper part of the normal range, are among the determinants of blood pressure and glucose tolerance in adulthood. In this group of men fetal programming of the HPA axis was more important than the effect of current socioeconomic position. While it seems likely that both fetal growth and experiences during the life course will turn out to be of importance in shaping neuroendocrine function in later life, an outstanding question is whether apparently adverse cortisol responses are directly responsible for future ill health, or an epiphenomenon. Related to this is the issue of reversibility. If HPA funtion is on the pathway to disease, to what extent can it be modified in adult life? Longitudinal studies are needed to clarify the relative importance of the neuroendocrine, behavioural, and early life hypotheses. Such findings will shed light on the feasibility of intervention.

From an evolutionary standpoint, humans are adapted to meet the challenge of external, potentially lethal, but short-term threats, perhaps from wild animals or from one another. Frequent and prolonged activation of the "fight or flight" or defence reaction appears to be maladaptive,[36] and may prove to be central to an understanding of the distribution of cardiovascular and other diseases. Added to our evolved predisposition to build up stores of body fat in times of plenty,[37,38] the defence reaction seems to be a double edged sword in modern times. The interaction of these two archetypal tendencies may lead to insulin resistance, type II diabetes, and other pathological changes.

Metabolic syndrome

Neuroendocrine stress mechanisms may be important in the causation of coronary heart disease. At this stage, lacking direct evidence in human populations, there are related findings which lend support to the psychosocial hypothesis.[39] Among these is the prospective observation from the Whitehall II study that adverse psychosocial conditions at work predict reports of newly incident coronary heart disease.[40] In this large cohort of middleaged civil servants in London, working conditions were able to account statistically for much of the gradient in coronary events across the employment grade hierarchy.[41]

In the same study population, the biological evidence is consistent with a psychosocial and neuroendocrine interpretation. Central obesity and features of the metabolic syndrome, with the exception of resting blood pressure, increase in prevalence with each step down the British civil service employment grade strata.[30] The findings (Figure 12.3) are evidence for a distinctive socially patterned clustering of coronary risk factors corresponding to the inverse social gradient in coronary heart disease seen in the first Whitehall study,[42] and generally in industrialised countries. As we shall see, several lines of evidence suggest that stress mechanisms may contribute to this risk gradient. Before describing this, a brief detour into the historical background is necessary to set the scene.

In the first Whitehall study, started by Rose and Reid in 1968, the three classic risk factors accounted for about a third of the steep gradient in incident premature heart disease across employment grades.[42] It appeared that differences in smoking rate, blood pressure, and plasma cholesterol level, although important influences on an individual's risk, did not provide

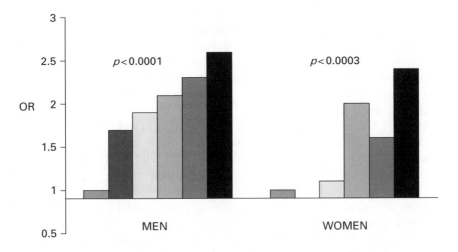

Figure 12.3   Prevalence of the metabolic syndrome by employment grade in the Whitehall II study. Employment grade is stratified into six levels. Odds ratios (OR) adjusted for age and (in women) menopausal status; p values are tested for trend across grades. From Brunner et al.[30]

a good explanation for the cardiovascular mortality differences between social classes. In fact, social differences in blood cholesterol level and blood pressure were and continue to be small, while smoking rates are strongly related, inversely, to social position and in relative terms social differences in smoking have tended to grow. The Whitehall II study, with its baseline survey in 1985–1988, was set up by Marmot, Stansfeld and others to investigate the specific explanation for the disease gradient, of which smoking was clearly a part.[16]

A key proposal was that the psychosocial environment, particularly working conditions at different levels in the civil service hierarchy, would provide new insights. As we have seen above this approach turned out to be fruitful, since the gradient in self reported coronary heart disease is largely accounted for by differences in reported low control at work across employment grades.[41] The metabolic syndrome findings are an important element in developing an understanding of the means by which the psychosocial environment might exert its effects on health. Confirmation of this biological mechanism as an important mediator of the social gradient in coronary heart disease would strengthen considerably the case for a "stress effect" in general, as well as in relation to social inequalities.

The metabolic syndrome is a well known precursor state to coronary heart disease.[43] Central, or abdominal, obesity predicts coronary heart disease in men[44] and women,[45,46] and is linked with increased risk of non-insulin-dependent diabetes.[47,48] The main components of the metabolic syndrome, or Reaven's syndrome X[29]—namely impaired glucose tolerance, insulin resistance, and disturbances of lipoprotein metabolism

189

characterised by raised concentrations of serum triacylglycerols and low HDL cholesterol—are associated both with increased coronary risk and with central obesity.[49-51] There is a well established link between the metabolic syndrome and coronary heart disease. Less certain is the upstream link between psychosocial factors and the metabolic syndrome, and the extent to which it might be generated by central neural drive and neuroendocrine mechanisms.

Support for a mediating role for the metabolic syndrome in the social gradient in coronary heart disease comes from detailed studies of a different social hierarchy: that of baboons in the wild.[52] The neuroscientist Sapolsky, who has conducted a longterm study of the behaviour and physiology of wild baboon troops in the Serengeti, argues that these animals are ideal subjects for investigating psychosocial factors.[52] Food is plentiful, predators are scarce, and infant mortality is low. Only some 4 hours per day are required for foraging, leaving the animals, who live in groups of fifty to a hundred, plenty of time to engage in social activity. Attainment and maintenance of social rank is a preoccupation that determines access to a variety of resources. On the basis of these behaviours, Sapolsky classified males of the troop into dominants and subordinates. Analysis of blood obtained following anaesthesia under controlled conditions produced fascinating parallels with the results from men in the Whitehall II study.

Lipid and lipoprotein profiles showed striking similarities according to rank position in the two study samples. Total and low density lipoprotein cholesterol and apolipoprotein B concentrations were similar across the hierarchies in both groups. Serum HDL cholesterol and apolipoprotein A-I levels were higher in the dominant male baboons compared with the subordinates, again mirroring findings in civil servants.[53] Further, subordinate baboons were found to have higher resting blood cortisol levels, and levels of the hormone were inversely correlated with serum HDL cholesterol.

The latter finding is consistent with the proposal that metabolic syndrome is at least in part a psychosocial effect, in this case an effect in some way connected with lower social position. Cushing's syndrome, a condition of great cortisol excess, provides an extreme example of the chronic effects of glucocorticoids on lipoprotein metabolism and glucose tolerance.[54] Cushing's syndrome is characterised by central obesity and increased risks for diabetes, hypertension, and coronary disease. Central obesity is a feature of low socioeconomic status in many healthy populations,[55] and it may be that less extreme changes in HPA function than those encountered in Cushing's syndrome have less pronounced but still significant effects on disease risk.

Comparing baboons with civil servants is a speculative exercise, but it has one particular strength. Baboons have "clean" lifestyles: they neither smoke nor drink, nor spend much time slumped in front of a television set. We can infer from these facts that systematic lifestyle differences across the hierarchy are unlikely to account for the metabolic syndrome pattern of risk factors among subordinate baboons. It may be that psychosocial factors contribute to the physiological differences related to hierarchy in both primate species, though the psychosocial factors in question are probably not the same.

Having established some evidence for links between stress, HPA function, and metabolic syndrome, we turn to the mediating role of the autonomic nervous system, and the sympathetic branch in particular. This mechanism has been proposed primarily because hypertension is commonly associated with abnormalities of glucose, insulin, and lipoprotein metabolism.[56] It is unclear, however, whether the initial event is an increase in sympathetic activity, leading subsequently to raised blood pressure and insulin resistance, or whether insulin resistance may occur initially, as animal studies have found, before the onset of hypertension. Importantly, hypertension does not develop in all individuals with insulin resistance, and not all hypertensive individuals are insulin resistant.[56] Differential activation of the HPA axis and sympathetic nervous system may explain the apparent paradox of similar mean resting blood pressures, but a marked inverse gradient in metabolic syndrome prevalence according to occupational position in the Whitehall II study.[30]

Further investigations in the Whitehall II study will help to answer some of the important but unresolved questions raised here. In particular, we are in the process of examining the proposed roles of psychosocial factors at work and other domains in the genesis of the metabolic syndrome, and whether altered neuroendocrine function, indexed by heart rate variability and measures of cortisol secretion, output, and glucocorticoid sensitivity may be related to the distinct clustering of coronary risk factors we have identified.

Haemostasis and fibrinogen

Haemostasis is of interest in the study of stress mechanisms in coronary heart disease for two major reasons. First, there is a thrombotic component both in the slow process of atherosclerotic plaque development and in acute coronary events.[57] Second, haemostatic function is altered in the acute phase response to infection and other stressors. Considerable attention has been devoted to the study of fibrinogen for these reasons.

Fibrinogen is a large protein synthesised by the liver, and comprises some 5% of total plasma protein. Stimuli including injury activate the clotting cascade with the effect that soluble fibrinogen is converted enzymatically to fibrin, an insoluble polymer matrix which is the structural component of blood clots. A raised fibrinogen level has been shown to be associated with increased risk of coronary heart disease and stroke in several Western populations.[58–61] Other haemostatic variables, including factor VII, plasma viscosity, and fibrinolytic activity, predict coronary heart disease, but the evidence is less extensive.[58,62,63]

Fibrinogen is an acute phase reactant, and the circulating level increases in response to infection and other exposures including smoking. Moderate alcohol consumption and habitual vigorous exercise are each linked with lower fibrinogen levels.[53]

Plasma fibrinogen concentration is related to several social and psychosocial factors in adulthood. This is consistent with a contribution of haemostasis to the high rates of coronary disease experienced by people in unfavourable socioeconomic circumstances, which, as we have seen in the previous section, are poorly explained by the traditional coronary risk factors. Mean fibrinogen levels are strongly and inversely related to grade of employment in the British civil service,[33] (Figure 12.4) and to social class based on occupation in a stratified sample of the population of England and Wales. Among civil servants, approximately half of the inverse association with social position was accounted for by health related behaviours and degree of obesity.

Control over work, a measure of the psychosocial environment, was inversely related to fibrinogen level in both sexes when assessed by personnel managers at the baseline of the Whitehall II study.[33] A parallel effect with self rated control, based on the Karasek–Theorell job strain questionnaire, was seen among men but not women (Table 12.1). These findings have been reinforced by the results of another cross-sectional study in Stockholm County, Sweden, in a working population sample of 1018 men and 490 women.[64] Using the same Karasek questionnaire to measure self reported job characteristics and additionally inferring job characteristics using a standard job exposure matrix, the study showed the expected effects of job control on plasma fibrinogen level, although in this population the evidence was more consistent for women than for men. The Stockholm study provides support for Karasek's job strain model, in that inferred high demands together with low control were linked with higher fibrinogen levels in both sexes even after adjustment for covariates such as smoking.

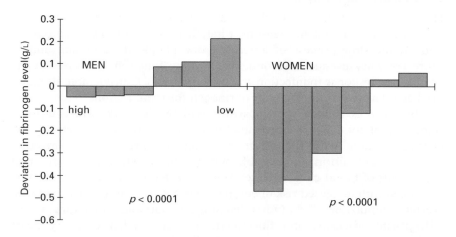

Figure 12.4 Plasma fibrinogen level by employment grade in the Whitehall II study. Data given as deviations in fibrinogen concentration from the overall mean for men (2.64 g/L) and women (2.84 g/L) with 95% confidence intervals. Means are adjusted for age and ethnic origin, and menopausal status in women. Employment grade is stratified into six levels. From Brunner et al.[30]

Table 12.1 Plasma fibrinogen concentrations (in g/L) in men and women according to self rating and external rating of degree of job control; values in parentheses are standard error.

Self rated	Externally rated		
	Low	Medium	High
Men (n = 1788)*			
Low	2·76 (0·04)	2·65 (0·05)	2·65 (0·05)
Medium	2·66 (0·05)	2·61 (0·03)	2·63 (0·03)
High	2·67 (0·05)	2·64 (0·03)	2·59 (0·03)
Women (n = 1012)**			
Low	2·86 (0·03)	2·87 (0·05)	2·78 (0·07)
Medium	2·91 (0·06)	2·83 (0·06)	2·71 (0·08)
High	2·76 (0·07)	2·82 (0·07)	2·84 (0·08)

*Low/low–high/high contrast: $p < 0.001$. Adjusted for age and ethnicity.
**Low/low–high/high contrast: not significant. Adjusted for age, ethnicity, and menopausal status.

An established acute effect of stress is the increased platelet stickiness in the "fight or flight" response, mediated by an increase in circulating catecholamines. There is growing evidence that psychosocial factors may exert longterm effects on the haemostatic system and thereby influence disease risk. Prospective population based studies are needed to confirm such mechanisms.

Inflammation and immunity

Infectious disease appears to contribute to short-term variations in morbidity and mortality from coronary heart disease,[65] and there is evidence that fibrinogen may be a mediator.[66] Some evidence for the role of chronic inflammatory processes in heart disease comes from a case–control study showing an association between coronary events and chronic gastric *Helicobacter pylori* infection.[67] Such asymptomatic infections, acquired in childhood and linked with the stress of deprivation and overcrowded housing, may produce a longterm low level systemic inflammatory response which enhances atherogenesis. Supporting this, a meta-analysis found consistently moderate to high prospective associations between levels of inflammatory markers (fibrinogen, C-reactive protein, albumin, and leucocyte count) and risk of coronary disease.[68] Against the infection hypothesis, a further systematic review found no consistent link between *H. pylori* seropositivity and the same set of inflammatory markers.[69]

Although the link between chronic infection and coronary disease appears weak, the strength of the prospective associations between inflammatory markers and coronary disease suggests that stress mechanisms may be involved, through inflammatory processes. Consistent with this suggestion, the brain is known to influence immune function. There is autonomic innervation of the relevant tissues (bone marrow, thymus, spleen, and lymph nodes); there are neuroendocrine controls on inflammatory mechanisms; and glucocorticoids have large effects on the immune system. In the Whitehall II study, employment grade and chronic low control at work were linked with raised concentrations of fibrinogen,[33] suggesting that inflammatory processes may mediate the effect of psychosocial circumstances on disease risk.

The possibility of an acute psychosocial effect on fibrinogen levels is suggested by a study of astronauts.[70] Space flight evoked raised urinary interleukin 6 (IL-6) levels on the first day, but not on other days before or after launch, consistent with a psychological explanation, since infection would not appear to be implicated. Cytokine release in response to psychosocial stimuli, and thereby increased fibrinogen synthesis, is feasible in view of the observation that messenger RNA for IL-6 is expressed within the brain. Over decades, such small effects may add to the formation of arterial plaques to increase risks of heart disease and stroke.

Genes and susceptibility

Evolutionary perspectives on stress are intended to shed light on the similarity of individuals who make up the species, including the shared predispositions to react to psychological demands in particular ways. In contrast to this is the new study of genetic polymorphisms, which underlie variation in biological responses to the same external stimulus. Commonly occurring polymorphisms potentially contribute to the social distribution of coronary and other disease through gene–environment interactions (see Chapter 15). While no gene has been shown to exhibit a social pattern, it is certainly possible that social and cultural differences in environmental exposures may interact with genetic variants to produce susceptibility to certain categories of disease.

The hypothetical interaction between repeated exposure to work or other stresses and the β-fibrinogen polymorphism (Figure 12.5) illustrates this possibility. The polymorphism may result in distinctive variation in the stress response, mediated by IL-6, in terms of amplitude and duration of plasma fibrinogen increase. This mechanism could, over time, increase coronary risk among high responders.

Conclusion

There is increasing concern about the effects that psychological aspects of modern life may have on health, particularly coronary disease risk. Social and biological epidemiology provides an important means to evaluate this link. Biological theories of stress are plausible, given what is known is about the physiology and anatomy of the human mind–body. Largescale prospective studies of neurohormonal functioning in coronary disease are lacking, and are required to provide evidence for the importance of direct stress effects.

Central drive may modify function of the hypothalamic–pituitary–adrenal axis in response to chronic stress, with the effect that insulin resistance

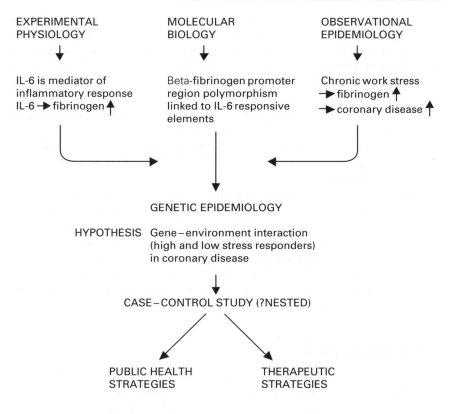

Figure 12.5 Hypothetical gene–environment interaction. Beta-fibrinogen polymorphism and chronic work stress. IL-6, interleukin 6.

develops and the circulating level of triglyceride rich lipoproteins increases. Such metabolic disturbances are related to abdominal adiposity. The relation between abdominal adiposity and insulin resistance, and hypothalamic–pituitary–adrenal function, is likely to be reflexive, so that physical inactivity and overeating may interact with psychological stress to increase the risks of coronary disease and diabetes. The link between the metabolic syndrome and coronary heart disease is well established. Less certain is the nature of the upstream link between psychosocial factors and the metabolic syndrome.

Mechanisms involving haemostasis and thrombosis may contribute to coronary risk associated with psychosocial effects. In the Whitehall II study, for example, lower employment grade and chronic low control at work were linked with raised plasma fibrinogen concentration. Loss of control is not only encountered at work. Raised fibrinogen levels in adults are seen among those with poor childhood socioeconomic circumstances, and in tenants compared with owner occupiers.[33]

195

From an evolutionary perspective, humans are adapted to respond to the challenge of external threats with an autonomic reaction, followed by a rise in cortisol secretion. This mechanism, if repeatedly activated, may lead to development of the metabolic syndrome, as we saw above.[36] The thrifty genotype hypothesis,[37] on the other hand, proposes that type II diabetes is the product of a genetic predisposition to store fat efficiently in preparation for times of scarcity, leading all too often to obesity and insulin resistance when food is abundant and prolonged physical activity unnecessary, as is the case for most people today. It may be that these two mechanisms interact to produce glucose intolerance and atherosclerosis, both precursors of coronary heart disease.

Research on the interrelationship of psychosocial, hormonal, metabolic, and disease processes is valuable for advancing scientific understanding and public health policy. It remains to be seen whether prevalence of the metabolic syndrome identifies those who later develop coronary disease, and if it accounts for differences in coronary disease incidence according to measures of chronic stress. If hypothalamic–pituitary–adrenal function is on the pathway to the disease, a question that follows is to what extent this function might be modified in adult life.

Acknowledgements

Parts of this chapter have been published previously in *Social Epidemiology*, edited by LF Berkman and I Kawachi, Oxford University Press, New York, 2000. The author is supported by the British Heart Foundation.

The Whitehall II study has been supported by grants from the Medical Research Council; British Heart Foundation; Health and Safety Executive; Department of Health; National Heart Lung and Blood Institute (HL36310), US, NIH: National Institute on Aging (AG13196), US, NIH; Agency for Health Care Policy Research (HS06516); and the John D and Catherine T MacArthur Foundation Research Networks on Successful Midlife Development and Socioeconomic Status and Health. Thanks are due to all participating civil service departments and their welfare, personnel, and establishment officers; the Occupational Health and Safety Agency; the Council of Civil Service Unions; all participating civil servants in the study; and all members of the Whitehall II study team.

References

1   Aveyard P, Cheng KK, Almond J et al. Cluster randomised controlled trial of expert system based on the transtheoretical ("stages of change") model for smoking prevention and cessation in schools. *BMJ* 1999;**319**:948–53.
2   Selye H. *The stress of life*. New York: McGraw-Hill, 1956.
3   McEwen BS. Protective and damaging effects of stress mediators. *N Engl J Med* 1998; **338**:171–9.
4   Seeman TE, Singer BH, Rowe JW, Horwitz RI, McEwen BS. Price of Adaptation – Allostatic Load and Its Health Consequences. *Arch Intern Med* 1997;**157**:2259–68.

5 Grossman AB. Regulation of human pituitary responses to stress. In: Brown MB, Koob GF, Rivier C, eds. *Stress: neurobiology and neuroendocrinology*. New York: Marcel Dekker, 1991.

6 McCarty R, Gold PE. Catecholamines, Stress, and Disease: A Psychobiological Perspective. *Psychosom Med* 1996;**58**:590–7.

7 Baum A, Grunberg N. Measurement of stress hormones. In: Cohen S, Kessler RC, Gordon LU, eds. *Measuring stress: a guide for health and social scientists*. New York: Oxford University Press, 1995.

8 White IR, Brunner EJ, Barron JL. A comparison of overnight and 24 Hour collection to measure urinary catecholamines. *J Clin Epidemiol* 1995;**48**:263–7.

9 Kawachi I, Sparrow D, Vokonas PS, Weiss ST. Decreased heart rate variability in men with phobic anxiety (data from the normative aging study). *Am J Cardiol* 1995;**75**:882–5.

10 Bigger JT, Fleiss JL, Steinman RC, Rolnitzky LM, Kleiger RE, Rottman JN. Frequency domain measures of heart period variability and mortality after myocardial infarction. *Circulation* 1992;**85**:164–71.

11 Bigger JT, Fleiss JL, Rolnitzky LM, Steinman RC. The ability of several short-term measures of RR variability to predict mortality after myocardial infarction. *Circulation* 1993;**88**:927–34.

12 Liao D, Cai J, Rosamond WD *et al.* Cardiac autonomic function and incident coronary heart disease: a population-based case-cohort study. The ARIC Study. Atherosclerosis Risk in Communities Study. *Am J Epidemiol* 1997;**145**:696–706.

13 Algra A, Tijssen JGP, Roelandt JRTC, Pool J, Lubsen J. Heart rate variability from 24-hour electrocardiography and the 2-year risk for sudden death. *Circulation* 1993;**88**:180–5.

14 Checkley S. The neuroendocrinology of depression and chronic stress. *Br Med Bull* 1996; **52**:597–617.

15 Hemingway H, Marmot M. Psychosocial factors in the aetiology and prognosis of coronary heart disease: systematic review of prospective cohort studies. *BMJ* 1999;**318**:1460–7.

16 Marmot MG, Davey Smith G, Stansfeld SA *et al.* Health inequalities among British Civil Servants: the Whitehall II study. *Lancet* 1991;**337**:1387–93.

17 Molijn GJ, Spek JJ, van Uffelen JC. Differential adaptation of glucocorticoid sensitivity of peripheral blood mononuclear leukocytes in patients with sepsis or septic shock. *J Clin Endocrinol Metab* 1995;**80**:1799–803.

18 Steptoe A, Cropley M, Joekes K. Job strain, blood pressure, and responsivity to uncontrollable stress. *J Hypertension* 1999;**17**:193–200.

19 Kirschbaum C, Prussner JC, Stone AA *et al.* Persistent high cortisol responses to repeated psychological stress in a subpopulation of healthy men. *Psychosom Med* 1995;**57**:468–74.

20 Seeman TE, Berkman LF, Gulanski BI *et al.* Self-esteem and neuroendocrine response to challenge: MacArthur studies of successful aging. *J Psychosom Res* 1995;**39**:69–84.

21 Ockenfels MC, Porter L, Smyth J, Kirschbaum C, Hellhammer DH, Stone AA. Effect of chronic stress associated with unemployment on salivary cortisol: overall cortisol levels, diurnal rhythm and acute stress reactivity. *Psychosom Med* 1995;**57**:460–7.

22 Hellhammer DH, Buchtal J, Gutberlet I, Kirschbaum C. Social hierarchy and adrenocortical stress reactivity in men. *Psychoneuroendocrinology* 1997;**22**:643–50.

23 Kirschbaum C, Hellhammer D. Salivary cortisol in psychoneuroendocrine research: recent developments and applications. *Psychoneuroendocrinology* 1994;**19**:313–33.

24 Van Eck M, Berkhof H, Nicolson N, Sulon J. The effects of perceived stress, traits, mood states and stressful daily events on salivary cortisol. *Psychosom Med* 1996;**58**:447–58.

25 Walker BR, Best R, Shackleton CHL, Padfield PL, Edwards CRW. Increased vaso-constrictor sensitivity to glucocorticoids in essential hypertension. *Hypertension* 1996;**27**: 190–6.

26 Walker BR, Seckl JR, Phillips DIW. Increased dermal glucocorticoid sensitivity is associated with insulin resistance and related cardiovascular risk factors. *J Hypertens* 1996;**14**:142.

27 Bjorntorp P. Visceral fat accumulation: the missing link between psychosocial factors and cardiovascular disease? *J Intern Med* 1991;**230**:195–201.

28 Brunner EJ. Stress and the biology of inequality. *BMJ* 1997;**314**:1472–6.

29 Reaven GM. Role of insulin resistance in human disease (syndrome X): an expanded definition. *Ann Rev Med* 1993;**44**:121–31.

30 Brown RE. *An introduction to neuroendocrinology*. Cambridge: Cambridge University Press; 1994.

31 Brunner EJ, Marmot MG, Nanchahal K *et al.* Social inequality in coronary risk: central obesity and the metabolic syndrome. Evidence from the Whitehall II study. *Diabetologia* 1997;**40**:1341–9.

32 Hautanen A, Adlercreutz H. Altered adrenocorticotropin and cortisol secretion in abdominal obesity: implications for the insulin resistance syndrome. *J Intern Med* 1993; **234**:461–9.

33 Brunner EJ, Davey Smith G, Marmot MG, Canner R, Beksinska M, O'Brien J. Childhood social circumstances and psychosocial and behavioural factors as determinants of plasma fibrinogen. *Lancet* 1996;**347**:1008–13.

34 Brunner EJ, Shipley MJ, Blane D, Davey Smith G, Marmot MG. When does cardiovascular risk start? Past and present socioeconomic circumstances and risk factors in adulthood. *J Epidemiol Community Health* 1999;**53**:757–64.

35 Phillips DIW, Barker JP, Fall CHD *et al*. Elevated plasma cortisol concentrations: A link between low birth weight and insulin resistance syndrome? *J Clin Endocrinol Metab* 1998;**83**:757–60.

36 Sapolsky RM. Endocrinology alfresco: psychoendocrine studies of wild baboons. *Recent Prog Horm Res* 1993;**48**:437–68.

37 Neel JV. Diabetes mellitus: a "thrifty" genotype rendered detrimental by "progress"? *Am J Hum Genet* 1962;**14**:353–62.

38 O'Dea K. Obesity and diabetes in "the land of milk and honey". *Diabetes Metab Rev* 1992;**8**:373–88.

39 Blane D, Brunner EJ, Wilkinson RG. *Health and Social Organization*. London: Routledge, 1996.

40 Bosma H, Marmot MG, Hemingway H, Nicholson A, Brunner EJ, Stansfeld S. Low job control and risk of coronary heart disease in the Whitehall II (prospective cohort) study. *BMJ* 1997;**314**:558–65.

41 Marmot M, Bosma H, Hemingway H, Brunner EJ, Stansfeld SA. Contribution of job control and other risk factors to social variations in coronary heart disease incidence. *Lancet* 1997;**350**:235–9.

42 Marmot MG, Rose G, Shipley M, Hamilton PJS. Employment grade and coronary heart disease in British civil servants. *J Epidemiol Community Health* 1978;**32**:244–9.

43 Vague J. The degree of masculine differentiation of obesities: a factor determining predisposition to diabetes, atherosclerosis, gout, and uric calculous disease. *Am J Clin Nutr* 1956;**4**:20–34.

44 Larsson B, Svardsudd K, Welin L, Wilhelmsen L, Bjorntorp P, Tibblin G. Abdominal adipose tissue distribution, obesity, and risk of cardiovascular disease and death: 13 year follow up of participants in the study of men born in 1913. *BMJ* 1984;**288**:1401–4.

45 Lapidus L, Bengtsson C, Larsson B, Pennert K, Rybo E, Sjostrom L. Distribution of adipose tissue and risk of cardiovascular disease and death: a 12 year follow up of participants in the population study of women in Gothenburg, Sweden. *BMJ* 1984;**289**:1257–61.

46 Folsom AR, Kaye SA, Sellers TA *et al*. Body fat distribution and 5-year risk of death in older women. *JAMA* 1993;**269**:483–7.

47 Ohlson LO, Larsson B, Svardsudd K *et al*. The influence of body fat distribution on the incidence of diabetes mellitus. 13.5 years of follow-up of the participants in the study of men born in 1913. *Diabetes* 1985;**34**:1055–8.

48 McKeigue PM, Shah B, Marmot MG. Relation of central obesity and insulin resistance with high diabetes prevalence and cardiovascular risk in South Asians. *Lancet* 1991;**337**:382–6.

49 Kissebah AH, Vydelingum N, Murray R *et al*. Relation of body fat distribution to metabolic complications of obesity. *J Clin Endocrinol Metab* 1982;**54**:254–60.

50 Folsom AR, Burke GL, Ballew C, Jacobs DR, Haskell WL, Donahue RP. Relation of body fatness and its distribution to cardiovascular risk factors in young blacks and whites. *Am J Epidemiol* 1989;**130**:911–24.

51 Seidell JC, Bjorntorp P, Sjostrom L, Kvist H, Sannerstedt R. Visceral fat accumulation in men is positively associated with insulin, glucose, and C-peptide levels, but negatively with testosterone levels. *Metabolism* 1990;**39**:897–901.

52 Sapolsky RM, Mott GE. Social subordinance in wild baboons is associated with suppressed high density lipoprotein-cholesterol concentrations: the possible role of chronic social stress. *Endocrinology* 1987;**121**:1605–10.

53 Brunner EJ, Marmot MG, White IR *et al*. Gender and employment grade differences in blood cholesterol, apolipoproteins and haemostatic factors in the Whitehall II study. *Atherosclerosis* 1993;**102**:195–207.

54 Johnston DG, Alberti KGMM, Nattrass M, Barnes AJ, Bloom SR, Joplin GF. Hormonal and metabolic rhythms in Cushing's syndrome. *Metabolism* 1980;**29**:1047–51.

55 Brunner EJ, Juneja M, Marmot MG. Adbominal obesity and disease are linked to social position. *BMJ* 1998;**316**:508–9.

198

56 Reaven GM, Lithell H, Landsberg L. Hypertension and associated metabolic abnormalities—the role of insulin resistance and the sympathoadrenal system. *N Engl J Med* 1996;**334**:374–81.
57 Rabbani LE, Loscalzo J. Recent observations on the role of hemostatic determinants in the development of the atherothrombotic plaque. *Atherosclerosis* 1994;**105**:1–7.
58 Meade TW, Ruddock V, Stirling Y, Chakrabarti R, Miller GJ. Fibrinolytic activity, clotting factors, and long-term incidence of ischaemic heart disease in the Northwick Park Heart Study. *Lancet* 1993;**342**:1076–9.
59 Wilhelmsen L, Svardsudd K, Korsan-Bengsten K *et al*. Fibrinogen as a risk factor for stroke and myocardial infarction. *N Engl J Med* 1984;**311**:501–5.
60 Kannel WB, Wolf PA, Castelli WP, D'Agostino RB. Fibrinogen and risk of cardiovascular disease. *JAMA* 1987;**258**:1183–6.
61 Woodward M, Lowe GDO, Rumley A, Tunstall-Pedoe H. Fibrinogen as a risk factor for coronary heart disease and mortality in middle-aged men and women. *Eur Heart J* 1998; **19**:55–62.
62 Yarnell JWG, Baker IA, Sweetnam PM *et al*. Fibrinogen, viscosity and white blood cell count are major risk factors for ischemic heart disease. The Caerphilly and Speedwell Collaborative Heart Disease Studies. *Circulation* 1991;**83**:836–44.
63 Heinrich J, Balleisen L, Schulte H, Assmann G, van de Loo J. Fibrinogen and factor VII in the prediction of coronary risk: results from the PROCAM study in healthy men. *Arteriosclerosis Thromb* 1994;**14**:54–9.
64 Tsutsumi A, Theorell T, Hallqvit J, Reuterwall C, de Faire U. Association between job characteristics and plasma fibrinogen in a normal working population: a cross sectional analysis in referents of the SHEEP study. *J Epidemiol Community Health* 1999;**53**:348–54.
65 Vallance P, Collier J, Bhagat K. Infection, inflammation, and infarction: does acute endothelial dysfunction provide a link? *Lancet* 1997;**349**:1391–2.
66 Woodhouse PR, Khaw KT, Plummer M, Foley A, Meade TW. Seasonal variations of plasma fibrinogen and factor VII activity in the elderly: winter infections and death from cardiovascular disease. *Lancet* 1994;**343**:435–9.
67 Mendall MA, Goggin PM, Molineaux N *et al*. Relation of *Helicobacter pylori* infection and coronary heart disease. *Br Heart J* 1994;**71**:437–9.
68 Danesh J, Collins R, Appleby P, Peto R. Association of fibrinogen, C-reactive protein, albumin, or leukocyte count with coronary heart disease. *JAMA* 1998;**279**:1477–81.
69 Danesh J, Peto R. Risk factors for coronary heart disease and infection with *Helicobacter pylori*: meta-analysis of 18 studies. *BMJ* 1998;**316**:1130–2.
70 Stein TP, Schluter MD. Excretion of IL-6 by astronauts during spaceflight. *Am J Physiol* 1994;**266**:E448–552.

13: Arterial and myocardial structure and function: contributions of socioeconomic status and chronic psychosocial factors

HARRY HEMINGWAY

Coronary heart disease is visible to the naked eye at operation or post mortem. By the time coronary heart disease becomes clinically manifest as an acute myocardial infarction, unstable or stable angina, sudden cardiac death, or heart failure, there are usually macroscopic changes in the coronary and other arteries. Plaques may be visible, and thickening and hardening of the arterial walls may be palpable. However, disease of the coronary arteries is not the only pathological process in coronary heart disease; the "end tissue" damage—be it ischaemia, infarction, or poor function—occurs in the myocardium. It is increasingly recognised that increased left ventricular mass, macroscopically visible in its gross pathological forms, may be of aetiological importance in coronary heart disease.[1]

Formerly invisible in living general populations, arterial and myocardial disease processes can now be imaged using non-invasive techniques. These represent important new tools in investigating coronary heart disease aetiology. Ultrasonography allows, for the first time, direct measurements of arterial wall thickness (denoted by intima–media thickness) and left ventricular mass. Furthermore, as arterial pathophysiology is increasingly understood in terms of changes in arterial regulatory function, rather than the artery being a passive conduit, ultrasound techniques measuring endothelial dysfunction have been developed which are suitable for use in healthy populations.[2]

Established coronary heart disease is the end stage of a prolonged process in which abnormalities of arterial and myocardial structure and function precede by some decades the onset of clinically manifest disease. The first histological signs of atheroma involve lipid deposits in the intima of systemic arteries; fatty streaks are found in the aortas of children older than 3 years and in the coronary arteries of adolescents.[3,4] Investigating early subclinical changes in intima–media thickness, endothelial dysfunction, and left ventricular mass allows pathophysiological questions to be addressed separately from questions of clinical expression. Furthermore, these techniques offer potential methodological advantages compared with studying relationships with coronary heart disease events such as angina or myocardial infarction. Subclinical measures of coronary heart disease can be studied from early through to late life, and patterns of progression and regression investigated. Subclinical measures do not share the problems of using clinical events to infer the temporal sequence between putative risk factor and outcome. Thus low socioeconomic status and depression may be a cause and a consequence of myocardial infarction; yet associations with intima–media thickness, which increases without symptoms, most plausibly lie in only one direction. Subclinical measures also remove the potential bias in reporting symptoms and accessing medical care and, as continuous measures, have enhanced statistical power.

Educational level and other markers of socioeconomic status, such as occupation and income, consistently show inverse associations with the incidence of clinically manifest cardiovascular disease.[5] Social status may influence coronary risk through the behavioural coronary risk factors of smoking, exercise, diet, and alcohol. However, the finding that socioeconomic status gradients in heart disease are observed among non-smokers, and are independent of the classical risk factors of cholesterol and blood pressure,[6–9] suggests another possibility—that aspects of the psychosocial environment related to socioeconomic status may be involved.[10,11] Evidence from prospective epidemiological studies,[12] supported by non-human primate data,[13] suggests that psychosocial factors—such as anxiety, depression, hostility, type A behaviour, social supports, and work characteristics—show consistent, independent, dose–response relations with coronary heart disease.

However, such associations do not establish causation. Prospective cohort studies have related a single questionnaire based measure of chronic psychosocial stressors to coronary heart disease death or non-fatal myocardial infarction some years later. Investigating pathophysiological pathways, by which the psychosocial factors investigated in these studies may be associated with coronary heart disease, further tests the hypothesis that the psychosocial–coronary heart disease association is causal. Furthermore, understanding how socioeconomic status and psychosocial factors affect different pathological processes may yield fundamental insights into the pathogenesis of coronary heart disease. Ultimately, the purpose of this inquiry is to design the nature (for example, population or individual), timing (for example, maternal nutrition), and setting (for example, medical care) of interventions designed to prevent the onset or progression of coronary heart disease.

This chapter reviews the evidence from epidemiological, clinical, and animal studies indicating that socioeconomic status and psychosocial factors influence arterial structure (using carotid intima–media thickness and coronary angiography as markers of atherosclerosis), arterial function (endothelial function and arterial stiffness), and myocardial structure (left ventricular mass).

Method

Articles were included in this chapter if they related a measure of arterial or myocardial structure or function to a chronic psychosocial factor. Identification of relevant articles in English language, peer reviewed journals was carried out using NIH PubMed from 1970 to October 1999 (www.ncbi.nlm.nih.gov/). As well as using MeSH headings, articles were also identified by searching on any author who had contributed one relevant article and by using the "Related Articles" function in PubMed. The bibliographies of all retrieved articles were hand searched for further relevant articles. It is acknowledged that the reproducibility of these methods for reviewing non-randomised trial literature spanning widely different types of studies has not been empirically tested.

Arterial structure and function

Structurally, atherosclerosis involves a thickening of the arteries, particularly in the subintimal layer where depositions of lipid laden macrophages occur. While the invasive technique of coronary angiography is able to detect only focal lesions that protrude into the lumen, ultrasound measures of the carotid intima–media thickness are able to measure arterial wall thickening in the absence of luminal protrusion. Functionally, diseased arteries become stiff, and abnormalities of dilation in response to flow—mediated by the endothelium—are considered early markers of atherosclerosis. Table 13.1 summarises the interrelatedness of the different measures and the evidence that socioeconomic status or psychosocial factors are involved; Table 13.2 summarises the 15 studies investigating intima–media thickness.

Carotid intima–media thickness

Acute myocardial infarction is usually due to thrombus occluding the lumen of the coronary artery at the (mural) site of a ruptured atherosclerotic plaque. The importance of luminal phenomena, such as thrombus formation, is suggested by the lack of change in prevalence of coronary artery disease during a period of increasing or decreasing

Table 13.1 Published findings (reference numbers) of interrelations between socioeconomic status, psychosocial factors, and arterial and myocardial pathophysiology in epidemiological, clinical, and animal studies.

	1	2	3	4	5	6	7	8
1 Socioeconomic status								
2 Psychosocial factors	107*							
3 Parasympathetic/ sympathetic balance	108	108						
4 Left ventricular mass	99	99, 105, 106	96–102					
5 Endothelial function	109	75–81	34, 66–69	73, 74	74			
6 Arterial stiffness	0	49	88, 110	111–115				
7 Arterial wall thickness	41, 45, 116–118	43, 46–49, 119–122	34, 35, 46, 123, 124	27, 39, 40, 125	72, 74, 126, 127	123, 128		
8 Angiographic CAD	0	50–52	129	130	64, 67	0	24–26	
9 CHD mortality, non-fatal MI	5*	12*	131	93	0	84, 86, 111, 132	28–31	133
10 Sudden cardiac death	108*	108*	108*	93, 134–136	0	0	0	133

All studies identified in a search of Pub Med 1970–1999 are cited except where too numerous; 0 denotes no studies identified.
*Denotes reviews or illustrative publication, where there were numerous publications.
CAD, coronary artery disease; CHD, coronary heart disease; MI, myocardial infarction.

Table 13.2 Socioeconomic status, psychosocial factors and carotid intimal and medial layer thickness.

Study	Total sample (% women)	Age at entry (yr)	Psychosocial factor	Follow up (yr)	Measures	No. of adjustments	Results
Diez-Roux et al. (1995)[42]	14 266 (55)	45–64	SES: education, income, occupation	0	IMT	13: age, sex, smoking, SBP, antihypertensive Rx, LDL, HDL, diabetes, waist–hip ratio, Keys score, leisure index, sport index, fibrinogen	Inverse linear associations in each sex, race group for each SES measure. Multivariate adjustment: significant associations for whites for education only; the same adjustments did not abolish the association with clinical CHD
Helminen et al. (1995)[120]	4853(0)	50–60	Social networks, social supports	0	IMT	5: age, smoking, health status, education, saturated fat	Men living alone had higher IMT; emotional adequacy and social anchorage were particularly important
Lynch et al. (1995)[41]	1140(0)	42–60	SES: education, income, occupation	0	IMT	14: age, smoking, SBP, antihypertensive Rx, HDL, apoB, lipid lowering Rx, diabetes, alcohol, BMI, physical activity, fitness, family history, fibrinogen	Mean IMT 0·96, 0·04, 0·82 mm in those with primary school, some high school and completed high school respectively Effects present in the whole sample, and in those without CVD, or without stenosis or non-stenotic plaque
Agewall et al. (1996)[120]	97(0)	50–72	Negative feelings (discontent)	3.3	Change in mean IMT	2: cholesterol, CVD	Change in IMT associated with discontent

Study							
Barnett et al. (1997)[124]	351	24–78	Acute psychosocial stressor (Stroop colour word interference task)	2	Change in plaque area	2: age, baseline plaque area	Among the 136 untreated subjects with range of atherosclerotic disease, greater change in SBP during the task was associated with progression
Everson et al. (1997)[47]	942(0)	42–60	Hopelessness	4	Change in mean and max. IMT, plaque height and surface roughness	2: age, baseline IMT 11: age, baseline IMT, education, smoking, SBP, antihypertensive Rx, HDL, LDL, lipid lowering Rx, BMI, alcohol	High levels of hopelessness associated with faster progression of atherosclerosis; greatest effects among men with baseline IMT at or above the median Little effect of multivariate adjustment
Everson et al. (1997)[124]	591(0)	42–60	Workplace demands and reactivity of SBP in anticipation of maximal exercise ECG	4	Change in mean and max. IMT and plaque height	16: age, baseline IMT, education, smoking, SBP, antihypertensive Rx, HDL-2, apoB, antilipid Rx, fasting glucose, diabetes, BMI, alcohol, US zooming depth, sonographer, trial placebo status	High reactors (20 mmHg SBP or greater) with high job demands had 10–40% greater progression of mean (0·138 v 0·123 mm) and maximum (0·320 v 0·261 mm) IMT and plaque height (0·347 v 0·264) than men who were less reactive and had fewer job demands

continued

Table 13.2 continued

Study	Total sample (% women)	Age at entry (yr)	Psychosocial factor	Follow up (yr)	Measures	No. of adjustments	Results
Kamarck et al. (1997)[46]	901(0)	42–60	Acute psychosocial stressor: reactivity of SBP in anticipation of maximal exercise ECG	0	IMT	5: age, resting BP, smoking, lipids, fasting glucose	Stress related SBP and DBP reactivity was associated with higher IMT, particularly in those aged 46 or 52 years
Lynch et al. (1997)[117]	1022(0)	42–60	SES: education, income	4.1	Change in mean and max. IMT and plaque height	10: age, baseline IMT, smoking, SBP, antihypertensive R_X, HDL, LDL, lipid lowering R_X, BMI, alcohol	0·28 mm for primary schooling, 0·24 mm increase for those who completed high school Effects present in whole sample, and in those without CVD, or without stenosis or non-stenotic plaque
Lynch et al. (1997)[43]	940(0)	42–60	Workplace demands, economic rewards	4	Ditto	11: age, baseline IMT, smoking, SBP, antihypertensive R_X, HDL, LDL, triglycerides, lipid lowering R_X, BMI, alcohol	Greatest progression in those with high demands, low rewards Association did not differ by SES or social supports and was not altered by multivariate adjustment
Lynch et al. (1998)[118]	882(0)	42–60	SES: childhood circumstances, education, income; reactivity of SBP in anticipation of maximal exercise ECG	4	Ditto	2: age, baseline IMT 11: age, baseline IMT, smoking, SBP, antihypertensive R_X, HDL-2, apoB, triglycerides, lipid lowering R_X, BMI, alcohol	Those who had exaggerated SBP responses and had low SES in childhood or adulthood had the highest progression Not altered by multivariate adjustment

Study	N (N[a])	Age	Exposure measure		Outcome	Adjustments	Results
Matthews et al. (1998)[123]	200(100)	42–50	Hostility (Cook–Medley) and anxiety (Spielberger)	1.5–10	IMT	3: pulse pressure, smoking, triglycerides	Higher IMT associated with holding anger in, being self aware, having hostile attitudes
Matthews et al. (1998)[49]	254(100)	42–50	Acute psychosocial stressor: BP and HR change to public speaking and mirror image tracing	1.5–10	IMT	6: age, hormone replacement therapy, resting pulse pressure, smoking, triglycerides	Higher IMT associated with greater pulse pressure during stress
Muntaner et al. (1998)[48]	10801 (51)	45–64	Ecological assessment of work complexity, physical demand, job insecurity, skill discretion, decision authority, physical exertion	0	IMT	7: age, income, smoking, SBP, HDL, LDL, BMI	Low complexity and low skill discretion associated with high IMT; associations substantially reduced by RF adjustment
Ebrahim et al. (1999)[45]	800(47)	56–77	SES: social class	0	IMT at bifurcation, IMT at CCA, plaques	1: age	Non-manual participants had lower CCA IMT in men and women (non-significantly), IMT bifurcation in men and plaque prevalence in women

apoB, apolipoprotein B; BMI, body mass index; BP, blood pressure; CCA, common carotid artery; CHD, coronary heart disease; CVD, cardiovascular disease; DBP, diastolic BP; ECG, electrocardiogram; HDL, high density lipoprotein; HR, heart rate; IMT, intima–media thickness; LDL, low density lipoprotein; R_x, prescription; SBP, systolic BP; SES, socioeconomic status; US, ultrasound.

coronary heart disease incidence.[14,15] Indeed, socioeconomic status and psychosocial factors are associated with haemostatic factors involved in thrombus formation, particularly fibrinogen and platelet activity.[16–18] What, then, is the contribution of psychosocial factors to the mural phenomenon of atherosclerosis? The ability to measure atherosclerosis directly allows this question to be addressed.

Measurement and pathological significance

Atherosclerosis of the coronary and carotid arteries is highly correlated in postmortem studies.[19,20] The carotid arteries offer a convenient target for imaging, since their proximity to the skin allows an adequate acoustic window. In contrast, non-invasive imaging of the coronary arteries using computerised tomographic scanning or magnetic resonance angiography,[21] considerably more difficult techniques still in their infancy, are of uncertain prognostic importance,[22] and have not yet been used in investigating psychosocial factors. The validity of carotid intima–media thickness as a measure of generalised atherosclerotic process affecting the coronary arteries is suggested by cross-sectional associations with coronary risk factors,[23] angiographically defined coronary disease,[24–26] electrocardiographic evidence of ischaemia,[27] and prospective associations with incident myocardial infarction.[28–31]

Plausibility of psychosocial associations

Dominant male cynomolgus monkeys develop more extensive atherosclerosis than subordinate males when housed in unstable (but not stable) social groups; in contrast, subordinate females develop greater atherosclerosis (assessed postmortem) than dominant females, and do so irrespective of the conditions of social housing.[32] These effects are reduced by β-blockade, suggesting the importance of the sympathetic nervous system.[33–35] In humans, intima–media thickness is associated with biological markers which are themselves associated with psychosocial factors, such as insulin,[36] glucose,[37,38] and waist–hip ratio, while the presence of carotid plaque and increased intima–media thickness is associated with left ventricular mass.[27,39,40]

Table 13.2 summarises the 15 published studies identified, which investigated effects of socioeconomic status or psychosocial factors on intima–media thickness and its change. All were positive. This body of work, largely based on the Atherosclerosis Risk in Communities (ARIC) study and middleaged men in the Kuopio Ischaemic Heart Disease Risk Factor study, constitutes the best evidence that socioeconomic status and psychosocial factors have independent effects on subclinical measures of atherosclerosis.

Evidence of socioeconomic status/psychosocial associations

There is a strong inverse association between socioeconomic status and intima–media thickness.[41–45] In the ARIC study, among 14 266 middleaged men and women (black and white), there was a linear inverse association of intima–media thickness with each of three different measures of socioeconomic status (education, income, and occupation) for each sex and race group.[42] Furthermore, adjustment for 13 atherosclerotic risk factors explained this association with intima–media thickness, but not the inverse association with coronary heart disease observed in the same population, suggesting the importance of additional factors involved in the clinical expression of disease. In the Kuopio study, age adjusted mean intima–media thickness was 0.96 mm in men who had only primary schooling and 0.82 mm in men those who had completed high school.[41] The size of this effect was estimated to correspond to a 15.4% increase in the risk of myocardial infarction in the low education group. This effect size is smaller than the observed differences in myocardial infarction event rates by educational level, suggesting that other processes involving the lumen or the ventricular myocardium may be operating. Furthermore, adjustment for a similar group of 14 risk factors did not abolish this association. The progression of atherosclerosis, marked by increases in intima–media thickness or plaque height, was also associated with childhood and adult socioeconomic status,[44] providing strong evidence against the "downward drift" social selection hypothesis.

Carotid intima–media thickness studies provide evidence of the involvement of the sympathetic nervous system in linking socioeconomic status and psychosocial factors with subclinical atherosclerosis and its progression. Men anticipating an exercise electrocardiogram (an acute stressor, with a psychosocial component) vary in the degree to which their blood pressure rises, a marker of sympathetic activity. Men who had an exaggerated blood pressure response had higher baseline intima–media thickness;[46] men who also had low socioeconomic status experienced greater progression of intima–media thickness than those of high socioeconomic status.[44] Similarly, men with high job demands who were also high blood pressure reactors had worse intima–media thickness progression than those with low demands or who were less reactive.[47] In the ARIC study, psychosocial work characteristics were assessed ecologically, based on the classification of occupations, rather than on self reports. The observation that these measures of work characteristics affect intima–media thickness makes reporting bias unlikely.[48] Among postmenopausal women, pulse pressure change during public speaking was found to predict intima–media thickness.[49]

Coronary angiography

The invasive technique of coronary angiography offers direct visualisation of the luminal diameter of coronary arteries rather than imaging of the intimal and medial layers of the arterial wall at peripheral sites. While both positive and negative studies may be biased by the selection of patients for coronary angiography, there is increasing interest in angiographic or intravascular ultrasound characteristics of plaque morphology which may predict rupture or thrombus formation and therefore clinical expression.

The potential for such coronary angiographic studies to address the question of how socioeconomic status and psychosocial factors influence the conversion of subclinical to clinical phenomena awaits exploration.

Evidence of psychosocial associations

In a study of 131 women, Orth-Gomer *et al.* investigated the association of social supports with the severity (stenosis greater than 50% in at least one coronary artery) and extent (number of stenoses greater than 20% within the coronary tree) of coronary artery disease measured by computer assisted quantitative coronary angiography.[50] After adjustment for age, lack of social support was associated with both measures of coronary artery disease. The risk ratio for stenosis greater than 50% in women with poor versus strong social support was 2.5 (95% confidence interval 1.2–5.3), when adjustment was made for age, smoking, education, menopausal status, hypertension, high density lipoprotein (HDL), and body mass index.

Among 119 men and 40 women undergoing coronary angiography, Seeman and Syme found that functional aspects of social supports were more important than structural aspects.[51] Thus measurements of network instrumental support and feelings of being loved were better predictors of coronary atherosclerosis than network size, independent of age, sex, income, hypertension, serum cholesterol, smoking, angina, diabetes, family history of heart disease, type A behaviour pattern, and hostility. In a separate study, psychosocial work characteristics were not associated with the presence and severity of coronary artery disease at the time of angiography.[52]

No study has directly tested whether socioeconomic status or psychosocial factors affect the progression of angiographically demonstrated coronary disease. However, in a randomised trial of lifestyle changes including stress management (28 patients) versus usual care (20 patients) in people with angiographically demonstrated coronary artery disease, the average percentage diameter stenosis regressed from 40.0% (SD 16.9%) to 37.8% (SD 16.5%) in the experimental group, yet progressed from 42.7% (SD 15.5%) to 46.1% (SD 18.5%) in the control group at 1-year follow up.[53] These findings persisted and were associated with lower event rates at 5-year follow up.[54]

Endothelial dysfunction

If arterial structural changes indicative of atherosclerosis are associated with psychosocial factors in middle age, what are the antecedent or consequent functional changes? Arterial endothelial dysfunction is one of the earliest manifestations of atherosclerosis, preceding the development of plaques.[55] The endothelium plays a crucial physiological role in regulating local vasomotion (by nitric oxide), and pro- and antithrombotic and inflammatory processes. As well as being involved in early stages of atherosclerosis, abnormalities of endothelial function—such as paradoxical vasoconstriction in response to acetylcholine—are found among those with established coronary artery disease.

Measurement and pathological significance

A simple non-invasive marker of endothelial dysfunction has been developed using high resolution ultrasound measurements of the brachial artery diameter in response to reactive hyperaemia (with increased flow causing endothelium dependent dilation) and after glyceryl trinitrate (endothelial independent dilation). This technique has the major advantage of being suitable for use in healthy populations, including children. In the absence of clinically apparent coronary heart disease, impaired flow mediated dilation is associated with cardiovascular risk factors,[56-58] ageing,[59,60] low birthweight and HDL cholesterol in children,[61] and passive smoking in young adults.[62] Although endothelial dysfunction assessed at peripheral artery sites correlates well with that in the coronary circulation,[63-65] there are no prospective studies relating flow mediated dilation to incident myocardial infarction.

Plausibility of psychosocial associations

Endothelial dysfunction occurs in association with markers of sympathetic activity in animals,[34,66] and in humans.[67-69] Markers of insulin resistance have been associated with endothelial dysfunction.[70-72] Left ventricular mass is associated with endothelial dysfunction.[73,74]

Evidence of psychosocial associations

Endothelial dysfunction has been observed in response to psychosocial stressors in non-human primates (cynomolgus monkeys) using a variety of techniques. Introduction of a stranger into a social group of monkeys was associated with higher endothelial cell replication in the coronary arteries, and endothelial incorporation of immunoglobulin G in the thoracic aorta, in monkeys who had not been treated with a β-blocker.[75] This finding has been replicated.[76] Chronic social disruption was associated with relative coronary artery vasoconstriction in response to acetylcholine,[77] and recent psychosocial stress was associated with impaired endothelium mediated vasodilation of atherosclerotic iliac arteries.[78] Rat studies also show effects of stressors (air jet stress) on coronary artery function.[79-81]

There are no studies of chronic psychosocial stressors and endothelial dysfunction in humans. In the Whitehall II study, there is a strong inverse association between von Willebrand factor—a marker of endothelial damage with prothrombotic effects—and employment grade.[82] Yeung *et al.* studied the effects of acute mental stress (mental arithmetic) in 26 patients undergoing coronary angiography. Mental stress was associated with a paradoxical constriction of coronary arteries caused by a focal failure of endothelium dependent dilation at points of stenosis.[83]

Arterial stiffness

A further change in arterial function, which may be present in early and late stages of atherosclerosis, is stiffening of the arteries; the very term "sclerosis" denotes a hardening of the arteries.

Measurement and pathological significance

The simplest measurement of arterial stiffness is the pulse pressure (the difference between systolic and diastolic arterial pressure); pulse pressure rises with stiffness. Pulse pressure, independent of systolic or diastolic blood pressure, predicts coronary heart disease events in healthy populations,[84] and in those with hypertension[85] or after myocardial infarction.[86] Using ultrasound measurements of arterial diameter in systole and diastole, direct measurements of stiffness may be made, indexing change in cross-sectional area (distensibility) or volume (compliance) to the pulse pressure; increasing arterial stiffness is indeed a correlate of advancing age, other cardiovascular risk factors, and coronary heart disease.[87]

Plausibility of psychosocial associations

Autonomic function is associated with arterial stiffness.[88] The underlying cellular mechanism of arterial stiffening is likely to involve arterial smooth muscle cell proliferation and collagen deposition. Both may be associated with psychosocial stressors. For example, the serum of humans who have recently faced an episodic psychological challenge can stimulate a significant increase in c-*myc* RNA in cultured smooth muscle cells, compared with prestressor serum.[89]

Evidence of psychosocial associations

No study was identified.

Myocardial mass and function

Coronary heart disease is a disease of the myocardium involving ischaemia (angina, unstable angina), infarction (heart attack), poor function (heart failure), or electrical instability (sudden cardiac death). While for decades the research emphasis has been on disease of the coronary arteries, increasingly attention is being paid to pathological processes directly in the myocardium.

Measurement and pathological significance

Left ventricular hypertrophy may be measured using electrocardiography,[90] chest X-radiography,[91] echocardiography, or magnetic resonance imaging. Of all the risk factors obtained in the Framingham Heart Study, electrocardiographic left ventricular hypertrophy was the most consistently and strongly associated with clinical cardiovascular endpoints.[92] However, left ventricular hypertrophy as dichotomised is an uncommon finding and important aetiological information may be missed. Thus increased left ventricular mass measured on a continuous scale with electrocardiographic or echocardiographic techniques predicts incident coronary heart disease independently of blood pressure[93] or baseline coronary artery disease.[94] The mechanism by which greater cardiac mass is associated with myocardial infarction may involve increased myocardial oxygen demand and reduced coronary blood flow reserve, causing a mismatch in oxygen supply and demand; furthermore, hypertrophic hearts are predisposed to ventricular arrhythmia. Not only have prospective studies shown that the left ventricular mass associations with disease are independent of blood pressure, some have suggested that changes in left ventricular mass precede elevations of blood pressure.[95]

Plausibility of psychosocial associations

Low heart rate variability and cardiovascular reactivity, which is largely sympathetically mediated, are associated with left ventricular mass.[96-102] Diabetes and components of the insulin resistance syndrome[103,104] are associated with raised left ventricular mass and, in separate studies, with socioeconomic status.[17] Among normotensive men waist–hip ratio is a strong ($r = 0.71$) correlate of left ventricular mass, a stronger association than with body mass index. The pathophysiological mechanisms that control left ventricular mass are poorly understood, but roles for insulin resistance have been suggested.

Evidence of psychosocial associations

Job strain has been linked with left ventricular mass, independent of key confounders.[105] In a case–control study in employed men (87 cases of hypertension and a random sample of 128 controls), Schnall found an effect of the psychosocial work characteristic, job strain, on left ventricular mass, which was independent of blood pressure, body mass index, alcohol, type A behaviour, smoking, 24 hour urinary sodium, education, and physical demands of the job. This effect was, however, confined to those aged 30 to 40 years.

Siegrist has proposed that psychosocial factors may interact with (electrocardiographic) left ventricular hypertrophy in conferring risk of coronary heart disease.[106] Among 416 middleaged "blue collar" men followed up for 6.5 years, an imbalance between high effort and low reward was assessed. Expected probabilities of cardiovascular events were elevated if the combined effects of left ventricular hypertrophy and psychosocial risks are analysed.

However, there are important negative studies. Among 3742 young adults in the Coronary Artery Risk Development in Young Adults (CARDIA) study, echocardiographic measurement of left ventricular mass was examined in relation to cardiovascular reactivity to physical and psychological stressors (treadmill exercise, cold pressor, video game, and star tracing tasks) and psychosocial characteristics (hostility, anger suppression, anxiety, depressive symptoms, and education).[99] Systolic blood pressure reactivity to exercise was significantly related to left ventricular mass in both black and white men; left ventricular mass was 10% greater in white men with exaggerated (upper quintile) peak exercise systolic blood pressure than in other white men. Otherwise, reactivity to other stressors or psychosocial variables accounted for no more than 1% of the variance in left ventricular mass.

Conclusion

All 15 of the identified studies using carotid intimal and medial thickness to investigate effects of socioeconomic status or psychosocial factors were positive, suggesting that subclinical atherosclerotic mechanisms are involved in the socioeconomic status or psychosocial association with coronary heart disease. The demonstration of pathological processes unbiased by reporting of clinical events or "downward drift" selection gives further support to the idea that the associations between psychosocial factors and clinical coronary heart disease events are causal. Since the size of the effect on intima–media thickness is not sufficient to explain socioeconomic status differences in coronary heart disease, other factors should be investigated which may explain how the lesions become clinically expressed.

Future studies might benefit from a systematic approach across psychosocial exposures and pathophysiological outcomes. Further work is required to elucidate the interrelationships between arterial functional changes, and luminal, myocardial, and electrical factors. As Table 13.1 demonstrates, the measures of vascular and myocardial pathophysiology are importantly interrelated. Since most studies investigate only one process, such as the mural manifestations of atherosclerosis, there is the attendant risk of missing pathophysiological insights. Markers of autonomic nervous system function are related to arterial and myocardial structure and function as well as psychosocial factors, and this may represent an important mechanism by which psychosocial factors are related to structural changes. Furthermore, there are important gaps in the range of psychosocial factors that have been examined. Depression, for example, is one of the psychosocial factors with the most consistent prospective evidence of independent association with coronary heart disease events, yet there are no studies of depression and progression of intima–media thickness.

References

1 Chambers J. Left ventricular hypertrophy—an underappreciated coronary risk factor. *BMJ* 1995;**311**:273–4.
2 Celermajer DS, Sorensen KE, Gooch VM, *et al.* Non-invasive detection of endothelial dysfunction in children and adults at risk of atherosclerosis. *Lancet* 1992;**340**:1111–15.
3 Anonymous. Relationship of atherosclerosis in young men to serum lipoprotein cholesterol concentrations and smoking. A preliminary report from the Pathobiological Determinants of Atherosclerosis in Youth (PDAY) Research Group [see comments]. *JAMA* 1990;**264**:3018–24.
4 Stary HC. Changes in components and structure of atherosclerotic lesions developing from childhood to middle age in coronary arteries. *Basic Res Cardiol* 1994; **89**(suppl.1):17–32.
5 Kaplan GA, Keil JE. Socioeconomic factors and cardiovascular disease: a review of the literature. *Circulation* 1993;**88**:1973–98.

6   Marmot MG, Rose G, Shipley M, Hamilton PJS. Employment grade and coronary heart disease in British civil servants. *J Epidemiol Community Health* 1978;**32**:244–9.
7   Pocock SJ, Shaper AG, Cook DG, Phillips AN, Walker M. Social class differences in ischaemic heart disease in British men. *Lancet* 1987;**ii**:197–201.
8   Liu K, Cedres LB, Stamler J, *et al.* Relationship of education to major risk factors and death from coronary heart disease, cardiovascular diseases and all causes. *Circulation* 1982;**66**:1308–14.
9   Buring JE, Evans DA, Fiore M, Rosner B, Hennekens CH. Occupation and risk of death from coronary heart disease. *JAMA* 1987;**258**:791–2.
10 Marmot M, Bosma H, Hemingway H, Brunner E, Stansfeld S. Contribution of job control and other risk factors to social variations in coronary heart disease. *Lancet* 1997;**350**:235–40.
11 Wamala SP, Mittleman MA, Schenck-Gustafsson K, Orth-Gomer K. Potential explanations for the educational gradient in coronary heart disease: a population-based case-control study of Swedish women [published erratum appears in *Am J Public Health* 1999;**89**:785]. *Am J Public Health* 1999;**89**:315–21.
12 Hemingway H, Marmot M. Psychosocial factors in the aetiology and prognosis of coronary heart disease: systematic review of prospective cohort studies. *BMJ* 1999;**318**:1460–7.
13 Manuck SB, Marsland AL, Kaplan JR, Williams JK. The pathogenicity of behavior and its neuroendocrine mediation: an example from coronary artery disease. *Psychosom Med* 1995;**57**:275–83.
14 Morris JN. Recent history of coronary disease. *Lancet* 1951;**i**:1–7.
15 Enriquez-Sarano M, Klodas E, Garratt KN, Bailey KR, Tajik AJ, Holmes DR. Secular trends in coronary atherosclerosis—analysis in patients with valvular regurgitation [see comments]. *N Engl J Med* 1996;**335**:316–22.
16 Markowe HLJ, Marmot MG, Shipley MJ, *et al.* Fibrinogen: a possible link between social class and coronary heart disease. *BMJ* 1985;**291**:1312–14.
17 Brunner EJ, Davey Smith G, Marmot MG, Canner R, Beksinska M, O'Brien J. Childhood social circumstances and psychosocial and behavioural factors as determinants of plasma fibrinogen. *Lancet* 1996;**347**:1008–13.
18 Kamarck T, Jennings JR. Biobehavioral factors in sudden cardiac death. *Psychol Bull* 1991;**109**:42–75.
19 Mathur KS, Kashyap SK, Kumar V. Correlation of the extent and severity of atherosclerosis in the coronary and cerebral arteries. *Circulation* 1963;**27**:929–34.
20 Young W, Gofman JW, Tandy R, Malamud N, Waters ESG. The quantitation of atherosclerosis III. The extent of correlation of degrees of atherosclerosis within and between the coronary and cerebral vascular beds. *Am J Cardiol* 1969;**6**:300–8.
21 Manning WJ, Li W, Edelman RR. A preliminary report comparing magnetic resonance coronary angiography with conventional angiography [see comments] [published erratum appears in *N Engl J Med* 1993;**330**:152]. *N Engl J Med* 1993;**328**:828–32.
22 Detrano RC, Wong ND, Doherty TM, *et al.* Coronary calcium does not accurately predict near-term future coronary events in high-risk adults [see comments]. *Circulation* 1999;**99**:2633–8.
23 Sharrett AR, Sorlie PD, Chambless LE, *et al.* Relative importance of various risk factors for asymptomatic carotid atherosclerosis versus coronary heart disease incidence: the Atherosclerosis Risk in Communities Study. *Am J Epidemiol* 1999;**149**:843–52.
24 Craven TE, Ryu JE, Espeland MA, *et al.* Evaluation of the associations between carotid artery atherosclerosis and coronary artery stenosis. A case-control study. *Circulation* 1990;**82**:1230–42.
25 Geroulakos G, O'Gorman DJ, Kalodiki E, Sheridan DJ, Nicolaides AN. The carotid intima-media thickness as a marker of the presence of severe symptomatic coronary artery disease. *Eur Heart J* 1994;**15**:781–5.
26 Crouse JR, Craven TE, Hagaman AP, Bond MG. Association of coronary disease with segment-specific intimal–medial thickening of the extracranial carotid artery. *Circulation* 1995;**92**:1141–7.
27 Okin PM, Roman MJ, Devereux RB, Kligfield P. Association of carotid atherosclerosis with electrocardiographic myocardial ischemia and left ventricular hypertrophy. *Hypertension* 1996;**28**:3–7.
28 Salonen JT, Salonen R. Ultrasound B-mode imaging in observational studies of atherosclerotic progression. *Circulation* 1993;**87**:II56–65.

215

29 Bots ML, Hoes AW, Koudstaal PJ, Hofman A, Grobbee DE. Common carotid intima-media thickness and risk of stroke and myocardial infarction: the Rotterdam Study. *Circulation* 1997;**96**:1432–7.

30 Chambless LE, Heiss G, Folsom AR, *et al.* Association of coronary heart disease incidence with carotid arterial wall thickness and major risk factors: the Atherosclerosis Risk in Communities (ARIC) Study, 1987-1993. *Am J Epidemiol* 1997;**146**:483–94.

31 O'Leary DH, Polak JF, Kronmal RA, Manolio TA, Burke GL, Wolfson SK. Carotid-artery intima and media thickness as a risk factor for myocardial infarction and stroke in older adults. Cardiovascular Health Study Collaborative Research Group. *N Engl J Med* 1999;**340**:14–22.

32 Kaplan JR, Manuck SB, Clarkson TB, Lusso FM, Taub DM. Social status, environment, and atherosclerosis in cynomolgus monkeys. *Arteriosclerosis* 1982;**2**:359–68.

33 Kaplan JR, Manuck SB, Adams MR, Weingand KW, Clarkson TB. Inhibition of coronary atherosclerosis by propranolol in behaviorally predisposed monkeys fed an atherogenic diet. *Circulation* 1987;**76**:1364–72.

34 Kaplan JR, Pettersson K, Manuck SB, Olsson G. Role of sympathoadrenal medullary activation in the initiation and progression of atherosclerosis. *Circulation* 1991;**84**:VI23–32.

35 Manuck SB, Adams MR, McCaffery JM, Kaplan JR. Behaviorally elicited heart rate reactivity and atherosclerosis in ovariectomized cynomolgus monkeys (Macaca fascicularis). *Arteriosclerosis Thromb Vasc Biol* 1997;**17**:1774–9.

36 Suzuki M, Shinozaki K, Kanazawa A, *et al.* Insulin resistance as an independent risk factor for carotid wall thickening. *Hypertension* 1996;**28**:593–8.

37 Yamasaki Y, Kawamori R, Matusushima H *et al.* Asymptomatic hyperglycaemia is associated with increased intimal plus medial thickness of the carotid artery. *Diabetologia* 1995;**38**:585–91.

38 Hanefeld M, Koehler C, Schaper F, Fuecker K, Henkel E, Temelkova-Kurktschiev T. Postprandial plasma glucose is an independent risk factor for increased carotid intima-media thickness in non-diabetic individuals. *Atherosclerosis* 1999;**144**:229–35.

39 Roman MJ, Pickering TG, Pini R, Schwartz JE, Devereux RB. Prevalence and determinants of cardiac and vascular hypertrophy in hypertension. *Hypertension* 1995;**26**:369–73.

40 Aronow WS, Kronzon I, Schoenfeld MR. Left ventricular hypertrophy is more prevalent in patients with systemic hypertension with extracranial carotid arterial disease than in patients with systemic hypertension without extracranial carotid arterial disease. *Am J Cardiol* 1995;**76**:192–3.

41 Lynch J, Kaplan GA, Salonen R, Cohen RD, Salonen JT. Socioeconomic status and carotid atherosclerosis. *Circulation* 1995;**92**:1786–92.

42 Diez-Roux AV, Nieto FJ, Tyroler HA, Crum LD, Szklo M. Social inequalities and atherosclerosis. *Am J Epidemiol* 1995;**141**:960–72.

43 Lynch J, Krause N, Kaplan GA, Salonen R, Salonen JT. Workplace demands, economic reward, and progression of carotid atherosclerosis. *Circulation* 1997;**96**:302–7.

44 Lynch JW, Everson SA, Kaplan GA, Salonen R, Salonen JT. Does low socioeconomic status potentiate the effects of heightened cardiovascular responses to stress on the progression of cartoid atherosclerosis? *Am J Public Health* 1998;**88**:389–94.

45 Ebrahim S, Papacosta O, Whincup P *et al.* Carotid plaque, intima media thickness, cardiovascular risk factors, and prevalent cardiovascular disease in men and women: the British Regional Heart Study. *Stroke* 1999;**30**:841–50.

46 Kamarck TW, Everson SA, Kaplan GA, *et al.* Exaggerated blood pressure responses during mental stress are associated with enhanced carotid atherosclerosis in middle-aged Finnish men: findings from the Kuopio Ischemic Heart Disease Study. *Circulation* 1997;**96**:3842–8.

47 Everson SA, Kaplan GA, Goldberg DE, Salonen R, Salonen JT. Hopelessness and 4-year progression of carotid atherosclerosis. The Kuopio Ischemic Heart Disease Risk Factor Study. *Arteriosclerosis Thromb Vasc Biol* 1997;**17**:1490–5.

48 Muntaner C, Nieto FJ, Cooper L, Meyer J, Szklo M, Tyroler HA. Work organization and atherosclerosis: findings from the ARIC study. Atherosclerosis Risk in Communities. *Am J Prev Med* 1998;**14**:9–18.

49 Matthews KA, Owens JF, Kuller LH, Sutton-Tyrrell K, Lassila HC, Wolfson SK. Stress-induced pulse pressure change predicts women's carotid atherosclerosis. *Stroke* 1998;**29**:1525–30.

50 Orth-Gomer K, Horsten M, Wamala SP, et al. Social relations and extent and severity of coronary artery disease. The Stockholm Female Coronary Risk Study [see comments]. Eur Heart J 1998;19:1648–56.

51 Seeman TE, Syme SL. Social networks and coronary artery disease: a comparison of the structure and function of social relations as predictors of disease. Psychosom Med 1987;49:341–54.

52 Hlatky MA, Lam LC, Lee KL, et al. Job strain and the prevalence and outcome of coronary artery disease. Circulation 1995;92:327–33.

53 Ornish D, Brown SE, Scherwitz LW, Billings JH, Armstrong WT, Ports TA. Can lifestyle changes reverse coronary heart disease? The Lifestyle Heart Trial. Lancet 1990;336:129–33.

54 Ornish D, Scherwitz LW, Billings JH, et al. Intensive lifestyle changes for reversal of coronary heart disease [published erratum appears in JAMA 1999;281:1380] [see comments]. JAMA 1998;280:2001–7.

55 McLenachan JM, Williams JK, Fish RD, Ganz P, Selwyn AP. Loss of flow-mediated endothelium-dependent dilation occurs early in the development of atherosclerosis. Circulation 1991;84:1273–8.

56 Celermajer DS, Sorensen KE, Bull C, Robinson J, Deanfield JE. Endothelium-dependent dilation in the systemic arteries of asymptomatic subjects relates to coronary risk factors and their interaction. J Am Coll Cardiol 1994;24:1468–74.

57 Jensen-Urstad K, Johansson J, Jensen-Urstad M. Vascular function correlates with risk factors for cardiovascular disease in a healthy population of 35-year-old subjects. J Intern Med 1997;241:507–13.

58 Clarkson P, Celermajer DS, Powe AJ, Donald AE, Henry RM, Deanfield JE. Endothelium-dependent dilatation is impaired in young healthy subjects with a family history of premature coronary disease. Circulation 1997;96:3378–83.

59 Celermajer DS, Sorensen KE, Spiegelhalter DJ, Georgakopoulos D, Robinson J, Deanfield JE. Aging is associated with endothelial dysfunction in healthy men years before the age-related decline in women. J Am Coll Cardiol 1994;24:471–6.

60 Gerhard M, Roddy MA, Creager SJ, Creager MA. Aging progressively impairs endothelium-dependent vasodilation in forearm resistance vessels of humans. Hypertension 1996;27:849–53.

61 Leeson P, Thorne S, Donald A, Mullen M, Clarkson P, Deanfield J. Non-invasive measurement of endothelial function: effect on brachial artery dilatation of graded endothelial dependent and independent stimuli. Heart 1997;78:22–7.

62 Celermajer DS, Adams MR, Clarkson P, et al. Passive smoking and impaired endothelium-dependent arterial dilatation in healthy young adults. N Engl J Med 1996;334:150–4.

63 Anderson HR, Limb ES, Bland JM, Ponce de Leon A, Strachan DP, Bower JS. Health effects of an air pollution episode in London, December 1991. Thorax 1995;50:1188–93.

64 Neunteufl T, Katzenschlager R, Hassan A, et al. Systemic endothelial dysfunction is related to the extent and severity of coronary artery disease. Atherosclerosis 1997;129:111–18.

65 Takase B, Uehata A, Akima T, et al. Endothelium-dependent flow-mediated vasodilation in coronary and brachial arteries in suspected coronary artery disease. Am J Cardiol 1998;82:1535–9, A7–8.

66 Pettersson K, Bejne B, Bjork H, Strawn WB, Bondjers G. Experimental sympathetic activation causes endothelial injury in the rabbit thoracic aorta via beta 1-adrenoceptor activation. Circ Res 1990;67:1027–34.

67 Vita JA, Treasure CB, Yeung AC, et al. Patients with evidence of coronary endothelial dysfunction as assessed by acetylcholine infusion demonstrate marked increase in sensitivity to constrictor effects of catecholamines. Circulation 1992;85:1390–7.

68 Corretti MC, Plotnick GD, Vogel RA. Correlation of cold pressor and flow-mediated brachial artery diameter responses with the presence of coronary artery disease. Am J Cardiol 1995;75:783–7.

69 Treiber F, Papavassiliou D, Gutin B, et al. Determinants of endothelium-dependent femoral artery vasodilation in youth. Psychosom Med 1997;59:376–81.

70 Petrie JR, Ueda S, Webb DJ, Elliott HL, Connell JM. Endothelial nitric oxide production and insulin sensitivity. A physiological link with implications for pathogenesis of cardiovascular disease. Circulation 1996;93:1331–3.

71 Steinberg HO, Chaker H, Leaming R, Johnson A, Brechtel G, Baron AD. Obesity/insulin resistance is associated with endothelial dysfunction. Implications for the syndrome of insulin resistance. J Clin Invest 1996;97:2601–10.

72 Thalhammer C, Balzuweit B, Busjahn A, Walter C, Luft FC, Haller H. Endothelial cell dysfunction and arterial wall hypertrophy are associated with disturbed carbohydrate metabolism in patients at risk for cardiovascular disease. *Arteriosclerosis Thromb Vasc Biol* 1999;**19**:1173–9.

73 Treasure CB, Klein JL, Vita JA, *et al*. Hypertension and left ventricular hypertrophy are associated with impaired endothelium-mediated relaxation in human coronary resistance vessels. *Circulation* 1993;**87**:86–93.

74 Lind L, Sarabi M, Millgard J, Kahan T, Edner M. Endothelium-dependent vasodilation and structural and functional changes in the cardiovascular system are dependent on age in healthy subjects [in process citation]. *Clin Physiol* 1999;**19**:400–9.

75 Strawn WB, Bondjers G, Kaplan JR, *et al*. Endothelial dysfunction in response to psychosocial stress in monkeys. *Circ Res* 1991;**68**:1270–9.

76 Skantze HB. Psychosocial stress causes endothelial injury in cynomolgus monkeys via beta 1-adrenoceptor activation. *Atherosclerosis* 1998;**136**:153–61.

77 Williams JK, Vita JA, Manuck SB, Selwyn AP, Kaplan JR. Psychosocial factors impair vascular responses of coronary arteries [see comments]. *Circulation* 1991;**84**:2146–53.

78 Williams JK, Kaplan JR, Manuck SB. Effects of psychosocial stress on endothelium-mediated dilation of atherosclerotic arteries in cynomolgus monkeys. *J Clin Invest* 1993;**92**:1819–23.

79 Fuchs LC, Landas SK, Johnson AK. Behavioral stress alters coronary vascular reactivity in borderline hypertensive rats. *J Hypertens* 1997;**15**:301–7.

80 Fuchs LC, Hoque AM, Clarke NL. Vascular and hemodynamic effects of behavioral stress in borderline hypertensive and Wistar-Kyoto rats. *Am J Physiol* 1998;**274**:R375–82.

81 Giulumian AD, Clark SG, Fuchs LC. Effect of behavioral stress on coronary artery relaxation altered with aging in BHR. *Am J Physiol* 1999;**276**:R435–40.

82 Kumari M, Marmot M, Brunner E. Social determinants of von Willebrand factor: the Whitehall II study. *Arteriosclerosis Thromb Vasc Biol* 2000;**20**:1842–7.

83 Yeung AC, Barry J, Orav J *et al*. Effects of asymptomatic ischemia on long-term prognosis in chronic stable coronary disease. *Circulation* 1991;**83**:1598–604.

84 Franklin SS, Khan SA, Wong ND, Larson MG, Levy D. Is pulse pressure useful in predicting risk for coronary heart disease? The Framingham heart study. *Circulation* 1999;**100**:354–60.

85 Verdecchia P, Schillaci G, Borgioni C, Ciucci A, Pede S, Porcellati C. Ambulatory pulse pressure: a potent predictor of total cardiovascular risk in hypertension. *Hypertension* 1998;**32**:983–8.

86 Mitchell GF, Moye LA, Braunwald E, *et al*. Sphygmomanometrically determined pulse pressure is a powerful independent predictor of recurrent events after myocardial infarction in patients with impaired left ventricular function. SAVE investigators. Survival and Ventricular Enlargement. *Circulation* 1997;**96**:4254–60.

87 Arnett DK, Evans GW, Riley WA. Arterial stiffness: a new cardiovascular risk factor? *Am J Epidemiol* 1994;**140**:669–82.

88 Kosch M, Hausberg M, Barenbrock M, Kisters K, Rahn KH. Studies on cardiac sympathovagal balance and large artery distensibility in patients with untreated essential hypertension. *J Hum Hypertens* 1999;**13**:315–19.

89 Cui Y, Gutstein WH, Jabr S, Hsieh TC, Wu JM. Control of human vascular smooth muscle cell proliferation by sera derived from "experimentally stressed" individuals. *Oncol Rep* 1998;**5**:1471–4.

90 Rautaharju PM, Lacroix AZ, Savage DD, *et al*. Electrocardiographic estimate of left ventricular mass versus radiographic cardiac size and the risk of cardiovascular disease mortality in the epidemiologic follow-up study of the first national health and nutrition examination survey. *Am J Cardiol* 1988;**62**:59–66.

91 Chikos PM, Figley MM, Fisher L. Correlation between chest film and angiographic assessment of left ventricular size. *Am J Roetgenol* 1977;**128**:367–73.

92 Kannel WB, Cobb J. Left ventricular hypertrophy and mortality—results from the Framingham study. *Cardiology* 1992;**81**:291–8.

93 Levy D, Garrison RJ, Savage DD, Kannel WB, Castelli WP. Prognostic implications of echocardiographically determined left ventricular mass in the Framingham Heart Study. *N Engl J Med* 1990;**322**:1561–6.

94 Ghali JK, Liao Y, Simmons B, Castaner A, Guichan C, Cooper RS. The prognostic role of left ventricular hypertrophy in patients with or without coronary artery disease. *Ann Intern Med* 1992;**117**:831–6.

95 Iso H, Kiyama M, Doi M *et al.* Left ventricular mass and subsequent blood pressure changes among middle aged men in rural and urban Japanese populations. *Circulation* 1994;**89**:1717–24.

96 Mandawat MK, Wallbridge DR, Pringle SD, *et al.* Heart rate variability in left ventricular hypertrophy [see comments]. *Br Heart J* 1995;**73**:139–44.

97 Petretta M, Marciano F, Bianchi V *et al.* Power spectral analysis of heart period variability in hypertensive patients with left ventricular hypertrophy. *Am J Hypertens* 1995;**8**:1206–13.

98 Kohara K, Hara-Nakamura N, Hiwada K. Left ventricular mass index negatively correlates with heart rate variability in essential hypertension. *Am J Hypertens* 1995;**8**:183–8.

99 Markovitz JH, Raczynski JM, Lewis CE *et al.* Lack of independent relationships between left ventricular mass and cardiovascular reactivity to physical and psychological stress in the Coronary Artery Risk Development in Young Adults (CARDIA) Study [see comments]. *Am J Hypertens* 1996;**9**:915–23.

100 Perkiomaki JS, Ikaheimo MJ, Pikkujamsa SM, *et al.* Dispersion of the QT interval and autonomic modulation of heart rate in hypertensive men with and without left ventricular hypertrophy. *Hypertension* 1996;**28**:16–21.

101 Papavassiliou DP, Treiber FA, Strong WB, Malpass MD, Davis H. Anthropometric, demographic, and cardiovascular predictors of left ventricular mass in young children. *Am J Cardiol* 1996;**78**:323–6.

102 Murdison KA, Treiber FA, Mensah G, Davis H, Thompson W, Strong WB. Prediction of left ventricular mass in youth with family histories of essential hypertension. *Am J Med Sci* 1998;**315**:118–23.

103 Sharp SD, Williams RR. Fasting insulin and left ventricular mass in hypertensives and normotensive controls. *Cardiology* 1992;**81**:207–12.

104 Sasson Z, Rasooly Y, Bhesania T, Rasooly I. Insulin resistance is an important determinant of left ventricular mass in the obese. *Circulation* 1993;**88**:1431–6.

105 Schnall PL, Pieper C, Schwartz JE *et al.* The relationship between 'job strain,' workplace diastolic blood pressure, and left ventricular mass index. Results of a case-control study [published erratum appears in *JAMA* 1992;**267**:1209] [see comments]. *JAMA* 1990;**263**:1929–35.

106 Siegrist J, Peter R, Motz W, Strauer BE. The role of hypertension, left ventricular hypertrophy and psychosocial risks in cardiovascular disease: prospective evidence from blue-collar men. *Eur Heart J* 1992;**13**(suppl. D):89–95.

107 Marmot MG, Davey Smith G, Stansfeld SA, *et al.* Health inequalities among British Civil Servants: the Whitehall II study. *Lancet* 1991;**337**:1387–93.

108 Hemingway H. Social influences on sudden cardiac death, arrhythmias and heart rate variability. In: Malik M, ed. *Arrhythmia risk*. London: BMJ Books, 2000.

109 Strawn WB, Bondjers G, Kaplan JR, *et al.* Endothelial dysfunction in response to psychosocial stress in monkeys. *Circulation* 1991;**68**:1270–9.

110 Jensen-Urstad K, Reichard P, Jensen-Urstad M. Decreased heart rate variability in patients with type 1 diabetes mellitus is related to arterial wall stiffness. *J Intern Med* 1999;**245**:57–61.

111 Gatzka CD, Cameron JD, Kingwell BA, Dart AM. Relation between coronary artery disease, aortic stiffness, and left ventricular structure in a population sample. *Hypertension* 1998;**32**:575–8.

112 Rajkumar C, Cameron JD, Christophidis N, Jennings GL, Dart AM. Reduced systemic arterial compliance is associated with left ventricular hypertrophy and diastolic dysfunction in older people [see comments]. *J Am Geriatr Soc* 1997;**45**:803–8.

113 Resnick LM, Militianu D, Cunnings AJ, Pipe JG, Evelhoch JL, Soulen RL. Direct magnetic resonance determination of aortic distensibility in essential hypertension: relation to age, abdominal visceral fat, and in situ intracellular free magnesium. *Hypertension* 1997;**30**:654–9.

114 Boutouyrie P, Laurent S, Girerd X, *et al.* Common carotid artery stiffness and patterns of left ventricular hypertrophy in hypertensive patients. *Hypertension* 1995;**25**:651–9.

115 Dart A, Silagy C, Dewar E, Jennings G, McNeil J. Aortic distensibility and left ventricular structure and function in isolated systolic hypertension [see comments]. *Eur Heart J* 1993;**14**:1465–70.

116 Diez-Roux AV, Nieto FJ, Tyroler HA, Crum LD, Szklo M. Social inequalities and atherosclerosis. The atherosclerosis risk in communities study. *Am J Epidemiol* 1995;**141**:960–72.

117 Lynch J, Kaplan GA, Salonen R, Salonen JT. Socioeconomic status and progression of carotid atherosclerosis. Prospective evidence from the Kuopio Ischemic Heart Disease Risk Factor Study. *Arteriosclerosis Thromb Vasc Biol* 1997;**17**:513–19.
118 Lynch JW, Everson SA, Kaplan GA, Salonen R, Salonen JT. Does low socioeconomic status potentiate the effects of heightened cardiovascular responses to stress on the progression of carotid atherosclerosis? [see comments]. *Am J Public Health* 1998;**88**:389–94.
119 Helminen A, Rankinen T, Mercuri M, Rauramaa R. Carotid atherosclerosis in middle-aged men. Relation to conjugal circumstances and social support. *Scand J Soc Med* 1995;**23**:167–72.
120 Agewall S, Wikstrand J, Dahlof C, Fagerberg B. Negative feelings (discontent) predict progress of intima-media thickness of the common carotid artery in treated hypertensive men at high cardiovascular risk. *Am J Hypertens* 1996;**9**:545–50.
121 Everson SA, Lynch JW, Chesney MA, *et al.* Interaction of workplace demands and cardiovascular reactivity in progression of carotid atherosclerosis: population based study. *BMJ* 1997;**314**:553–8.
122 Matthews KA, Owens JF, Kuller LH, Sutton-Tyrrell K, Jansen-McWilliams L. Are hostility and anxiety associated with carotid atherosclerosis in healthy postmenopausal women? *Psychosom Med* 1998;**60**:633–8.
123 Matthews KA, Owens JF, Kuller LH, Sutton-Tyrrell K, Lassila HC, Wolfson SK. Stress-induced pulse pressure change predicts women's carotid atherosclerosis. *Stroke* 1998;**29**:1525–30.
124 Barnett PA, Spence JD, Manuck SB, Jennings JR. Psychological stress and the progression of carotid artery disease. *J Hypertens* 1997;**15**:49–55.
125 Kronmal RA, Smith VE, O'Leary DH, Polak JF, Gardin JM, Manolio TA. Carotid artery measures are strongly associated with left ventricular mass in older adults (a report from the Cardiovascular Health Study). *Am J Cardiol* 1996;**77**:628–33.
126 Enderle MD, Schroeder S, Ossen R, *et al.* Comparison of peripheral endothelial dysfunction and intimal media thickness in patients with suspected coronary artery disease. *Heart* 1998;**80**:349–54.
127 Ghiadoni L, Taddei S, Virdis A, *et al.* Endothelial function and common carotid artery wall thickening in patients with essential hypertension. *Hypertension* 1998;**32**:25–32.
128 Farrar DJ, Bond MG, Sawyer JK, Green HD. Pulse wave velocity and morphological changes associated with early atherosclerosis progression in the aortas of cynomolgus monkeys. *Cardiovasc Res* 1984;**18**:107–18.
129 Huikuri HV, Jokinen V, Syvanne M, *et al.* Heart rate variability and progression of coronary atherosclerosis. *Arteriosclerosis Thromb Vasc Biol* 1999;**19**:1979–85.
130 Liao Y, Cooper RS, McGee DL, Mensah GA, Ghali JK. The relative effects of left ventricular hypertrophy, coronary artery disease, and ventricular dysfunction on survival among black adults. *JAMA* 1995;**273**:1592–7.
131 Liao D, Cai J, Rosamond WD, *et al.* Cardiac autonomic function and incident coronary heart disease: a population-based case-cohort study. The ARIC Study. Atherosclerosis Risk in Communities Study. *Am J Epidemiol* 1997;**145**:696–706.
132 Domanski MJ, Mitchell GF, Norman JE, Exner DV, Pitt B, Pfeffer MA. Independent prognostic information provided by sphygmomanometrically determined pulse pressure and mean arterial pressure in patients with left ventricular dysfunction. *J Am Coll Cardiol* 1999;**33**:951–8.
133 Holmes DR, Davis K, Gersh BJ, Mock MB, Pettinger MB. Risk factor profiles of patients with sudden cardiac death and death from other cardiac causes: a report from the Coronary Artery Surgery Study (CASS). *J Am Coll Cardiol* 1989;**13**:524–30.
134 Koyanagi S, Eastham C, Marcus ML. Effects of chronic hypertension and left ventricular hypertrophy on the incidence of sudden cardiac death after coronary artery occlusion in conscious dogs. *Circulation* 1982;**65**:1192–7.
135 Algra A, Tijssen JGP, Roelandt JRTC, Pool J, Lubsen J. Heart rate variability from 24-hour electrocardiography and the 2-year risk for sudden death. *Circulation* 1993;**88**:180–5.
136 Haider AW, Larson MG, Benjamin EJ, Levy D. Increased left ventricular mass and hypertrophy are associated with increased risk for sudden death [see comments]. *J Am Coll Cardiol* 1998;**32**:1454–9.

14: Social and psychosocial influences on sudden cardiac death, ventricular arrhythmia, and cardiac autonomic function

HARRY HEMINGWAY

The importance of better understanding of arrhythmic risk lies, in public health terms, in the prevention of sudden cardiac death. Approximately 50% of all coronary deaths are sudden, occurring within 1 hour of the onset of symptoms.[1] Most cases of sudden cardiac death have coronary artery disease present at autopsy,[2,3] although in approximately 50% this will not have been clinically apparent prior to death.[4] Sudden cardiac death is most often due to ventricular fibrillation, and cardiac autonomic function may play an important role in setting arrhythmic threshold.[5,6] Figure 14.1 illustrates this simple model of arrhythmic risk.

Sudden cardiac death is not, however, distributed equally in society. In one study of 1608 cases of sudden cardiac death, the age adjusted rates of sudden cardiac death were higher among those with less education, an effect that was stronger than for people dying of non-sudden cardiac death.[1] Educational level and other markers of socioeconomic status, such as occupation and income, consistently show inverse associations with the incidence of cardiovascular disease.[7] Social status may influence coronary risk through the behavioural coronary risk factors of smoking, exercise, diet, and alcohol. However, the finding that socioeconomic status gradients in heart disease are observed among non-smokers and are independent of the classical risk factors of cholesterol and blood pressure suggests another possibility, that aspects of the psychosocial environment related to socioeconomic status may be involved.[8,9]

Evidence from prospective epidemiological studies,[10] supported by non-human primate data,[11] suggests that psychosocial factors—such as anxiety,

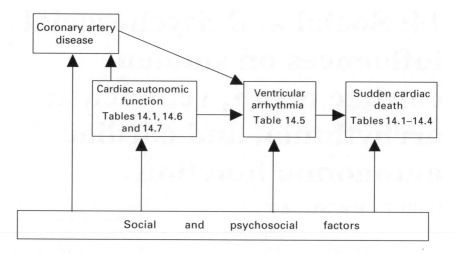

Figure 14.1 Possible pathways by which social and psychosocial factors may influence sudden cardiac death, ventricular arrhythmia, and cardiac autonomic function (the evidence is reviewed in the tables listed).

depression, hostility, type A behaviour, social supports, and work characteristics—may play a direct causal role in coronary heart disease. The majority of these studies relate a single questionnaire measurement of a psychosocial factor to incident coronary events many years ago. Such measurements may reflect chronic exposure to an adverse psychosocial environment which is relatively stable over time. The risk observed in these studies tends to be distributed in a dose–response fashion and is not confined to the extremes of the distribution. Since sudden cardiac death is a common mode of coronary death, such assessments of psychosocial factors may predict sudden cardiac death simply because they predict atherothrombotic disease of coronary arteries.

Acute psychosocial stressors—defined as events producing demands likely to tax or exceed an individual's adaptive responses over minutes, hours, and days—may represent more proximate "triggers" of sudden cardiac events. Such acute psychosocial stressors may trigger ischaemia or infarction.[12] While laboratory based measures of acute psychological stress have been extensively studied, the challenge lies in determining the effects of acute stressors in real life.

Determining the causality of putative psychosocial factors in arrhythmic risk may yield important insights into the pathogenesis of arrhythmic risk itself: mechanisms by which psychosocial factors might cause coronary heart disease (in which electrophysiological pathways are one of a number under consideration) and, ultimately, strategies for prevention of sudden cardiac death. As numerous reviews demonstrate, the clinical and biological plausibility for social and psychosocial factors being associated with arrhythmic risk is not at issue. The debate is over the quality and consistency of the totality of evidence that psychosocial factors play a causal role. Given the possibility that both chronic and acute psychosocial stressors affect arrhythmic risk, the evidence for a causal association has to be considered across a range of study designs. In prospective studies of psychosocial factors and sudden cardiac death, distinguishing acute from chronic effects may not be possible.

Previous reviews of this area have not been systematic in the identification of literature for review, the method of describing individual study results, or in the method of summarising findings from diverse types of study. For these reasons, gaps in current understanding are not clearly defined and non-contributory studies continue to be published. It is the objective, therefore, of this chapter to determine the strength of evidence for associations between social and psychosocial factors and sudden cardiac death, ventricular arrhythmia, and cardiac autonomic function. The structure of this review (outlined in Figure 14.1) is based on each of the measured outcomes: sudden cardiac death, ventricular arrhythmia, and cardiac autonomic function.

Method

Relevant articles in English language peer reviewed journals were identified using PubMed from 1970 to 1999 (www.ncbi.nlm.nih.gov/PubMed). As well as using MeSH headings (psychosocial, social, sudden death, autonomic nervous system, and arrhythmia), articles were also identified by searching on any author who had contributed one relevant article and by using the "Related Articles" function in PubMed. The bibliographies of all retrieved articles were hand searched for further relevant articles. Each study was categorised as positive if one or more measure of socioeconomic status or psychosocial factors showed a significant ($p < 0.05$) association with sudden cardiac death, ventricular arrhythmia, or cardiac autonomic function. A positive study is denoted by a plus sign in the last column of Tables 14.1 to 14.7. The methodological quality of studies, the direction of associations, and issues of multiple comparisons are considered in the text. In the absence of any previous systematic review in this area, a relaxed definition of a positive study was deliberately chosen, and no study was excluded on the grounds of methodological quality.

Animal studies

Animal studies, unlike human studies, offer the important advantages of direct study of arrhythmia precipitation; manipulation of psychosocial stressors which are observable; and not relying on language based self reports which have a potential for bias. However, in animals and humans, ventricular fibrillation and sudden death remain rare events and most animal models have, therefore, concentrated on proxies, such as the threshold for repetitive ventricular activity. All of the 12 identified studies (Table 14.1) were positive

223

Table 14.1 Socioeconomic status and psychosocial factors: associations with sudden cardiac death, ventricular arrhythmia, and cardiac autonomic function in experimental animal studies.

Study	Animal	Experimental setting	Acute psychosocial factor	Relieving factor	Outcome	Results	Summary
Lown et al.[55] (1973)	Dog	Conscious	Pavlovian sling; tension on leash and sound of switch preceding electrical shock	Cage in sound attenuated room	Threshold for repetitive ventricular response	Lowered in sling dogs	+
Corbalan et al.[56] (1974)	Dog	Conscious; coronary occlusion	Ditto	Ditto	Threshold for repetitive ventricular responses VPB, VT	Lowered before coronary occlusion in the sling group 7/8 dogs placed in sling developed VPB or VT; none in cage group	+
Johansson et al.[57] (1974)	Pig	Conscious	Psychological (restraint stress)		Ventricular arrhythmias Cardiomyopathy	Cardiomyopathy consistent with reflex catecholamine release	+
Skinner et al.[13] (1975)	Pig	Conscious; coronary occlusion	Unfamiliar (laboratory) v familiar surroundings	Adaptation to laboratory Propranolol	Latency to VF	VF delayed or prevented by adaptation or β-blockade	+

Reference	Species		Stimulus	Control	Outcome measure	Findings	
Corley et al. (1977)[58]	Squirrel monkey	11 pairs (1 avoidance 1 yoked)	Electrical shock: yoked monkey had no control	Avoidance monkey could make a lever response	Autopsy findings Sudden death	Avoidance monkeys showed more myofibrillar degeneration and 3 died suddenly after bradycardia	+
Liang et al. (1979)[59]	Dog	Conscious	Pavlovian sling	Cage	Threshold for repetitive ventricular response	Associated with circulating catecholamines	+
Natelson and Cagin (1979)[60]	Guinea pig		Restraint stress	Unrestrained	VPB, VT	Ventricular arrhythmias occurred in 7/7 restrained guinea pigs; couplets and VT in 3; no arrhythmia in unrestrained guinea pigs	+
Skinner and Reed (1981)[14]	Pig	Coronary occlusion	Unfamiliar laboratory Electrical shock	Adaptation to laboratory cryoblockade of frontal cortical brainstem pathways Central propranolol	VF	Reduce risk of VF by frontal blockade of frontal cortical brainstem pathways	+

continued

Table 14.1 *continued*

Study	Animal	Experimental setting	Acute psychosocial factor	Relieving factor	Outcome	Results	Summary
Verrier and Lown (1982)[61]	Dog	Coronary occlusion	Pavlovian sling	Cage Atropine β-blockade Stellectomy	Threshold for repetitive ventricular response	Vagal blockade with atropine reduced threshold in sling; propranolol prevented the decrease; bilateral stellectomy afforded only partial protection	+
Sgoifo et al. (1994)[62]	Rat (Wistar male)		12 males (intruders), aggressive lactating female rats (residents)		Telemetric ECG for HRV (time domain) and VPB, VT	VT in 12/12 male rats, preceded by periods of low R–R variability; more marked than controls (exposed only to novel environment)	+
Sgoifo et al. (1997)[63]	Rat (wild type)		Social stressor (defeat) non-social stressor (restraint)		Ditto	Social stressor associated with more sympathetic changes and VPB than the non-social stressor	+
Sgoifo et al. (1998)[64]	Rat (Wistar and wild type)		Defeat		Ditto	Higher sympathetic tone, low parasympathetic antagonism and more VPB in wild type rats	+

ECG, electrocardiogram; HRV, heart rate variability; VF, ventricular fibrillation; VPB, ventricular premature beat; VT, ventricular tachycardia.

and all examined acute psychosocial stressors. Taken as a whole these studies provide important evidence for a model of sudden cardiac death causation in which central and autonomic (sympathetic and parasympathetic) nervous system influences on ventricular arrhythmias are mediated by environmental, presumably psychosocial, stressors. Studies in pigs with coronary occlusion in an unfamiliar laboratory setting found that latency to ventricular fibrillation was lengthened by adaptation, β-blockade or blockade of frontal cortical brainstem pathways.[13,14] A study of 12 male rats faced with aggressive lactating female rats found that all the male rats developed ventricular tachycardia, preceded by periods of low R–R variability (using telemetrically recorded electrocardiograms).

There is an important role for further animal work, particularly when observations are made in the natural environment (for example, using telemetrically recorded electrocardiograms), and social factors that are real life (such as dominance) or long term can be studied. For example, Eisermann studied rabbits in a seminatural environment and found that a measure of socioeconomic status (dominance) was associated with radiotelemetric heart rate recordings over 1500 days; subordinate rabbits had chronically elevated heart rates not explained by limited access to burrow shelter.[15] Similar findings have been made in squirrel monkeys,[16] macaques and baboons,[17] and tree shrews.[18]

Sudden cardiac death

Death occurring within 1 hour of the onset of symptoms, in the absence of a non-cardiac cause, may be termed "sudden cardiac death". Compared with non-sudden cardiac death, sudden cardiac death is less frequently associated acute coronary thrombosis, plaque rupture, or acute myocardial infarction.[2] This observation has stimulated the enquiry that there might be differences in the risk factors for acute myocardial infarction and sudden cardiac death, and supports the importance of electrical events that leave no postmortem clues.

Methodological issues

There are major methodological challenges facing studies of sudden cardiac death. Definition of sudden cardiac death remains problematic. More recent studies have defined death as "sudden" if it occurs less than 1 hour from the onset of symptoms, but earlier studies included deaths up to 24 hours from symptom onset. Since up to a third of sudden unexplained deaths have a non-cardiac cause revealed at autopsy (such as cerebral haemorrhage or pulmonary embolus),[2] studies without autopsy confirmation of presumed cardiac cause are subject to considerable misclassification, which will tend to bias results to the null. Despite the assumption that sudden cardiac death is arrhythmic in origin, none of the identified studies directly measured arrhythmias. The largest number of sudden cardiac death events in prospective studies was 98,[19] and some were considerably smaller, leading to wide confidence intervals and the possibility of type II error.[20,21] Studies of sudden cardiac death share a bias of differences in access to community resuscitation. Retrospective studies, in seeking to determine the recent antecedents of sudden cardiac death, are subject to recall bias, since the next of kin may give unreliable accounts and researchers may be offered more explanation for a sudden than a non-sudden death. Conversely, prospective studies are not subject to recall bias but, with long periods of follow up, are able to examine the effects only of chronic measures of psychosocial stress.

Retrospective and postmortem studies

Fourteen out of 15 identified retrospective studies of sudden cardiac death were positive (Table 14.2). Cebelin and Hirsch studied the autopsies of 497 homicide victims, 15 of whom had no internal injuries or blood loss to explain death.[22] In 10 of these 15 there was myofibrillar degeneration, which was not present in 15 people who had been killed in road traffic accidents. The authors inferred that this was consistent with the fear of imminent injury in the assault (absent in the road traffic accidents) leading to a catecholamine induced stress cardiomyopathy and sudden cardiac death. Talbott et al. compared 80 cases of sudden cardiac death in women with live age, race, and sex matched neighbourhood controls, and found an excess of psychiatric history and death of a significant other among the cases.[23] Community wide stressors offer the opportunity to study the impact on sudden cardiac death in the absence of next of kin questionnaires, thus removing the potential for recall bias, but raising the problem of ecological fallacy, since the psychosocial stressor for the individual who died is inferred not measured. Increases in the number of cases of sudden cardiac death on the day of an earthquake,[24] or during the threat of missile attack,[25,26] have been reported.

Prospective studies in healthy populations

Distinguishing psychosocial effects on sudden cardiac death in patients with established coronary disease separately from healthy populations is important. If effects are seen in healthy populations where prolonged periods of follow up are required to accrue sufficient events, then this argues against psychosocial factors acting purely as triggers. Of all the cardiovascular disease cohort studies, only a proportion have incorporated psychosocial questionnaires in their risk factor measurements, and only a proportion of the latter studies have obtained data on the suddenness of cardiac death. The effect of psychosocial factors on total cardiac death separately in healthy and patient populations has been systematically reviewed.[10] Since approximately 50% of cardiac deaths are sudden, it is likely that psychosocial factors will in addition predict sudden cardiac death. Five out of six identified studies were positive (Table 14.3). No prospective study of sudden cardiac death in women was identified. The two studies by Kawachi et al. are particularly important: anxiety measured

Table 14.2 Socioeconomic status and psychosocial factors: associations with sudden cardiac death in retrospective studies.

Study	Sudden cardiac deaths			Comparison group	Psychosocial factor*	Results	Summary
	Number (% women)	Autopsy (%)	Age (yr)	SCD timing (from onset of symptoms)			
Greene et al. (1972)[65]	25 (0)	NS	55.6	NS	None	A, C	Acute anger or anxiety superimposed on a background of depression	+
Rahe et al. (1973)[66]	126 (18)	NS	56	<1 h	279 AMI survivors	A, C: 42 life change questions	SCD increase in magnitude of life changes in prior 6 months	+
Myers and Dewar (1975)[67]	100 (0)	100	NS	<24 h	100 AMI survivors	A, C: SES (social class)	SCD had more intense stress 30 min prior to onset of symptoms and had lower social class	+
Talbott et al. (1977)[68]	64 (100)	23	55.6	<24 h	64 live age related neighbourhood controls	C	Less married, more educational incongruity with spouses, fewer children: 12/64 (v 0) had definite psychiatric history	+

continued

Table 14.2 continued

| Study | Sudden cardiac deaths | | | | Comparison group | Psychosocial factor* | Results | Summary |
	Number (% women)	Autopsy (%)	Age (yr)	SCD timing (from onset of symptoms)				
Rissanen et al. (1978)[69]	118 (20)	100	31–83	<24 h	None	A, C: longstanding stress including troubles at work, family acute stress (emotional + physical)	30 had longstanding stress, leading to death within 2–24 h from symptom onset, with definite AMI; 23 patients had acute stress, death occurred less than 2 h from symptom onset and uncommonly had AMI	+
Cebelin and Hirsch (1980)[22]	15 (40)	100	1–82	Murder victims	15 road traffic accident deaths	A: inferred	15/497 had no evidence of internal injury, in whom 10 had myofibrillar degeneration (v 0/15 of comparison group)	+
Talbott et al. (1981)[23,70]	80 (100)	52.5	25–64	<24 h	80 live age, race, sex matched controls	A, C: 28 recent life events, SES (education)	SCD cases had more psychiatric history, smoking, death of significant other within last 6 months and less education compared with controls	+

Study							
Beard et al. (1982)[28]	1054 (33) NS	NS	<24h	None	A: inferred	SCD peak on Saturday: in men decreasing trend through to Friday regardless of baseline disease	+
Kirschner et al. (1986)[71]	18 (0) 100	19–51	Unexplained nocturnal deaths	None	C: inferred, refugees from SE Asia	Case series of unexplained nocturnal deaths noted among refugees	+
Strogatz et al. (1988)[72]	133 (0) NS	25–75	Fatal and non-fatal primary cardiac arrest	133 male controls chosen by random digit dialling	C: SES (wife's level of education)	Men with wives who had more than 12 years education v less education had odds ratio 0·80 (95% CI 0·5–1·3) for primary cardiac arrest	−
Meisel et al. (1991)[25]	41 (NS) NS	NS	NS	January 1990 (not under missile threat)	A: inferred, threat of war	41 sudden deaths in January 1991 v 22 in January 1990	+
Sexton et al. (1993)[73]	155 (0) 72	30–69	<1h	Expected numbers based on all CHD deaths in men aged 30–69	C: SES (occupation)	Observed v expected cases of SCD among those not working was 56 v 30 (p< 0·0001). No differences in observed/expected in non-manual or manual occupations	+

continued

Table 14.2 *continued*

Study	Sudden cardiac deaths			Comparison group	Psychosocial factor*	Results	Summary
	Number (% women)	Autopsy (%)	Age (yr)	SCD timing (from onset of symptoms)			
Escobedo and Zack *et al.* (1996)[1]	1608 (43)	NS	25->85	<1h	1585 non-sudden CHD deaths and 1053 CHD deaths, unknown timing	C: SES (education)	Age adjusted rates of SCD by decreasing educational categories were 88·9, 95·2, 129·2 per 100 000 (16%, 26%, 54% of SCD); *v* 99·4, 111·2, and 123·8 for non-sudden cardiac death	+
Leor *et al.* (1996)[24]	24 (24)	100	38–92	<1h	Mean daily rate of SCD prior to earthquake	A: inferred, Northridge earthquake	24 cases of SCD on day of earthquake *v* daily mean of 4·6 prior to earthquake	+
Weisenberg *et al.* (1996)[26]	68 (44)	NS	76.3	NS	213 cases in 5 control periods	A: inferred, threat of war	Higher rate of SCD during threat of war but not significant; no association with degree of threat in different geographical regions	+

* Source of psychosocial data was next of kin interviews, except where psychosocial factor was inferred.
A, acute; AMI, acute myocardial infarction; C, chronic; CHD, coronary heart disease; CI, confidence interval; NS, not stated; SCD, sudden cardiac death; SES, socioeconomic status.

Table 14.3 Socioeconomic status and psychosocial factors: associations with sudden cardiac death in prospective studies in healthy populations.

Study	Total sample (% women)	Age at entry (yr)	Psychosocial factor	Follow up (yr)	SCD number	SCD timing	Results	Summary
Rabkin et al. (1980)[27]	3983 (0)	25–34 (69%)	A: inferred from day of week	29	152	<24h	Excess of SCD on Mondays; only in those without previous CHD	+
Salonen (1982)[122]	2455 (0)	25–59	C: SES (education ≤7yr) and continuous psychosocial stress ≥ 1yr	6.5	27	NS	RR = 5·0 for the effect of education No significant effect of psychosocial stress	+
Hinkle et al. (1988)[74]	301 (0)	54–62	C: SES (education), type A, type B, hostility	20	65	Direct observation of sudden loss of consciousness	Low education was associated and psychosocial factors were not	+
Kagan et al. (1989)[19]	7591 (0)	46–68	C: SES (occupation)	18	131 98	1–24 h <1h	Blue collar protective	–
Kawachi et al. (1994)[20]	33 999 (0)	42–77	C: anxiety (Crown–Crisp)	2	16	<1h	Phobic anxiety associated with SCD (RR 6·08, 95% CI 2·35–15·73) not nonfatal MI	+
Kawachi et al. (1994)[21]	2280 (0)	21–80	C: anxiety (Cornell Medical Index)	32	26	<1h	RR = 5·73 (95% CI 1·26–26·1)	+

A, acute; C, chronic; CHD, coronary heart disease; CI, confidence interval; NS, not stated; RR, relative risk; SCD, sudden cardiac death; SES, socioeconomic status.

in men in the Health Professionals Study and in the Normative Aging Study using two different validated instruments was associated with sudden cardiac death.[20,21] Although the number of sudden cardiac death events was small, the effects were large, specific for sudden cardiac death, independent of other risk factors, and demonstrated dose–response effects.

The chronobiology of sudden cardiac death has been interpreted as being consistent with a psychosocial mechanism. Thus some,[27] but not all,[28] studies find a Monday excess of sudden cardiac death, consistent with the threat of returning to a stressful work environment. Sudden cardiac death and non-fatal myocardial infarction show a marked circadian rhythm, being more common in the morning. This circadian rhythm may be masked by treatment with β-blockers, suggesting that the morning excess may be mediated by the sympathetic nervous system.[29]

Prospective studies in coronary heart disease patient populations

Five out of six identified studies were positive (Table 14.4). All studies were in postmyocardial infarction populations, rather than other patient groups at high risk of sudden cardiac death (for example, patients resuscitated from near sudden death, undergoing electrophysiological studies, or with implantable defibrillators). All the studies made assessments of chronic psychosocial factors; there were no diary studies with prospective records of a patient's acute and chronic psychosocial state. Ruberman found effects of low education and low social supports on sudden cardiac death in a group of men following myocardial infarction, although in a retrospective study none of the four factors identified on interview with the patient's wife accounted for the education differences in survival.[30] Brackett and Powell examined 1012 survivors of myocardial infarction in the Recurrent Coronary Prevention Project and found an effect for type A behaviour and other psychosocial factors on sudden cardiac death but not on non-sudden cardiac death.[31]

Ventricular arrhythmia

Ventricular arrhythmias are important because they are the most common proximate cause of sudden cardiac death; they are electrical "accidents" which with appropriate treatment may be terminated and the risk of recurrence lowered. The morbidity associated with non-fatal ventricular arrhythmias is also considerable. Better understanding of the role of psychosocial factors in the ventricular arrhythmias may, therefore, offer insights into prevention and treatment.

Methodological issues

Because of the rarity and seriousness of ventricular tachycardia or ventricular fibrillation, many studies use proxy measures of arrhythmic risk, such as ventricular premature beats or QT interval. While this may offer

Table 14.4 Socioeconomic status and psychosocial factors: associations with sudden cardiac death in prospective studies in coronary heart disease patient populations.

Study	Total sample (% women)	Age at entry (yr)	Patient group	Psychosocial factor	Follow up (yr)	SCD number	SCD timing	Results	Summary
Bruhn et al. (1974)[75]	67 (21)	25–80	MI survivors and 67 healthy age, sex, type of job matched controls	C: Sisyphus type A, depression	10	23	NS	Sisyphus pattern and type A behaviour more frequent among cases than controls and predicted SCD	+
Weinblatt et al. (1978)[76]	1739 (0)	30–69	MI survivors	C: SES (education), life stress, social isolation, type A, depression	3	NS	<1 h	Among those with complex VPB low education had 33% mortality v 9% in better educated; not present among those without complex VPB	+
Ruberman et al. (1983)[30]	1684 (0)	35–74	MI survivors	C: wife assessed mood, communication, anxiety/worry, striving	3·5	NS	<1 h	None of the four factors explained the large SES (education) differences in SCD rates	–
Ruberman et al. (1984)[77]	2062 (0)	30–69	MI survivors	C: SES (education), life stress, social isolation, type A, depression	3	68	<1 h	Isolation and stress combined to predict SCD in both those with and those without VPB	+

continued

Table 14.4 *continued*

Study	Total sample (% women)	Age at entry (yr)	Patient group	Psychosocial factor	Follow up (yr)	SCD number	SCD timing	Results	Summary
Brackett and Powell (1988)[31]	1012 (8)	53	MI survivors: mean 42 months	C: SES (education), Type A (videotaped interview)	4·5	23	<1h	Low education, type A behaviour and other psychosocial factors predicted SCD but not non-sudden cardiac death	+
Ahern et al. (1990)[78] Thomas et al. (1990)[79]	331 (NS)	NS	≥ 10 VPB per h or ≥ 5 non-sustained VT 6–60 days post MI	C: anxiety, depression, type A, B, social support and desirability	NS	NS	Cardiac arrest	Depression, type B behaviour	+

C, chronic; MI, myocardial infarction; NS, not stated; SCD, sudden cardiac death; SES, socioeconomic status; VPB, ventricular premature beats; VT, ventricular tachycardia.

advantages in terms of statistical power and practicability, negative results may simply question the adequacy of the proxy rather than test the psychosocial–arrhythmia hypothesis.[32] There is a lack of population based studies and (in common with sudden cardiac death studies) there is a lack of studies examining real life acute psychosocial stressors measured in patient populations (0/21 studies) using prospective designs.

QT interval

All of four identified studies were positive (Table 14.5). Prolongation of the QT interval has been shown in prospective cohort studies to predict coronary heart disease mortality and sudden cardiac death in healthy populations. In the rare, genetic long QT syndrome, ventricular arrhythmias are common and lead to premature death; in 328 families, acute emotional stress was reported as the most common single precipitant of syncope or arrhythmia. Toivonen et al. found that in 30 healthy physicians subjected to the naturalistic acute stressor of an emergency call waking them from sleep, the QT interval was 59–67 ms longer than at equivalent heart rates during stable conditions.[33]

Ventricular premature beats

Nine of 11 identified studies were positive, but the negative studies are important (Table 14.5). In one of the few prospective studies designed to test the psychosocial–arrhythmia hypothesis, Follick et al. found no associations between a battery of carefully measured psychosocial factors (including depression, anxiety, type A behaviour, and anger) measured in state and trait form and ventricular premature beats on 24 hour electrocardiography carried out at 3, 6 and 12 month follow up.[32] One of the reasons for this may lie in the highly selected nature of the population; all participants were myocardial infarction survivors with ventricular arrhythmias, and in such a setting psychosocial factors may not further predict risk. However, the one population based study, in healthy civil servants, found no evidence that ventricular premature beats were related to socioeconomic status.[34] Thus the marker of ventricular arrhythmia, ventricular premature beats, may not be an appropriate proxy for ventricular arrhythmia.

Ventricular tachycardia and ventricular fibrillation

Eleven of 12 identified studies were positive (Table 14.5). Reich et al. found that 25 of 117 patients referred for antiarrhythmic management had experienced acute emotional disturbances during the 24 hours preceding the arrhythmias. Eighteen had two or more episodes associated with psychological disturbances. These 25 patients were distinguished from the rest of the series in having generally less severe structural heart disease.[35] Brodsky et al. selected 6 patients with lifethreatening ventricular tachyarrhythmia without underlying structural heart disease.[36] Five of

Table 14.5 Socioeconomic status and psychosocial factors: associations with ventricular premature beats, ventricular tachycardia, ventricular fibrillation and QT interval.

Study	Total sample (% Women)	Age (yr)	Patient group	Design	Psychosocial factor	Ventricular arrhythmia: type (n patients)	Results	Summary
Healthy populations								
Taggart et al. (1973)[80]	23 (91)	21–58	Healthy (17 hospital doctors)	Real life stressor	A: public speaking	VPB, catecholamines	VPB >6/min occurred in 6/23 subjects, but in 0/8 when treated with oxprenolol	+
Cook and Cashman (1982)[81]	14 (0)	39–63	Ship's pilots	Real life stressor	C: Eysenck neuroticism	VPB ≥ 1 (n = 8) on ambulatory ECG	v 6 ship's pilots without aberrant beats were more neurotic; aberrant beats occurred mainly at times of manoeuvring ships in hazardous conditions	+
Rainey et al. (1982)[82]	21 depressed	NS	Depressed and drug free	Controls (healthy 752, substance use 44)	C: depression	QT interval	Prolonged QT interval was more frequent and more severe among depressed than controls	+
Hijzen and Slangen (1985)[83]				Emotional and physical stress		QT interval	Shorter in physical rather than emotional stress	+
Katz et al. (1985)[84]	102 (37)	19–69	38 arrhythmia, 30 with > 30 VPB per h and no MI	34 age and sex matched general medical or surgical controls	C: personality inventories: 72 scales	VPB > 30/h and no MI	Depression more common than among controls	+
Huang et al. (1989)[85]	17	26–74		Laboratory stressor	A: inactivity, neutral discussion, stressful discussion, reassurance	QT interval	Shortened in most who responded with anger to the stressful situation; lengthened in 2 who reached with despondency	+
Toivonen et al. (1997)[33]	30 (30)	29–52	Healthy physicians	Real life stressor	A: awakening from emergency calls	QT interval, cycle length before and first 30 s after emergency call	QT interval 59–67 ms longer that at same heart rate during stable conditions	+
Hemingway et al. (1999)[34]	17 000 (0)	40–69	Population based, civil servants	Cross-sectional	C: SES (civil service employment grade)	VPB on resting ECG	Not related to employment grade	–

Patient populations

Lown et al. (1976)[86]	1 (0)	39	Patient with VF	Clinical stressor	A: recall of intense emotion	VF (2)	VF precipitated by recall of emotional stress	+
Lynch et al. (1977)[87]	225 (42)	59	Patients in CCU	Clinical stressor	A: pulse palpation on ward round	Ventricular arrhythmia	Reduced as a result of the ward round	+
Lown and DeSilva (1978)[88]	19 (10)		Ventricular arrhythmia	Laboratory stressor	A: mental arithmetic, reading task, emotional recall	VPB	11/19 showed an increase in VPB activity	+
Weinblatt et al. (1978)[76]	1739 (0)	30–69	MI survivors	Cross-sectional	C: SES (education), low social support	VPB on 3 h ECG	Among those with complex VPB low education had 33% mortality v 9% in better educated; not present among those without complex VPB	+
Donlon et al. (1979)[89]	1 (0)	38	MI	Laboratory stressor (62 min filmed psychiatric interview)	A: 2 independent ratings each minute of degree of stress the patient showed	VPB measured for each of 62 min	VPB > 4 per min were significantly more common during stress	+
Orth-Gomer et al. (1980)[90]	150 (0)	58	50 CHD 50 high risk 50 healthy	Cross-sectional	Emotions profile index depression type A	VPB on 24 h ECG	Depression in healthy men was associated with prognostically severe ventricular arrhythmia	+
Graboys (1981)[91]	1 (NS)	54	Avid Celtics basketball fan, 2 mo post MI	Real life stressor (watching a basketball play-off on television)	Celtic play-offs	VT, grade of VPB on 24 h ECG	Grade of VPB (couplets, salvos of VT) association with timing of the game	+
Reich et al. (1981)[35]	117	17–79	62 cardiac arrest survivors 55 symptomatic VT	Retrospective	Interviewed by cardiologist and psychiatrist for triggers	Cardiac arrests Symptomatic VT	25 patients were experiencing acute emotional disturbances during 24 h preceding arrhythmia	+

continued

Table 14.5 *continued*

Study	Total sample (% Women)	Age (yr)	Patient group	Design	Psychosocial factor	Ventricular arrhythmia: type (*n* patients)	Results	Summary
Krantz et al. (1982)[92]	26 (0)	38–68	Coronary artery bypass graft	Clinical stressor	Type A	VT or VF	4/12 type A and 0/6 non-type A	+
Freeman et al. (1984)[93]	104 (0)	54	Coronary artery bypass graft	Clinical stressor	Type A, depression, anxiety, competitive behaviour	Ventricular arrhythmia	Only competitive behaviour associated	+
Jennings and Follansbee (1984)[94]	22 (0)	57	11 CHD 11 healthy volunteers	Laboratory stressor	Type A and performance tasks	VPB	Type A was associated with higher prevalence of ectopy	+
Tavazzi et al. (1986)[95]	19 (0)	51	MI mean 37 d	Laboratory stressor	Mental arithmetic stressor	Mean ventricular refractory period, unsustained VT, VF	7 patients developed VT during stress; VF provoked in 2 patients with extra stimuli during stress	+
Brodsky et al. (1987)[36]	6 (100)	22–60	Ventricular tachyarrhythmia without structural disease	Prospective, 38 mo follow up	Psychological stress	VT	5/6 had marked psychological stress; VT related to sympathetic activity and improved by β-blocker during 38 mo follow up	
Kennedy et al. (1987)[37]	88 (39)	52·2	Programmed electrical stimulation for ventricular (66), supraventricular (12) arrhythmias or syncope (10)	Prospective	Depression and cognitive impairment	Programmed electrical stimulation of arrhythmias	Neither related to arrhythmia severity or treatment efficacy	–
Follick et al. (1988)[96]	125 (26)	54·5	MI survivors	Prospective, 12 mo follow up	Depression, SCL-90 sum of 9 scales	VPB over 1 yr follow up (*n* = 59) by transtelephonic ECG	Distress showed direct relation to VPB on follow up independent of cardiac risk and prescription of β-blockers	+

Hatton et al. (1989)[97]	17 (12)	27–74	Electro-physiological studies for VF (4) or VT (13)	Direct cardiac stimulation at catheterisation	Desire for control, locus of control and behaviour pattern	VT sustained or VF	Associated with desire for control	+
Follick et al. (1990)[32]	277 (17)	59	MI survivors 6–60 d ≥10 VPB per h or ≥5 runs of unsustained VT	Prospective, 12 mo follow up	Depression, anxiety, anger, type A	VPB on 24h ECG at baseline and 3, 6, 12 mo follow up	No effects	−
Moss et al. (1991)[98]	328 probands (69)	21 at first contact	Long QT syndrome	Retrospective	Acute emotional stress	Syncope and ventricular arrhythmia	Commonest precipitant was emotional stress	+
Carney et al. (1993)[99]	103 (82)	60	CAD	Cross-sectional	Depression on standardised interview	VT on 24h ECG	5/21 depressed v 3/82 non-depressed	+

A, acute; C, chronic; CAD, coronary artery disease; CCU, coronary care unit; CHD, coronary heart disease; ECG, electrocardiogram; MI, myocardial infarction; NS, not stated; SCL-90, Symptom Checklist 90; SES, socioeconomic status; VF, ventricular fibrillation; VPB, ventricular premature beats.

these 6 patients experienced marked psychological stress. Each of these 5 patients had recurrent rapid monomorphic ventricular tachycardia related to changes in tone of the sympathetic nervous system. Kennedy *et al.* prospectively examined 88 patients undergoing programmed electrical stimulation for the diagnosis and treatment of supraventricular and ventricular tachyarrhythmias or syncope of unknown origin.[37] While depression and cognitive impairment were related to mortality, they were not related to arrhythmia severity or treatment efficacy.

Cardiac autonomic function

Cardiac autonomic function is one of the most important predictors of sudden cardiac death and serious ventricular arrhythmia in patients with myocardial infarction.[38,39] But what in turn sets cardiac autonomic tone? One possibility is that social and psychosocial phenomena have an important role. The autonomic nervous system has for decades been considered a key putative pathway linking psychosocial to pathological processes. Social and psychosocial factors related to tonic and reflex sympathetic/parasympathetic balance may affect arrhythmic risk directly, by lowering the threshold for ventricular arrhythmia, or indirectly, by causing atherothrombotic disease in the coronary arteries (see Figure 14.1). Autonomic function is implicated in coronary heart disease aetiology through effects on the endothelium and platelet adhesiveness and on the risk factors that cluster together in the metabolic syndrome (systolic blood pressure, levels of high density lipoprotein, triglycerides, and glucose, and waist–hip ratio).[40] Socioeconomic status may be related to features of the metabolic syndrome.[41] The central nervous system is involved both in the conscious experience of psychosocial stressors and in mediating arrhythmic threshold.

Heart rate, a crude marker of autonomic function, is an independent predictor of coronary heart disease events and is higher in those of low socioeconomic status or having low levels of social support at work.[42,43] Heart rate variability measured in short (5 minute) or long (24 hour) electrocardiographic recordings offers potential advantages over simple measurements of heart rate at rest or in response to a laboratory stressor. Power spectral analysis of heart rate variability gives a valid measure of cardiac autonomic function, with the high frequency power a measure of parasympathetic tone and the low frequency power a measure of sympathetic/parasympathetic balance. Heart rate variability is clinically relevant, predicting prognosis following myocardial infarction,[44] coronary heart disease aetiology,[45] all cause mortality,[45] and ventricular tachycardia.[47] The "reactivity" of heart rate and blood pressure to psychosocial stress is outside the scope of this review because these measures have less clear relations with arrhythmic risk, do not measure vagal influences and (until recently at least) were not used in the study of real life psychosocial stressors.

Methodological issues

There was an important lack of standardised measurement protocols and complete reporting of heart rate variability measures.[47] Only five studies had more than 100 participants. Only two studies were population based and the remainder gave sparse details of the means of selection of their patients. There is thus a serious potential for selection bias. There was a lack of studies examining psychosocial stressors in a continuous or dose–response fashion, the majority treating the psychosocial factor as a qualitative (present or absent) variable. No study was identified that considered acute real life stressors applicable to a general population. Although there were seven studies that examined heart rate variability over a 24 hour period during "normal daily activities", none of these reported psychosocial stressors within these, using diary or other methods. None of the four studies in patients with coronary artery disease included measures of sympathetic/parasympathetic balance.

Cardiac autonomic function in healthy samples

Sixteen of 18 identified studies were positive (Table 14.6). Both of the negative studies involved aspects of the psychosocial work environment.[48,49] The study by Kawachi et al. is particularly important, being one of the few population based studies analysing a continuously distributed anxiety score.[50] It found an inverse linear relationship with heart rate variability; for Crown–Crisp scores of 0–1 (low anxiety), 2, 3, and 4 and over, the standard deviations of normal to normal R–R intervals (SDNN, a measure of parasympathetic activity) were, respectively, 3.54, 3.37, 3.35, and 3.11, after adjustment for age, heart rate, and body mass index. De Meersman et al. examined the effects of a real life stressor: research students giving a presentation in the setting of a (critical) audience, and without an audience.[51] There was lower low frequency and higher high frequency in the no audience recordings. In the only population based study of healthy women, Horsten et al. found that social isolation and inability to relieve anger by talking to others were associated with low heart rate variability.[52] In the Atherosclerosis Risk in Communities study there was an association between low educational attainment and low heart rate variability.[45]

Cardiac autonomic function in patients with psychiatric or coronary disease

Eleven of 12 identified studies were positive (Table 14.7). Seven of the 12 studies examined anxiety and panic disorder, and a mixed pattern emerged with some studies finding reduced low frequency, some increased low frequency, and some reduced high frequency. Eight studies examined depression; four of these were in patients with coronary artery disease, and all showed higher depression to be associated with lower standard deviation of the normal R–R intervals or other vagally mediated measures.

Baroreflex control of heart rate reflects largely reflex control of heart rate, rather than the tonic vagal activity reflected in heart rate variability.

Table 14.6 Socioeconomic status and psychosocial factors: associations with cardiac autonomic function in healthy populations.

Study	Total sample (% women)	Age (yr)	Study group	Design	Psychosocial factor	Cardiac autonomic function			Results	Summary
						Duration, setting of measurement	Time domain measures	Frequency domain measures		
Rohmert et al. (1973)[100]	21 (0)	NS	Air traffic controllers	Real life stressor	A: number of planes controlled	50 beats	SDNN	–	HR but not HRV associated with number of planes controlled	+/–
Sekiguchi et al. (1979)[101]	9 (0)	22–43	Pilots and air traffic controllers	Real life stressor	A: rest, tracking, air traffic control, flight simulation and actual flying	10 min	–	LF, HF	LF at first increased under moderate mental load and then decreased	+
Bronis et al. (1980)[102]			Radio broadcasters	Real life stressor	A: live broadcasts	After 3·5 h of work	SDNN	–	Decreased	+
Mulders et al. (1982)[103]			Professional drivers	Real life stressor	C: high v low absenteeism		SDNN	–	Lower HRV in those with high v low absenteeism	+
Kamada et al. (1992)[104]	19 (0)	21	Healthy students	Laboratory stressor (addition of 2 digit numbers)	C: type A and type B	5 min (9 episodes related to tasks)	–	LF, HF	LF/HF 3·9 for type A v 2·2 for type B (p < 0·05) resting and during tasks	+
Toivanen et al. (1993)[105]	98 (100)	23–60	50 hospital cleaners 48 bank employees	Prospective randomised trial	C: 15 min relaxation programme	2 min, sitting, Valsalva, deep breathing, standing	SDNN	–	At 3 mo and 6 mo follow up values were closer to "expected" based on Finnish reference values by age	+
Sloan et al. (1994)[106]	35 (13)	36	Volunteers, healthy	Normal daily activities (not specified)	C: hostility, sleep/wake	24 h	–	LF, HF	Hostility correlated inversely with HF and directly with LF/HF among <40 y (n = 19) during daytime only	+

Reference	n (%)	Age	Population	Design	Stressor/exposure	Protocol	Time domain	Frequency domain	Findings	
Kawachi et al. (1995)[50]	581 (0)	47–86	Volunteers, healthy	Cross-sectional	C: phobic anxiety (Crown-Crisp)	1 min supine, paced breathing	SDNN, max–min HR	–	SDNN inversely associated with Crown-Crisp score 0–1, 2, 3, ≥4, SDNN 3·54, 3·37, 3·35, 3·11 adjusted for age, heart rate and body mass index, p for trend 0·03	+
McCraty et al. (1995)[107]	24 (63)	24–47	Volunteers, healthy	Randomised trial	A: self induced appreciation or anger	5 min sitting	–	LF, MF, HF	LF increased in angry (0·025 to 0·072) and appreciation; HF increased in appreciation (0·019 to 0·031) only	+
De Meersman et al. (1996)[51]	15 (73)	23–48	Volunteer research students	Real life stressor (giving presentation of their own research)	A: anticipation of and presentation with and without audience	30 min before, during 30 min presentation	–	LF, HF	No audience had lower LF (7·6), LF/HF (0·23) and higher HF (32·5) v audience or anticipation phase	+
Myrtek et al. (1996)[108]	50 (100)	23	Students	Normal daily activities (not specified)	Stress of studying	23 h	–	–	Lower HRV during university activities	+
Liao et al. (1997)[45]	2252 (55)	54	Population based	Cross-sectional	C: SES (education)	2 min supine	SDNN	LF, HF, HF/LF	Low education monotonically; directly associated with LF; less consistent for HF, SDNN	+
Kageyama et al. (1998)[48]	223 (0)	30·8	White-collar workers	Cross-sectional	C: job stress	2 min supine and standing	–	LF, HF	Job stress not related to HRV	–
Kageyama et al. (1998)[109]	223 (0)	30·8	White-collar workers	Cross-sectional	C: commuting time, overtime	2 min supine and standing	–	LF, HF	Commuting >90 min or >60 h/mo overtime gave a sympathodominant state	+
Sato et al. (1998)[110]	16 (100)	20	Students	Laboratory stressor (psychomotor)	C: type A ($n = 8$) v type B ($n = 8$)	5 min (×8) recordings	–	LF, HF	LF and LF/HF increased after task in type A	+

continued

Table 14.6 *continued*

Study	Total sample (% women)	Age (yr)	Study group	Design	Psychosocial factor	Cardiac autonomic function			Results	Summary
						Duration, setting of measurement	Time domain measures	Frequency domain measures		
Watkins *et al.* (1998)[111]	93 (47)	25–44	Volunteers, healthy	Cross-sectional	C: anxiety (Spielberger)	5 min normal and paced breathing	–	BRC, RSA	Lower BRC and RSA in high trait anxiety (n = 23) than low (n = 22)	+
Horsten *et al.* (1999)[52]	300 (100)	57.5	Population based	Normal daily activities (not specified)	C: social isolation anger depression	24 h	SDNN	LF, HF, LF/HF	Social isolation and inability to relieve anger by talking to others were associated with low HRV; depression with LF/HF. Education not associated)	+
Myrtek *et al.* (1999)[49]	86	50	29 blue-collar 57 white-collar	Normal daily activities (not specified)	C: during home activities (not	23 h and work	–	–	No differences in HRV	–

A, acute; BRC, baroreflex control; C, chronic; HF, high frequency; HR, heart rate; HRV, heart rate variability; LF, low frequency; MF, mid frequency; RSA respiratory sinus arrhythmia; SDNN, standard deviation of normal to normal R–R interval; SES, socioeconomic status.

Table 14.7 Socioeconomic status and psychosocial factors: associations with cardiac autonomic function in patient populations.

Study	Total sample (% women)	Age (yr)	Study group	Design	Psychosocial factor	Cardiac autonomic function			Results	Summary
						Duration, setting of measurement	Time domain measures	Frequency domain measures		
Psychiatric patient populations										
Yeragani et al. (1991)[112]	49 (42)	33	19 major depression, 30 panic disorder	20 normal controls	C: depression	1 min supine, standing normal and deep breathing	MCR, SDC, MCDC, MCDSDC, PNN50	–	Panic disorder patients had lowest SDC, MCDC, MCD SDC, PNN50	+
Yeragani et al. (1993)[113]	21 (67)	20–44	Phobic anxiety	21 normal controls	C: depression (Hamilton) anxiety	5 min supine, standing, standing + deep breathing	SDNN	LF, MF, HF	Panic disorder had lower supine SDNN (3·7 v 4·9) and lower standing LF (1199 v 2211) than controls	+
Rechlin et al. (1994)[114]	80 (78)	31	16 major depression 16 panic disorder 16 reactive depression 16 amitriptyline treated	16 normal controls	C: depression, panic disorder	5 min supine, standing, paced breathing	CVr, RMSSDr, CVdr, RMSSDdr, MCR	LF, MF, HF	Panic disorder had increased LF (2·8 v 1·4 control); major depression had lower HF (0·6) v 1·2 controls and RMSSDr	+
Klein et al. (1995)[115]	10 (60)	32	Panic disorder	14 normal controls	C: panic disorder	5–10 min	–	LF, HF, Energy Ratio Index	Reduced HF	+

continued

Table 14.7 *continued*

Study	Total sample (% women)	Age (yr)	Study group	Design	Psychosocial factor	Cardiac autonomic function			Results	Summary
						Duration, setting of measurement	Time domain measures	Frequency domain measures		
Mezzacappa et al. (1996)[116]	175 (0)	15	7 aggressive, 6 anxious	8 normal controls	C: aggression and anxiety (prospective yearly reports since age 10)	1.5 min supine, standing		RSA	Aggression less RSA in supine	+
Thayer et al. (1996)[117]	34 (65)	36	Anxiety disorder	34 normal controls	C: anxiety	Baseline, relaxation and worry	–	LF, HF	Anxiety associated with lower HF than in controls; lower HF found under conditions of worry	+
Bonnet and Arand (1998)[118]	12 (ns)	18–50	Volunteer insomniacs	12 age, sex, weight matched controls	A: sleep	5 min (×100) during stages of sleep	SDNN	LF, HF, HF/TP	Higher LF, lower HF in insomniacs	+
Watkins et al. (1999)[53]	56 (70)	50–70	Volunteers with major depression	Cross-sectional	C: depression severity (Beck, Hamilton) anxiety (Spielberger)	5 min normal and paced breathing	–	BRC, RSA	Anxiety, but not depression associated with decreased baroreflex control	+

CAD patient populations

Study	n (%)	Age	Patients	Design/controls	Depression	Duration	HRV measure	Other measure	Findings	Result
Carney et al. (1988)[119]	77 (44)	58	CAD	Normal daily activities (not specified)	C: depression	24 h	SDNN		Decreased (non-significantly)	–
Carney et al. (1995)[120]	19 (37)	58	$n = 19$ CAD and depression	$n = 19$ age, sex, smoking matched controls	C: depression	24 h	SDNN, SDANN, SDNNIDX, pNN50, rMSSD	–	SDNN lower in depressed than controls 74 v 94	+
Krittayaphong et al. (1997)[121]	42 (21)	46–79	CAD	Normal daily activity (not specified)	C: depression (MMPI)	24 h	SDNN	–	Lower SDNN among those with MMPI depression scores above than below the median (114 v 135) and higher HR	+
Watkins et al. (1999)[53]	66 (13)	62	CAD	Cross-sectional	C: depressive symptoms (Beck)	10 min	–	BRC, RSA	Depression associated with decreased baroreflex control	+

BRC, baroreflex control of heart rate; CVdr, coefficient of variation during deep respiration; CVr, coefficient of variation while resting; HF, high frequency; LF, low frequency; MCDC, mean consecutive difference corrected for heart rate; MCDSDC, standard deviation of the mean consecutive difference; MCR, mean circular resultant; MF, mid frequency; MMPI, Minnesota Multiphasic Personality Interview; PNN50, percentage of all differences in R–R intervals 50 ms; RMSSDr, root mean square of successive differences during deep respiration; RMSSDr, root mean square of successive differences while resting; RSA, respiratory sinus arrhythmia; SDC, standard deviation of R–R intervals corrected for heart rate; SDNN, standard deviation of the normal R–R intervals.

Non-invasive measurements of baroreflex control in 56 men and women with major depression showed that state anxiety (measured using the Spielberger scale) was negatively correlated with levels of baroreflex control ($r = -0.32$, $p < 0.05$), whereas depression severity was not related to either respiratory sinus arrhythmia or baroreflex control.[53] Among 66 patients with coronary artery disease, high scores on the Beck Depression Inventory were associated with lower age adjusted baroreflex sensitivity compared with low depressive symptomatology: 4.5 (SD 2.7) ms/mmHg v 6.5 (SD 2.8) ms/mmHg.[54]

Summary of strength of evidence

Overall, 84 of 93 (90%) identified published studies investigating social and psychosocial aspects of arrhythmic risk were positive. Notwithstanding the quality of the studies, the proportions of positive studies were as follows. All 12 animal studies were positive across all outcomes. For human studies the proportions were:

- sudden cardiac death, retrospective (14/15), prospective healthy populations (5/6), and prospective patient populations (5/6)
- ventricular arrhythmia: QT interval (4/4), ventricular premature beats (9/11), and ventricular tachycardia or fibrillation (11/12)
- cardiac autonomic control in healthy populations (16/18) and patient populations (11/12).

This remarkable consistency across different populations and study designs lends cautious support to a causal association.

Future research

Given the public health and clinical importance of the association between psychosocial factors and arrhythmic risk, further research is required to reconcile important negative findings and address methodological limitations of existing studies and the possibility of publication bias. Complementary studies of populations at low and high risk of arrhythmic events are required. Investigation of social and psychosocial factors in high risk groups—such as patients resuscitated from near sudden death, undergoing electrophysiological studies, or with implantable defibrillators—has two main advantages. First, it provides an opportunity of accruing sufficient numbers of arrhythmic events. Second, it allows examination of real life acute psychosocial stressors (for example, using diary methods) alongside chronic psychosocial factors measured as continuous variables (for example, anxiety and depression). High and low risk population studies are required to identify which are the most important psychosocial factors. Existing studies have tended to make many measurements—risking spurious inferences from multiple comparisons—as well as neglecting certain factors, such as socioeconomic status, social supports, and psychosocial work characteristics, which may be causally related to coronary heart disease. Further development of appropriate outcome measures, indicating arrhythmic activity and threshold, and suitable for use in population studies, are required. Sudden cardiac death is a public health problem, yet few agencies have the ability to monitor its occurrence routinely. This should be redressed.

References

1 Escobedo LG, Zack MM. Comparison of sudden and nonsudden coronary deaths in the United States. *Circulation* 1996;**93**:2033–6.
2 Thomas AC, Knapman PA, Krikler DM, Davies MJ. Community study of the causes of "natural" death. *BMJ* 1988;**297**:1453–6.
3 Davies MJ, Thomas A. Thrombosis and acute coronary-artery lesions in sudden cardiac ischemic death. *N Engl J Med* 1984;**310**:1137–40.
4 Kannel WB, Anderson K, McGee DL, Degatano LS, Stampfer MJ. Nonspecific electrocardiographic abnormality as a predictor of coronary heart disease: the Framingham study. *Am Heart J* 1987;**113**:370–6.
5 Meredith IT, Broughton A, Jennings GL, Esler MD. Evidence of a selective increase in cardiac sympathetic activity in patients with sustained ventricular arrhythmias [see comments]. *N Engl J Med* 1991;**325**:618–24.
6 Barron HV, Lesh MD. Autonomic nervous system and sudden cardiac death [published erratum appears in *J Am Coll Cardiol* 1996;**28**:286]. *J Am Coll Cardiol* 1996;**27**:1053–60.
7 Kaplan GA, Keil JE. Socioeconomic factors and cardiovascular disease: a review of the literature. *Circulation* 1993;**88**:1973–98.
8 Marmot MG, Rose G, Shipley M, Hamilton PJS. Employment grade and coronary heart disease in British civil servants. *J Epidemiol Community Health* 1978;**32**:244–9.
9 Marmot MG, Bosma H, Hemingway H, Brunner E, Stansfeld S. Contribution of job control and other risk factors to social variations in coronary heart disease. *Lancet* 1997;**350**:235–40.
10 Hemingway H, Marmot M. Psychosocial factors in the aetiology and prognosis of coronary heart disease: systematic review of prospective cohort studies. *BMJ* 1999;**318**:1460–7.
11 Manuck SB, Marsland AL, Kaplan JR, Williams JK. The pathogenicity of behavior and its neuroendocrine mediation: an example from coronary artery disease. *Psychosom Med* 1995;**57**:275–83.
12 Mittleman MA, Maclure M, Nachnani M, Sherwood JB, Muller JE. Educational attainment, anger and the risk of triggering myocardial infarction onset. The Determinants of Myocardial Infarction Onset Study Investigators. *Arch Intern Med* 1997;**157**:769–75.
13 Skinner JE, Lie JT, Entman ML. Modification of ventricular fibrillation latency following coronary artery occlusion in the conscious pig. *Circulation* 1975;**51**:656–67.
14 Skinner JE, Reed JC. Blockade of frontocortical-brain stem pathway prevents ventricular fibrillation of ischemic heart. *Am J Physiol* 1981;**240**:H156–63.
15 Eisermann K. Long-term heart rate responses to social stress in wild European rabbits: predominant effect of rank position. *Physiol Behav* 1992;**52**:33–6.
16 Candland DK, Bryan DC, Nazar BL, Kopf KJ, Sendor M. Squirrel monkey heart rate during formation of status orders. *J Comp Physiol Psychol* 1970;**70**:417–23.
17 Cherkovich GM, Tatoyan SK. Heart rate (radiotelemetrical registration) in macaques and baboons according to dominant-submissive rank in a group. *Folia Primatol (Basel)* 1973;**20**:265–73.
18 Holst D. Social relations and their health impact in tree shrews. *Acta Physiol Scand* (suppl.) 1997;**640**:77–82.
19 Kagan A, Yano K, Reed DM, MacLean CJ. Predictors of sudden cardiac death among Hawaiian-Japanese men [see comments]. *Am J Epidemiol* 1989;**130**:268–77.
20 Kawachi I, Colditz GA, Ascherio A *et al*. Prospective study of phobic anxiety and risk of coronary heart disease in men. *Circulation* 1994;**89**:1992–7.
21 Kawachi I, Sparrow D, Vokonas PS, Weiss ST. Symptoms of anxiety and risk of coronary heart disease. *Circulation* 1994;**90**:2225–9.
22 Cebelin MS, Hirsch CS. Human stress cardiomyopathy. Myocardial lesions in victims of homicidal assaults without internal injuries. *Hum Pathol* 1980;**11**:123–32.
23 Talbott E, Kuller LH, Perper J, Murphy PA. Sudden unexpected death in women: biologic and psychosocial origins. *Am J Epidemiol* 1981;**114**:671–82.

24 Leor J, Poole WK, Kloner RA. Sudden cardiac death triggered by an earthquake [see comments]. *N Engl J Med* 1996;**334**:413–19.

25 Meisel SR, Kutz I, Dayan KI *et al*. Effect of Iraqi missile war on incidence of acute myocardial infarction and sudden death in Israeli civilians [see comments]. *Lancet* 1991;**338**:660–1.

26 Weisenberg D, Meisel SR, David D. Sudden death among the Israeli civilian population during the Gulf War—incidence and mechanisms. *Isr J Med Sci* 1996;**32**:95–9.

27 Rabkin SW, Mathewson FA, Tate RB. Chronobiology of cardiac sudden death in men. *JAMA* 1980;**244**:1357–8.

28 Beard CM, Fuster V, Elveback LR. Daily and seasonal variation in sudden cardiac death, Rochester, Minnesota, 1950–1975. *Mayo Clin Proc* 1982;**57**:704–6.

29 Willich SN, Maclure M, Mittleman M, Arntz HR, Muller JE. Sudden cardiac death. Support for a role of triggering in causation. *Circulation* 1993;**87**:1442–50.

30 Ruberman W, Weinblatt E, Goldberg JD, Chaudhary BS. Education, psychosocial stress and sudden cardiac death. *J Chronic Dis* 1983;**36**:151–60.

31 Brackett CD, Powell LH. Psychosocial and physiological predictors of sudden cardiac death after healing of acute myocardial infarction. *Am J Cardiol* 1988;**61**:979–83.

32 Follick MJ, Ahern DK, Gorkin L *et al*. Relation of psychosocial and stress reactivity variables to ventricular arrhythmias in the Cardiac Arrhythmia Pilot Study (CAPS). *Am J Cardiol* 1990;**66**:63–7.

33 Toivonen L, Helenius K, Viitasalo M. Electrocardiographic repolarization during stress from awakening on alarm call. *J Am Coll Cardiol* 1997;**30**:774–9.

34 Hemingway H, Shipley M, Macfarlane PW, Marmot M. Impact of socioeconomic status on coronary mortality in people with symptoms, electrocardiographic abnormalities, both or neither: the original Whitehall study 25 year follow up. *J Epidemiol Community Health* 2000;**54**:510–16.

35 Reich P, DeSilva RA, Lown B, Murawski BJ. Acute psychological disturbances preceding life-threatening ventricular arrhythmias. *JAMA* 1981;**246**:233–5.

36 Brodsky MA, Sato DA, Iseri LT, Wolff LJ, Allen BJ. Ventricular tachyarrhythmia associated with psychological stress. The role of the sympathetic nervous system. *JAMA* 1987;**257**:2064–7.

37 Kennedy GJ, Hofer MA, Cohen D, Shindledecker R, Fisher JD. Significance of depression and cognitive impairment in patients undergoing programmed stimulation of cardiac arrhythmias. *Psychosom Med* 1987;**49**:410–21.

38 Malik M, Camm AJ. Heart rate variability. *Clin Cardiol* 1990;**13**:570–6.

39 Farrell TG, Paul V, Cripps TR *et al*. Baroreflex sensitivity and electrophysiological correlates in patients after acute myocardial infarction. *Circulation* 1991;**83**:945–52.

40 Reaven GM, Lithell H, Landsberg L. Hypertension and associated metabolic abnormalities—the role of insulin resistance and the sympathoadrenal system. *N Engl J Med* 1996;**334**:374–81.

41 Brunner EJ, Marmot MG, Nanchahal K *et al*. Social inequality in coronary risk: central obesity and the metabolic syndrome. Evidence from the Whitehall II study. *Diabetologia* 1997;**40**:1341–9.

42 Gillum RF. The epidemiology of resting heart rate in a national sample of men and women: associations with hypertension, coronary heart disease, blood pressure, and other cardiovascular risk factors. *Am Heart J* 1988;**116**:163–74.

43 Unden AL, Orth-Gomer K, Elofsson S. Cardiovascular effects of social support in the work place: twenty-four-hour ECG monitoring of men and women. *Psychosom Med* 1991;**53**:50–60.

44 Bigger JT, Fleiss JL, Rolnitzky LM, Steinman RC. The ability of several short-term measures of R–R variability to predict mortality after myocardial infarction. *Circulation* 1993;**88**:927–34.

45 Liao D, Cai J, Rosamond WD *et al*. Cardiac autonomic function and incident coronary heart disease: a population-based case-cohort study. The ARIC Study. Atherosclerosis Risk in Communities Study. *Am J Epidemiol* 1997;**145**:696–706.

46 Dekker JM, Schouten EG, Klootwijk P, Pool J, Swenne CA, Kromhout D. Heart Rate Variability from Short Electrocardiographic Recordings Predicts Mortality from All Causes in Middle-aged and Elderly Men: The Zutphen Study. *Am J Epidemiol* 1997;**145**:899–908.

47 Heart rate variability: standards of measurement, physiological interpretation and clinical use. Task Force of the European Society of Cardiology and the North American Society of Pacing and Electrophysiology [see comments]. *Circulation* 1996;**93**:1043–65.

48   Kageyama T, Nishikido N, Kobayashi T, Kurokawa Y, Kaneko T, Kabuto M. Self-reported sleep quality, job stress, and daytime autonomic activities assessed in terms of short-term heart rate variability among male white-collar workers. *Ind Health* 1998;**36**:263–72.

49   Myrtek M, Fichtler A, Strittmatter M, Brugner G. Stress and strain of blue and white collar workers during work and leisure time: results of psychophysiological and behavioral monitoring. *Appl Ergon* 1999;**30**:341–51.

50   Kawachi I, Sparrow D, Vokonas PS, Weiss ST. Decreased heart rate variability in men with phobic anxiety (data from the Normative Aging Study). *Am J Cardiol* 1995;**75**:882–5.

51   De Meersman R, Reisman S, Daum M, Zorowitz R. Vagal withdrawal as a function of audience. *Am J Physiol* 1996;**270**:H1381–3.

52   Horsten M, Ericson M, Perski A, Wamala SP, Schenck-Gustafsson K, Orth-Gomer K. Psychosocial factors and heart rate variability in healthy women. *Psychosom Med* 1999;**61**:49–57.

53   Watkins LL, Grossman P, Krishnan R, Blumenthal JA. Anxiety reduces baroreflex cardiac control in older adults with major depression. *Psychosom Med* 1999;**61**:334–40.

54   Watkins LL, Grossman P. Association of depressive symptoms with reduced baroreflex cardiac control in coronary artery disease. *Am Heart J* 1999;**137**:453–7.

55   Lown B, Verrier R, Corbalan R. Psychologic stress and threshold for repetitive ventricular response. *Science* 1973;**182**:834–6.

56   Corbalan R, Verrier R, Lown B. Psychological stress and ventricular arrhythmias during myocardial infarction in the conscious dog. *Am J Cardiol* 1974;**34**:692–6.

57   Johansson G, Jonsson L, Lannek N, Blomgren L, Lindberg P, Poupa O. Severe stress-cardiopathy in pigs. *Am Heart J* 1974;**87**:451–7.

58   Corley KC, Shiel FO, Mauck HP, Clark LS, Barber JH. Myocardial degeneration and cardiac arrest in squirrel monkey: physiological and psychological correlates. *Psychophysiology* 1977;**14**:322–8.

59   Liang B, Verrier RL, Melman J, Lown B. Correlation between circulating catecholamine levels and ventricular vulnerability during psychological stress in conscious dogs. *Proc Soc Exp Biol Med* 1979;**161**:266–9.

60   Natelson BH, Cagin NA. Stress-induced ventricular arrhythmias. *Psychosom Med* 1979;**41**:259–62.

61   Verrier RL, Lown B. Experimental studies of psychophysiological factors in sudden cardiac death. *Acta Med Scand* (suppl.) 1982;**660**:57–68.

62   Sgoifo A, Stilli D, Aimi B, Parmigiani S, Manghi M, Musso E. Behavioral and electrocardiographic responses to social stress in male rats. *Physiol Behav* 1994;**55**:209–16.

63   Sgoifo A, De Boer SF, Westenbroek C *et al.* Incidence of arrhythmias and heart rate variability in wild-type rats exposed to social stress. *Am J Physiol* 1997;**273**:H1754–60.

64   Sgoifo A, De Boer SF, Buwalda B *et al.* Vulnerability to arrhythmias during social stress in rats with different sympathovagal balance. *Am J Physiol* 1998;**275**:H460–6.

65   Greene WA, Goldstein S, Moss AJ. Psychosocial aspects of sudden death. A preliminary report. *Arch Intern Med* 1972;**129**:725–31.

66   Rahe RH, Bennett L, Romo M, Siltanen P, Arthur RJ. Subjects' recent life changes and coronary heart disease in Finland. *Am J Psychiatry* 1973;**130**:1222–6.

67   Myers A, Dewar HA. Circumstances attending 100 sudden deaths from coronary artery disease with coroner's necropsies. *Br Heart J* 1975;**37**:1133–43.

68   Talbott E, Kuller LH, Detre K, Perper J. Biologic and psychosocial risk factors of sudden death from coronary disease in white women. *Am J Cardiol* 1977;**39**:858–64.

69   Rissanen V, Romo M, Siltanen P. Prehospital sudden death from ischaemic heart disease. A postmortem study. *Br Heart J* 1978;**40**:1025–33.

70   Cottington EM, Matthews KA, Talbott E, Kuller LH. Environmental events preceding sudden death in women. *Psychosom Med* 1980;**42**:567–74.

71   Kirschner RH, Eckner FA, Baron RC. The cardiac pathology of sudden, unexplained nocturnal death in Southeast Asian refugees. *JAMA* 1986;**256**:2700–5.

72   Strogatz DS, Siscovick DS, Weiss NS, Rennert G. Wife's level of education and husband's risk of primary cardiac arrest. *Am J Public Health* 1988;**78**:1491–3.

73   Sexton PT, Jamrozik K, Walsh J. Sudden unexpected cardiac death among Tasmanian men. *Med J Aust* 1993;**159**:467–70.

74   Hinkle LE, Thaler HT, Merke DP, Renier-Berg D, Morton NE. The risk factors for arrhythmic death in a sample of men followed for 20 years. *Am J Epidemiol* 1988;**127**:500–15.

75 Bruhn JG, Paredes A, Adsett CA, Wolf S. Psychological predictors of sudden death in myocardial infarction. *J Psychosom Res* 1974;**18**:187–91.

76 Weinblatt E, Ruberman W, Goldberg JD, Frank CW, Shapiro S, Chaudhary BS. Relation of education to sudden death after myocardial infarction. *N Engl J Med* 1978;**299**:60–5.

77 Ruberman W, Weinblatt E, Goldberg JD, Chaudhary BS. Psychosocial influences on mortality after myocardial infarction. *N Engl J Med* 1984;**311**:552–9.

78 Ahern DK, Gorkin L, Anderson JL *et al*. Biobehavioral variables and mortality or cardiac arrest in the Cardiac Arrhythmia Pilot Study (CAPS). *Am J Cardiol* 1990;**66**:59–62.

79 Thomas SA, Friedmann E, Wimbush F, Schron E. Psychological factors and survival in the cardiac arrhythmia suppression trial (CAST): a reexamination. *Am J Crit Care* 1997;**6**:116–26.

80 Taggart P, Carruthers M, Somerville W. Electrocardiogram, plasma catecholamines and lipids, and their modification by oxyprenolol when speaking before an audience. *Lancet* 1973;**ii**:341–6.

81 Cook TC, Cashman PM. Stress and ectopic beats in ships' pilots. *J Psychosom Res* 1982;**26**:559–69.

82 Rainey JM, Pohl RB, Bilolikar SG. The QT interval in drug-free depressed patients. *J Clin Psychiatry* 1982;**43**:39–40.

83 Hijzen TH, Slangen JL. The electrocardiogram during emotional and physical stress. *Int J Psychophysiol* 1985;**2**:273–9.

84 Katz C, Martin RD, Landa B, Chadda KD. Relationship of psychologic factors to frequent symptomatic ventricular arrhythmia. *Am J Med* 1985;**78**:589–94.

85 Huang MH, Ebey J, Wolf S. Responses of the QT interval of the electrocardiogram during emotional stress. *Psychosom Med* 1989;**51**:419–27.

86 Lown B, Temte JV, Reich P, Gaughan C, Regestein Q, Hal H. Basis for recurring ventricular fibrillation in the absence of coronary heart disease and its management. *N Engl J Med* 1976;**294**:623–9.

87 Lynch JJ, Thomas SA, Paskewitz DA, Katcher AH, Weir LO. Human contact and cardiac arrhythmia in a coronary care unit. *Psychosom Med* 1977;**39**:188–92.

88 Lown B, DeSilva RA. Roles of psychologic stress and autonomic nervous system changes in provocation of ventricular premature complexes. *Am J Cardiol* 1978;**41**:979–85.

89 Donlon PT, Meadow A, Amsterdam E. Emotional stress as a factor in ventricular arrhythmias. *Psychosomatics* 1979;**20**:233–40.

90 Orth-Gomer K, Edwards ME, Erhardt L, Sjogren A, Theorell T. Relation between ventricular arrhythmias and psychological profile. *Acta Med Scand* 1980;**207**:31–6.

91 Graboys TB. Celtics fever: playoff-induced ventricular arrhythmia [letter]. *N Engl J Med* 1981;**305**:467–8.

92 Krantz DS, Arabian JM, Davia JE, Parker JS. Type A behavior and coronary artery bypass surgery: intraoperative blood pressure and perioperative complications. *Psychosom Med* 1982;**44**:273–84.

93 Freeman AM, Fleece L, Folks DG, Cohen-Cole S, Waldo A. Psychiatric symptoms, type A behavior, and arrhythmias following coronary bypass. *Psychosomatics* 1984;**25**:586–9.

94 Jennings JR, Follansbee WP. Type A and ectopy in patients with coronary artery disease and controls. *J Psychosom Res* 1984;**28**:49–54.

95 Tavazzi L, Zotti AM, Rondanelli R. The role of psychologic stress in the genesis of lethal arrhythmias in patients with coronary artery disease. *Eur Heart J* 1986;**7**(suppl. A):99–106.

96 Follick MJ, Gorkin L, Capone RJ *et al*. Psychological distress as a predictor of ventricular arrhythmias in a post-myocardial infarction population. *Am Heart J* 1988;**116**:32–6.

97 Hatton DC, Gilden ER, Edwards ME, Cutler J, Kron J, McAnulty JH. Psychophysiological factors in ventricular arrhythmias and sudden cardiac death. *J Psychosom Res* 1989;**33**:621–31.

98 Moss AJ, Schwartz PJ, Crampton RS *et al*. The long QT syndrome. Prospective longitudinal study of 328 families. *Circulation* 1991;**84**:1136–44.

99 Carney RM, Freedland KE, Rich MW, Smith LJ, Jaffe AS. Ventricular tachycardia and psychiatric depression in patients with coronary artery disease. *Am J Med* 1993;**95**:23–8.

100 Rohmert W, Laurig W, Philipp U, Luczak H. Heart rate variability and work-load measurement. *Ergonomics* 1973;**16**:33–44.

101 Sekiguchi C, Handa Y, Gotoh M, Kurihara Y, Nagasawa Y, Kuroda I. Frequency analysis of heart rate variability under flight conditions. *Aviat Space Environ Med* 1979;**50**:625–34.

102 Bronis M, Vicenik K, Rosik V, Tysler M. Heart rhythm variability during work in radio speakers. *Act Nerv Super (Prague)* 1980;**22**:66–8.

103 Mulders HP, Meijman TF, O'Hanlon JF, Mulder G. Differential psychophysiological reactivity of city bus drivers. *Ergonomics* 1982;**25**:1003–11.

104 Kamada T, Miyake S, Kumashiro M, Monou H, Inoue K. Power spectral analysis of heart rate variability in Type As and Type Bs during mental workload. *Psychosom Med* 1992;**54**:462–70.

105 Toivanen H, Lansimies E, Jokela V, Hanninen O. Impact of regular relaxation training on the cardiac autonomic nervous system of hospital cleaners and bank employees. *Scand J Work Environ Health* 1993;**19**:319–25.

106 Sloan RP, Shapiro PA, Bigger JT, Bagiella E, Steinman RC, Gorman JM. Cardiac autonomic control and hostility in healthy subjects. *Am J Cardiol* 1994;**74**:298–300.

107 McCraty R, Atkinson M, Tiller WA, Rein G, Watkins AD. The effects of emotions on short-term power spectrum analysis of heart rate variability [published erratum appears in *Am J Cardiol* 1996;**77**:330]. *Am J Cardiol* 1995;**76**:1089–93.

108 Myrtek M, Weber D, Brugner G, Muller W. Occupational stress and strain of female students: results of physiological, behavioral, and psychological monitoring. *Biol Psychol* 1996;**42**:379–91.

109 Kageyama T, Nishikido N, Kobayashi T, Kurokawa Y, Kaneko T, Kabuto M. Long commuting time, extensive overtime, and sympathodominant state assessed in terms of short-term heart rate variability among male white-collar workers in the Tokyo megalopolis. *Ind Health* 1998;**36**:209–17.

110 Sato N, Kamada T, Miyake S, Akatsu J, Kumashiro M, Kume Y. Power spectral analysis of heart rate variability in type A females during a psychomotor task. *J Psychosom Res* 1998;**45**:159–69.

111 Watkins LL, Grossman P, Krishnan R, Sherwood A. Anxiety and vagal control of heart rate. *Psychosom Med* 1998;**60**:498–502.

112 Yeragani VK, Pohl R, Balon R *et al.* Heart rate variability in patients with major depression. *Psychiatry Res* 1991;**37**:35–46.

113 Yeragani VK, Pohl R, Berger R *et al.* Decreased heart rate variability in panic disorder patients: a study of power-spectral analysis of heart rate. *Psychiatry Res* 1993;**46**:89–103.

114 Rechlin T, Weis M, Spitzer A, Kaschka WP. Are affective disorders associated with alterations of heart rate variability? *J Affect Disord* 1994;**32**:271–5.

115 Klein E, Cnaani E, Harel T, Braun S, Ben-Haim SA. Altered heart rate variability in panic disorder patients. *Biol Psychiatry* 1995;**37**:18–24.

116 Mezzacappa E, Tremblay RE, Kindlon D *et al.* Relationship of aggression and anxiety to autonomic regulation of heart rate variability in adolescent males. *Ann NY Acad Sci* 1996;**794**:376–9.

117 Thayer JF, Friedman BH, Borkovec TD. Autonomic characteristics of generalized anxiety disorder and worry. *Biol Psychiatry* 1996;**39**:255–66.

118 Bonnet MH, Arand DL. Heart rate variability in insomniacs and matched normal sleepers. *Psychosom Med* 1998;**60**:610–15.

119 Carney RM, Rich MW, teVelde A, Saini J, Clark K, Freedland KE. The relationship between heart rate, heart rate variability and depression in patients with coronary artery disease. *J Psychosom Res* 1988;**32**:159–64.

120 Carney RM, Saunders RD, Freedland KE, Stein P, Rich MW, Jaffe AS. Association of depression with reduced heart rate variability in coronary artery disease. *Am J Cardiol* 1995;**76**:562–4.

121 Krittayaphong R, Cascio WE, Light KC *et al.* Heart rate variability in patients with coronary artery disease: differences in patients with higher and lower depression scores. *Psychosom Med* 1997;**59**:231–5.

122 Salonen JT. Socioeconomic status and risk of cancer, cerebral stroke and death due to coronary heart disease and any disease: a longitudinal study in eastern Finland. *J Epidemiol Community Health* 1982;**36**:294–7.

15: Stress and gene–environment interactions in coronary heart disease

HUGH MONTGOMERY, HARRY HEMINGWAY, AND STEVE HUMPHRIES

The human body is maintained in health through the integration of numerous complex homeostatic physiological processes operating at the level of the cell, tissue, and between organs. These processes rely on the production of appropriate quantities of structural proteins and enzymes, each coded for by a single gene. Many diseases, such as coronary heart disease, may be thought to result from a failure of adequate homeostasis within a physiological system, or a failure of integration of such processes. Such homeostatic failure may result from an imbalance between the scale of an environmental stimulus and the scale of the physiological response. In this way, a predisposition to the development of coronary heart disease may be the result of the interaction between the environment and the genes coding for homeostatic structural proteins and enzymes.

Rarely, coronary disease results from a major mutation in an important homeostatic gene such as that regulating lipoprotein lipase synthesis. The resulting abnormal lipid profile may cause aggressive early onset coronary disease. More commonly, however, minor variations in such genes exist. Many of these variations have no effects at all, while others may affect either the structure of the protein transcribed from the gene (for instance, the structure of a receptor protein which may influence agonist binding) or the quantity of protein that is synthesised when gene transcription is activated.

Each gene has its own "ignition key" and "accelerator pedal", which switch the gene on, and determines the rate at which it "revs" (or synthesises product). This "ignition–accelerator" module is known as the promoter region of the gene. Small variations in this region may thus have huge effects on the rate at which the gene makes its product: in other words, promoter polymorphisms may have significant functional effects. Such polymorphic variants may alter the synthetic responsiveness of a gene by influencing the attachment of "DNA binding" proteins.

These proteins represent the transduction mechanism through which an environmental stimulus produces a synthetic response. Some of these proteins will repress, and others activate, transcription. Small changes in DNA sequence in the promoter region may thus markedly influence binding of these proteins: promoter polymorphisms may strongly influence gene–environment interactions.

Gene variations such as these (which affect either the amount of product made by the gene, or the nature of the gene product) are known as *functional polymorphisms*. Such polymorphisms account for much of the biological diversity seen in homeostatic systems. Without them, all humans would respond in an identical way to every environmental challenge, and risk of disease development would be directly linked to the degree of exposure to an injurious environmental stimulus. We know this not to be the case, however: some individuals exposed to cigarette smoke, and with an otherwise identical risk factor profile, will go on to develop coronary heart disease, while others will not. The fact that this is so is largely due to common functional genetic polymorphisms as well as other environmental risk factors. Environmental factors other than cigarette smoke may interact with genetic factors to influence the risk of coronary heart disease development. One such set of environmental factors might include psychosocial stress.

Although much effort has been directed towards the physiological mechanisms activated in the stress response, little work has yet been directed towards the influence of genetic polymorphic variants on the magnitude of these responses. Such an effort would be well justified. First it might help establish risk profiles for individuals exposed to stress. Second, such studies might help identify other systems involved in the transduction of the stress response and the genesis of coronary heart disease.

Strategy for investigating the interaction of genes with psychosocial factors

In principle, such a strategy begins with the identification of a system that might have a role in the development of coronary heart disease in response to stress—a *candidate system*. Within this system, a key component is identified, and its gene (the candidate gene) targeted for investigation. As stated above, the structure of a gene is not constant within populations, with minor variations (polymorphisms) occurring. Initial studies are aimed at the identification of common functional polymorphisms in candidate genes, through the sequencing of gene structure in large numbers of individuals. Further studies are then conducted to show whether a common polymorphism in a candidate gene is indeed functional. This may be done in one of two ways.

- Measurements are made of a basal phenotypic characteristic (such as cardiac mass or serum fibrinogen levels) that might be influenced by the gene, and these measurements in a population are correlated with individual phenotypes for the polymorphism. Thus, if variant A (rather than variant B) of the fibrinogen gene is thought to be functional, are levels of fibrinogen higher in those with AA genotype (i.e. possessing two A alleles) than those of BB genotype? These investigations can again be performed by study of normal and patient samples.

- A phenotypic characteristic is measured upon stimulation. Thus, it might be that variant A of the fibrinogen gene is likely to control fibrinogen synthesis. Individuals of known genotype are exposed to a challenge that would normally be expected to stimulate fibrinogen synthesis. Changes in the phenotypic characteristic (in this case, levels of fibrinogen or, in other studies, perhaps changes in heart mass) are studied.

Finally, studies make use of the functional polymorphism of the candidate gene in the investigation of the cardiovascular disease state. If a gene variant A has been identified that causes greater activity of a given candidate system (for example, greater synthesis of fibrinogen in the coagulation process), and if the candidate system is indeed playing an important role in the development of coronary heart disease, then individuals of AA genotype are more likely to suffer coronary heart disease than those of BB genotype. Such studies, therefore, involve the correlation of an increased frequency of a particular genotype with the presence or severity of a given disease state. Let us thus suppose that a "highly responsive" polymorphism of the glucocorticoid receptor gene is identified. If we examine populations exposed to psychosocial stressors and find this polymorphism to be more common in those who have heart attacks than in those who do not, then this would strongly suggest the importance of the glucocorticoid receptor (and, indeed, the hypothalamic–pituitary–adrenal axis) in the genesis of coronary heart disease in response to stress.

How might gene–environment interactions link psychosocial stress and coronary heart disease?

Stress is a risk factor for the development of coronary heart disease. Indeed, emotional state may have a profound influence on the development of this disease.[1] Further, acute stress may lead to sudden death—even if merely caused by dreams.[2] Diverse environmental stimuli lead to a multifaceted collection of biological responses, which we refer to as a "stress response". These biological responses may modulate the homeostatic mechanisms maintaining normal coronary artery structure and function. The scale of the stress response, and of the alteration in coronary risk profile, will be dependent on the genetic milieu of the individual under examination. Gene–environment interactions underlie much of the development of coronary heart disease, and the gene–stress interaction is no different.

There are a paucity of published data investigating gene–environment interactions linking stress and coronary heart disease. This chapter looks at the systems linking stress and coronary heart disease and examines, by way of example, some of the candidate genes that may link the two. In principle, a genetic influence might operate in one of three ways:

- Genetic variation might be responsible for the predisposition to personality types who mount higher psychological stress responses. Twin and sibling studies suggest that genetic factors account for a substantial part of the causes of neurotic traits.[3,4] The influence of such genetic architecture seems to vary between the sexes.[5] Polymorphism in the human serotonin transporter gene contributes to up to 9% of the inherited variance in anxiety related personality traits.[6] Meanwhile, genetic markers of stress responsiveness have been identified in a mouse model,[7] the adenosine A2a receptor may play a role in aggression and anxiety in rodents,[8] and the rodent analgesic stress response may be regulated by a single gene.[9] Polymorphic variation of the human dopamine D2 receptor gene is associated with risk of development of post-traumatic stress disorder.[10] Other loci are being sought.
- Genetic variation might influence the behavioural response to stress, and propensity to risk behaviour. These, in turn, might influence coronary risk. The wish to smoke cigarettes or adopt a high alcohol intake (for instance),[11–13] to eat excessively and become obese, or to retreat to a sedentary life and withdraw from exercise, might all be genetically influenced. Thus, smoking is a well recognised risk factor for the development of coronary heart disease. People tend to smoke more under stressful situations.[14] A tendency to take up cigarette smoking may be influenced by genetic factors.[11] Whether this might increase smoking tendency under stress is not known, although genetic factors may influence tendency to smoke during pregnancy.[15]
- More commonly, however, the genes lie in systems regulating levels of conventional risk factors such as blood pressure, platelet numbers and function, the coagulation cascade, insulin sensitivity and the metabolic syndrome, and lipid profile, as well as the transduction of such risk factors. Regardless of whether a genetic predisposition to smoking under stress exists, the response to the cigarette smoking under stress may be so influenced. Fibrinogen is a major risk factor for the development of coronary heart disease; smoking causes a rise in plasma fibrinogen levels,[16] and the fibrinogen response to smoking[17–19] may be influenced by specific genetic polymorphisms.[20,21]

By way of example, we examine four risk factors for coronary heart disease: markers of inflammation, coagulation status, the metabolic syndrome, and blood pressure and left ventricular hypertrophy. Many of these factors are responsive to psychosocial stress, and the means by which genetic variation might have an impact on this response is discussed below. In some cases the data suggesting involvement are clear, but in others the suggestions are much more speculative. Nonetheless, it is to be hoped that the principles that they illustrate may inform future studies.

Stress and the inflammatory response

Inflammation is a risk factor for coronary heart disease

The physiological response to a wide variety of different inflammatory stimuli is qualitatively similar, with soluble inflammatory mediators known as cytokines—such as interleukins 1 and 6 (IL-1, IL-6) and tumour necrosis factor α (TNF-α)—playing a central role. These induce hepatic synthesis of acute phase proteins such as C-reactive protein (CRP) and fibrinogen.[17] This inflammatory response may be causal in the pathogenesis of progressive coronary atheroma and the transition to myocardial infarction or unstable angina.[22,23] Markers of inflammation are associated with the development of coronary disease, disease severity,[24-26] and with the occurrence of coronary events.[27] In addition, chronic gastric,[28-31] lung,[31-36] and gum[37-41] infections are associated with both a chronic inflammatory response and with the development of coronary heart disease. Systemic inflammatory responses may also play a role in the conversion of stable coronary disease to an unstable coronary syndrome. Unstable angina is associated with activation of systemic circulating neutrophils,[42] and with elevated inflammatory markers such as CRP and IL-6 levels.[43-45] The magnitude of this elevation predicts poor outcome,[46] and is not merely secondary to the presence of myocardial necrosis[46] or simple ischaemia.[45] More directly, severe exercise,[47] acute *Chlamydia pneumoniae* infection,[36,48,49] acute influenza-like illness,[39,50] and temperature change,[51,52] all cause an acute inflammatory response and are all associated with increased risk of acute myocardial infarction.[53,54]

The proinflammatory cytokine IL-6 may play a central role, being the only cytokine capable of inducing all the hepatic acute phase proteins. It is derived from diverse tissues including fibroblasts, monocytes, adipocytes, and endothelial cells.[55]

Both inflammatory stimuli themselves (such as smoking, severe exertion, and cold exposure[56,57]) and their associated hormonal or cytokine responses (such as catecholamines and tumour necrosis factor[58]) are associated with a rise in IL-6 levels.[59] Once produced, IL-6 has a key role in driving the acute inflammatory response, and orchestrates the production of acute phase proteins.[55] It may thus be pivotal in the putative inflammatory pathogenesis of coronary disease, through a direct role (such as induction of endothelial activation[60]) or an indirect role (for instance, through the stimulation of fibrinogen synthesis,[61,62] which may itself be directly pathogenic).

Stress may induce an "inflammatory" response

Psychological stress is known to alter immune function, and indeed may be associated with a response in many ways resembling that of acute inflammation. The fact that white cell count and fibrinogen levels rise with mental stress suggest that a classic acute phase response may in part be generated from psychological as well as physical stress. This may partly be driven by catecholamines.[63] Stress is thus associated with increased circulating levels of the proinflammatory cytokines IL-1, IL-6, and TNF-α.[64,65] Levels of IL-6 also rise in brain tissue.[66] Such responses may alter health through changes in immune function,[67] as well as in wound healing responses.[68]

The inflammatory response to stress may be influenced by genetic variation

Polymorphisms of many of the proinflammatory cytokines are likely to influence the "inflammatory" response to stress, and hence the consequent development of coronary heart disease. A functional polymorphism of the IL-6 gene has recently been identified in its promoter region.[69,70] Here, a single base pair of the gene is swapped from a cytosine to a guanine residue, and we thus can identify two versions of the gene: C or G. The polymorphism is common, with the frequency of the C allele being 0.41 in a group of 944 healthy men from the UK. When this gene is artificially expressed in cells in culture, the C version has 62% lower ($p = 0.005$) expression than the G version at baseline. However, when the gene is "switched on" by exposure to lipopolysaccharide (released in some forms of septic shock, for instance), expression of the C version is not significantly increased, while expression from the G variant rises two- or threefold ($p < 0.01$). Thus, the G allele seems to be associated with a significant increase in IL-6 response to inflammatory stimuli, at least in vitro. The situation in living humans is not clear and to date there have been conflicting reports regarding the association of these genotypes with plasma levels of IL-6, with initial studies (Figure 15.1) suggesting that the -174C allele was associated with lower mean plasma levels of IL-6 in healthy subjects,[69] but later studies finding higher levels in subjects with aneurysmal disease,[70] which is a strong inflammatory state, as evidenced by the considerably higher mean IL-6 levels in these patients. These data suggest that there is a genetically determined difference in the degree of the IL-6 response to a stressful or inflammatory situation that is influenced by this promoter variant. If this is the case, and bearing in mind the magnitude of the genotype effects seen, it is likely to be of biological significance in causing an elevated risk of atherosclerosis and thrombosis and greater predisposition to CHD. In support of this, the -174C allele was associated with 1.8 fold higher CHD mortality in the abdominal aortic aneurysms patients during 5 years follow-up[70] (independently of classical risk factors), and also with 1.54 (95%CI 1.0–2.23) higher CHD risk in middle aged

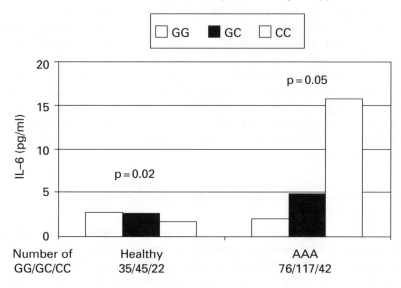

Figure 15.1 Association between interleukin 6 (IL-6) promoter G/C polymorphism and IL-6 levels in 102 healthy subjects (data from[69]), and from 235 Abdominal Aortic Aneurysm patients (data from[70]).

healthy UK men over a similar period, with this effect being greatest in smokers (2.66, 95%CI 1.64–4.32) (SE Humphries unpublished).

Stress and coagulation status

We have seen that the acute stress response might be influenced by genetic variation. In fact, the cytokine stress response may lead to coronary heart disease through effects on the coagulation system. The extent of this cytokine–coagulation interaction may also be subject to genetic variation.

Coagulation factors

Haemostatic variables have been consistently linked to the risk of development of ischaemic heart disease. Increased coagulation tendency—higher levels of factors VII, VIII, and von Willebrand factor—as well as reduced fibrinolytic tendency—lower activity of plasminogen activator inhibitor type 1 (PAI-1) and tissue plasminogen activating factor (t-PA)—are all prospectively associated with coronary risk.[71] The coagulation system may thus have a key role in the development and progression of coronary heart disease.[72]

Fibrinogen, in particular, has been strongly associated with the development of coronary heart disease. It is not merely a coagulation factor, but a hepatically derived acute phase protein,[73–75] whose synthesis is responsive to the cytokine IL-6.[61,62] Fibrinogen levels thus rise as part of any chronic or acute inflammatory process. Elevated serum fibrinogen concentrations represent an independent risk factor for ischaemic heart disease,[76,77] of greater magnitude than serum cholesterol level, body mass index, or blood pressure.[78–80] Levels correlate with cardiovascular disease severity and progression,[81–83] with the transition from stable coronary disease to unstable angina and myocardial infarction,[75,78] and with the risk of recurrent events.[84–86] Overall, a change in fibrinogen concentration of just 0.1 g/L might correspond to a cardiovascular risk alteration of 15%.[87] Given the responsiveness of fibrinogen levels to inflammation, it is likely that the risk associated with fibrinogen is underestimated: the rises in fibrinogen levels in response to inflammatory stimuli (which will vary between individuals) may be a much better marker of risk.[88]

A procoagulant state is known to result from psychological stress. Psychological stress and high job demands can influence coagulation status through changes in plasma fibrinogen, von Willebrand factor antigen, PAI-1 and t-PA activity.[89–91] High occupational demands are similarly independently associated with reduced t-PA activity.[90] Thus levels of factors I, VII, and VIII increase during cyclical periods of increased stress at work,[92] and a procoagulant state is seen in fighter pilots after flight activity.[93] In particular, fibrinogen levels rise acutely in response to psychological stress in animal models as well as humans,[94,95] and are higher in those facing high perceived stress, high effort, and low reward, at work.[96,97] Given the rise in fibrinogen levels with psychological stress, and the association of fibrinogen levels with coronary heart disease risk, it has been suggested that the increased risk of myocardial infarction associated with recent earthquake may be mediated though such alterations in coagulation status.[98,99]

This response of the coagulation system to acute stress may be strongly genetically influenced. The fibrinogen molecule comprises two identical subunits, each composed of three polypeptide chains (αa, Bβ, and γ) encoded by a different gene (*FGA*, *FGB*, and *FGG*, respectively).[100] Synthesis of the Bβ chain is responsive to IL-6,[61,62] and is the rate limiting step in fibrinogen synthesis.[62,101] Polymorphisms of the *FGB* (β-fibrinogen) gene might thus influence the fibrinogen response to inflammatory stimuli. The G→A substitution polymorphism at position 453 in the 5′ flanking sequence of the β-fibrinogen gene is one such variant.[21,74,102] It interacts strongly with environmental factors,[103] and lies in an IL-6 responsive element. The fibrinogen response to an inflammatory stimulus might thus be influenced by both IL-6 and fibrinogen genotype.

Severe exertion is an inflammatory stimulus associated with a rise in fibrinogen levels.[104,105] Levels remain raised for at least 4 days, allowing for continued stimulation of fibrinogen synthesis.[106]

This fibrinogen response to environmental stressors might thus be dependent upon both IL-6 and fibrinogen genotype. Provisional studies from our group support this hypothesis. The fibrinogen response to severe exercise was studied in 156 male British Army recruits. Cohorts were studied at the start of their 10 week physical training, and again 0.5–5 days after a strenuous 2 day military exercise undertaken in their final week of training. Compared with baseline values, fibrinogen concentrations were

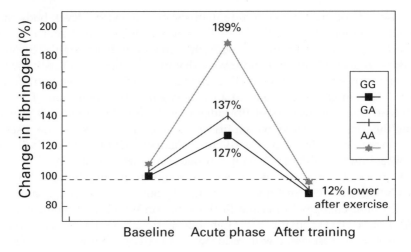

Figure 15.2   Mean percentage change in plasma fibrinogen concentration after severe exercise in men with different G/A genotype. Adapted from Montgomery *et al.* (1996).[47]

significantly higher on days 1–3 after the exercise, consistent with the acute inflammatory response to severe exercise, being maximal on days 1 and 2 (mean rise 27.2%, $p < 0.001$; 37.1%, $p < 0.001$, respectively). Despite no difference at baseline, the acute rise in fibrinogen concentrations (days 2 and 3) seemed to be influenced by the presence of the A allele, mean values being 26.7 (SE 5.4)%, 36.5 (SE 11.0)%, and 89.2 (SE 30.7)% for those of *GG*, *GA*, and *AA* genotype respectively ($p = 0.01$) (Figure 15.2). However, these data relate to very small numbers: there were only three of *AA* genotype in total. Intensive exercise thus generates an "acute phase" rise in fibrinogen levels, possibly influenced by the *G/A* polymorphism of the β-fibrinogen gene.[47]

Once again, it is plausible that the fibrinogen response to stress (and hence, possibly, coronary risk) may depend upon fibrinogen genotype. An interaction with the IL-6 polymorphism might also be possible: IL-6 levels rise with stress, and IL-6 drives fibrinogen synthesis. The responsiveness of the IL-6 gene and subsequent responsiveness of the β-fibrinogen gene may both be genotype dependent. Polymorphisms for other coagulation factors, which are known risk factors, may behave in a similar fashion.

Platelet action

Platelet aggregation is also a key factor in the development of thrombus. Given the association between coagulation status and coronary heart disease risk, it is no surprise that platelet number and function are risk factors for coronary heart disease. Platelet activation leads first to adhesion and then to degranulation, upon which numerous vasoactive peptides and growth factors are released. Through such mechanisms, platelets are

264

thought to play a role in the pathogenesis of progressive coronary atherosclerosis[107,108] and the acute coronary syndromes.[109–111]

The systemic inflammatory response is associated with an increase in platelet number and reactivity, mediated by cytokines including IL-6 acting on the hormone thrombopoietin and its receptor.[112–114] Indeed, the thrombopoietin receptor is itself a member of a family of cytokine receptors.[115] Part of the cardiovascular risk attributable to chronic or acute inflammation might thus be mediated through increases in platelet numbers and reactivity. Evidence supports this hypothesis. Mean platelet volume is a marker of platelet reactivity.[116] This volume is raised in those developing atherosclerosis,[117,118] and correlates with the severity of atherosclerotic stenosis.[119]

In keeping with a key role for platelet activation in the development of acute coronary syndromes, increasing mean platelet volume is a risk factor for the development of both unstable angina and myocardial infarction.[120–123] Meanwhile, myocardial infarction itself generates a systemic inflammatory response in which platelet size increases.[122,124,125] This rise is a strong predictor of a recurrent myocardial infarction within 2 years.[122]

The number and function of platelets are influenced by acute psychological stress. Platelets are activated by mental stress.[126–128] Platelet activation and secretion, therefore, increase prior to public speaking.[129] Even 10 minutes of mental arithmetic leads to a shortlived (30 minutes) increase in platelet aggregation induced by ADP, the formation of platelet aggregates, and an increase in plasma thromboxane B_2 levels.[130] The magnitude of the platelet response is variable, but tends to be higher in those with known coronary heart disease, suggesting a potentially causal association.[131] This response is carried forward into the workplace: thrombin and ADP induced platelet aggregation increase with cyclical increases in workplace stress.[92] Such effects may be partly mediated through the actions of catecholamines,[132] and partly through a secondary increase in shear stress.[133]

Just as for the coagulation factors discussed above, a variety of polymorphisms may influence the platelet response to stress, and thus the associated risk of coronary heart disease. These polymorphisms may affect the transduction of stress to altered platelet function in a number of ways. First, the increased heart rates and blood pressure generated as part of the stress response place the platelet under increased shear stress. This is a stimulus for platelet activation. The degree of shear stress may itself be related to polymorphic variants in other systems, which influence blood pressure and heart rate responses (see below), and the platelet activation it induces may also be influenced by polymorphic genetic variants. Thus, the platelet receptor for von Willebrand factor (vWF), the glycoprotein (GP) Ib/IX complex, mediates shear stress dependent platelet activation. A polymorphism of the α chain of this receptor (145 Thr/Met) influences activation. The 145 Met allele is associated with the development of coronary heart disease.[134]

Similarly, various coagulation factors cause platelet activation. As described above, stress is associated with a rise in fibrinogen levels, which may be dependent on β-fibrinogen genotype. The response of the platelets to the fibrinogen rise may also be dependent on a polymorphism of the GPIIIa *PLA/A2* gene and hence with coronary heart disease. The *PLA2* allele may be associated with coronary heart disease risk,[135] and myocardial infarction,[136] as well as stenosis after coronary stent placement.[137] Further, the *PLA2* polymorphism may be directly associated with fibrinogen levels, as well as with the ratio of very low density lipoprotein (VLDL) to high density lipoprotein (HDL) in a smoking dependent fashion—perhaps through linkage disequilibrium with neighbouring genes.[138,139] Other polymorphisms of the platelet thrombin receptor (GPIb-α) are also associated with the development of coronary heart disease.[140]

Stress is associated with raised catecholamine levels. The platelet α_2-adrenergic receptor is encoded by a gene on chromosome 10. Polymorphic variants of this gene influence adrenergically induced platelet aggregation.[141] Polymorphism of the serotonin transporter promoter may also affect platelet serotonin (5-HT) uptake.[142]

The metabolic syndrome and stress

Coronary heart disease risk factors are often clustered in given individuals. In particular, the metabolic syndrome (syndrome X) is identified as the coexistence of central obesity, insulin resistance, hypertension, dyslipidaemia, and coronary artery disease. In fact, components of this syndrome may be influenced by stress.

It is well established that specific lipid profiles are associated with raised coronary heart disease risk. In particular, raised levels of LDL cholesterol and high ratios of LDL to HDL cholesterol are detrimental. Levels of LDL cholesterol are elevated in those facing high work stresses.[96] Total cholesterol levels rise with stress and emotional burn-out[143–145] and are higher in those feeling frustration and aggression,[146] while lipid peroxidation may also be reduced by relaxation.[147] Lipid profile may also be adversely affected, with a relative fall in HDL levels, at least in animal models.[148] Additionally, an association of cardiovascular reactivity to stress with detrimental lipid profile has also been identified.[149]

The lipid profile response to stress may be influenced by genetic variation. A wealth of polymorphic variants in other genes controlling lipid metabolism have been identified, all of which may have a potential influence on lipid profile under stress conditions. However, variations in catecholamine and glucocorticoid receptors seem obvious candidates. Lipid metabolism is strongly influenced by catecholamine and glucocorticoid activity. At least in animal studies, the action of catecholamines may underlie the hyperlipidaemic response to stress.[150] The β_2-adrenergic receptor may play a particularly important role in this regard. The lipid stress response may be influenced by variation in β-adrenergic receptor activity,[151] expression,[152,153] or subtype numbers.[154] In theory, polymorphisms influencing structure, expression, or transduction of receptor activity could all modulate the lipid response to stress. Several such polymorphisms have been identified (for instance, in codons 16, 27, and 164),[155] some of which are associated with changes in agonist sensitivity or receptor expression.[156,157] Similarly, polymorphisms in glucocorticoid receptors have been identified. Although some of these seem not to influence glucocorticoid sensitivity,[158] this might not be the case for others.[159,160] Such functional variants might in theory modulate the lipid stress response.

Other components of the metabolic syndrome might also be responsive to stress, and genetically influenced. In rat models, for instance, incidence of phenotypic expression of the gene for type I diabetes is increased by psychological stress.[161] Whether such an effect on type II diabetes is possible is unclear. As discussed above, psychological stress can elevate circulating interleukin 6 levels,[162] and this response might be influenced by polymorphic variants of the IL-6 gene. As well as having potentially profound effects on the coagulation system, circulating IL-6 has stimulatory actions on the hypothalamic–pituitary–adrenal axis,[163] increasing hypothalamic secretion of corticotrophin releasing hormone, and responsiveness both of pituitary corticotrophin release and adrenal cortisol secretion. Through this mechanism, IL-6 may increase the tendency to central obesity, insulin resistance, and dyslipidaemia.[164] Tissue renin–angiotensin systems may influence fat metabolism,[165] insulin sensitivity,[166] and hypertension,[167,168] and as such, may be influenced by the angiotensin converting enzyme (ACE) gene insertion/deletion polymorphism described in detail below. Evidence is accumulating that insulin sensitivity and resistance may be under such control.[169–171] Finally, the polymorphisms of the β_2-adrenergic receptor and glucocorticoid receptor described above may modulate insulin sensitivity and fat distribution. Many other genes, however, are likely to play an integrated role.

Blood pressure and left ventricular hypertrophy

As a final example, we consider left ventricular hypertrophy. This condition is associated with poor outcome, an excess total mortality independent of systolic blood pressure, and increased risk of cardiovascular death and disease.[172] Overall, left ventricular hypertrophy is associated with a 10-fold increase in mortality rate,[173] and risk of developing congestive cardiac failure.[174] Risk of cerebrovascular accident and death, coronary heart disease, cerebral transient ischaemic attack, and intermittent claudication prevalence are all more frequent in those with left ventricular hypertrophy.[173]

Stress itself will increase the stimulus to hypertrophy through increasing cardiac work. Heart rate, and systolic and diastolic blood pressure all rise during acute psychological stress,[95] and are elevated after earthquake exposure.[98,99] An exaggerated pressor response to mental stress is associated with atherosclerosis, although it remains unproven as to whether this is causal.[175] Studies in cynomolgus monkeys suggest, however, that the heart rate response to stress is indeed causal in atherosclerotic disease.[176] This may be partly a direct effect. However, an association of cardiovascular reactivity to stress with detrimental lipid profile has also been identified.[149]

Studies suggest that the cardiac work response to stress (in terms of both blood pressure[177–179] and heart rate[175]) has a strong genetic component. So far, few candidate genes have been identified. Studies suggest that a polymorphism of the human ACE gene may be implicated in both the blood pressure response and the associated left ventricular hypertrophy.

The circulating human renin–angiotensin system plays an important role in circulatory homeostasis. Angiotensin converting enzyme degrades vasodilator kinins and generates vasoconstrictor angiotensin II.

A polymorphism of the human ACE gene has been identified in which the absence (deletion, D allele) rather than the presence (insertion, I allele) of a 287 base pair fragment is associated with higher tissue ACE activity.[180] Local tissue renin–angiotensin systems exist in diverse tissues including the vascular wall.[181] These may influence blood pressure responses. Although resting blood pressure may be unaffected by ACE genotype,[182] diastolic blood pressure rise during and after standardised physical stress is associated with the D allele.[183] Whether increases in blood pressure related to emotional stress are associated with the D allele is unclear, although ambulatory blood pressure derivatives (including circadian rhythm blood pressure changes) may be associated with this allele.[184,185]

This putative influence may be related to alterations in sympathetic neurotransmission. Angiotensin II might interact with the sympathetic nervous system at a number of different levels.[186]

- It facilitates presynaptic norepinephrine (noradrenaline) release through a specific action on angiotensin II type receptors.
- It facilitates adrenergic release from chromaffin cells of the adrenal medulla.
- It enhances the effects of catecholamines by acting synergistically on the same intracellular second messenger system (inositol triphosphate) in vascular smooth muscle cells.

Independently of whether stress related blood pressure is influenced by the human ACE gene I/D polymorphism, the left ventricular hypertrophic response may well be. Local myocardial renin–angiotensin systems may regulate left ventricular growth. Cardiac ACE and angiotensinogen gene expression increase during left ventricular hypertrophy, as do angiotensin receptor numbers. Angiotensin II increases physiological cardiac hypertrophy, while renin–angiotensin system antagonists impair such growth.[187]

Such data strongly support a role for the renin–angiotensin system in the control of both physiological and pathophysiological growth, and are supported by studies in humans. The magnitude of the left ventricular growth response associated with a 10 week exercise training programme is strongly influenced by ACE genotype: mean left ventricular mass increased by 2.0 g in those of II genotype, and by 42.3 g in those of DD genotype.[188] In those exposed to a hypertrophic stimulus (such as hypertension, or inherited hypertrophic cardiomyopathy), the D allele is also associated with the scale of hypertrophic response.[189] Tissue renin–angiotensin system activity may thus powerfully influence the left ventricular hypertrophic response.

Conclusion

Many disease states result from the interaction of environmental stimuli (whether of the internal or external environment) with genes. Coronary heart disease is no exception. The interaction of psychosocial stress (as an "environmental" stimulus) with the genetic milieu is, however, complex. Our genetic inheritance may lead to an altered level of basal emotional state both qualitatively (our basal expression of anxiety, depression, or anger) and quantitatively (how angry or depressed we are). The keenness of perception by an individual of a "stressful" situation will vary, as will the very nature of what might be perceived as stressful. Additionally, the sensitivity and responsiveness of the basal state to external stressful stimuli are partly genetically determined. Once a given level of "cerebral" stress has been reached, the nature and magnitude of each component of the biological response might also be genetically influenced. Finally, the effects of these changes on tissue physiology and pathophysiology will depend on genetic variation.

The study of the genetic interactions of genes with psychosocial stress in determining the onset of disease is thus difficult, but worth while. In the long term, it might be possible to predict the risk of coronary heart disease development in an individual exposed to a given environment. In the short term, genetic studies might prove our most powerful tool in unravelling the mechanisms linking psychosocial stress and disease. Genetic studies have this power simply because they offer a means of demonstrating causality rather than association. If levels of a cytokine are raised in response to stress and fluctuate wildly over time, how are we to demonstrate that they may be crucial in causing coronary heart disease over a lifetime? The demonstration that a "high responding cytokine gene" is found more frequently in those who develop coronary heart disease than in those who do not, when exposed to a similar work environment, strongly implicates that cytokine in causing coronary heart disease.

Sequencing of the entire human genome is now a reality. Advances in technology may allow us to "read" 100 000 genes at a time on one "chip". Such advances will amplify the power available to us in the realms of research into genetic physiology and psychosocial epidemiology. The insights that such novel approaches may yield are eagerly awaited.

References

1 Nemeroff CB, Musselman DL, Evans DL. Depression and cardiac disease. *Depress Anxiety* 1998;**8**(suppl. 1):71–9.

2 Parmar MS, Luque-Coqui AF. Killer dreams. *Can J Cardiol* 1998;**14**:1389–91.

3 Padersen NL, Plomin R, McClearn GE, Friberg L. Neuroticism, extraversion, and related traits in adult twins reared apart and reared together. *J Pers Soc Psychol* 1988;**55**:950–7.

4 Lynn R, Hampson S, Agahi E. Genetic and environmental mechanisms determining intelligence, neuroticism, extraversion and psychoticism: an analysis of Irish siblings. *Br J Psychol* 1989;**80**:499–507.

5 Eaves LJ, Heath AC, Neale MC, Hewitt JK, Martin NG. Sex differences and non-additivity in the effects of genes on personality. *Twin Res* 1998;**1**:131–7.

6 Lesch KP, Bengel D, Heils A *et al*. Association of anxiety-related traits with a polymorphism in the serotonin transporter gene regulatory region. *Science* 1996;**274**(5292):1527–31.

7 Roberts AJ, Phillips TJ, Belknap JK, Finn DA, Keith LD. Genetic analysis of the corticosterone response to ethanol in BXD recombinant inbred mice. *Behav Neurosci* 1995;**109**:1199–208.

8 Ledent C, Vaugeois JM, Schiffmann SN *et al*. Aggressiveness, hypoalgesia and high blood pressure in mice lacking the adenosine A2a receptor. *Nature* 1997;**388**(6643):674–8.

9 Sternberg WF, Liebeskind JC. The analgesic response to stress: genetic and gender considerations. *Eur J Anaesthesiol* 1995;**10**(suppl.):14–17.

10 Comings DE, Muhleman D, Gysin R. Dopamine D2 receptor (DRD2) gene and susceptibility to posttraumatic stress disorder: a study and replication. *Biol Psychiatry* 1996;**40**:368–72.

11 Boomsma DI, Koopmans JR, Van Doomen LJ, Orlebeke JF. Genetic and social influences on starting to smoke: a study of Dutch adolescent twins and their parents. *Addiction* 1994;**89**:219–26.

12 Blum K, Sheridan PJ, Wood RC, Braverman ER, Chen TJ, Comings DE. Dopamine D2 receptor gene variants: association and linkage studies in impulsive–addictive–compulsive behaviour. *Pharmacogenetics* 1995;**5**:121–41.

13 Hill SY, Locke J, Zezza N *et al*. Genetic association between reduced P300 amplitude and the DRD2 dopamine receptor A1 allele in children at high risk for alcoholism. *Biol Psychiatry* 1998;**43**:40–51.

14 Pomerleau OF, Pomerleau CS. Behavioural studies in humans: anxiety, stress and smoking. *Ciba Found Symp* 1990;**152**:225–35.

15 Magnus P, Berg K, Bjerkedal T, Nance WE. The heritability of smoking behaviour in pregnancy, and the birth weights of offspring of smoking-discordant twins. *Scand J Soc Med* 1985;**13**:29–34.

16 Rosengren A, Wilhelmsen L, Welin T, Tsipogianni A, Teger-Nilsson AC, Wedel H. Social influences and cardiovascular risk factors as determinants of plasma fibrinogen concentration in a general population sample of middle aged man. *BMJ* 1990;**300**:634–8.

17 De Maat MP, Pietersma A, Kofflard M, Sluiter W, Kluft C. Association of plasma fibrinogen levels with coronary artery disease, smoking and inflammatory markers. *Atherosclerosis* 1996;**121**:185–91.

18 Kannel WB, D'Agostino RB, Belanger AJ. Fibrinogen, cigarette smoking, and risk of cardiovascular disease: insights from the Framingham Study. *Am Heart J* 1987;**113**:1006–10.

19 Wilkes HC, Kelleher C, Meade TW. Smoking and plasma fibrinogen. *Lancet* 1988;**i**:307–8.

20 Behague I, Poirier O, Nicaud V *et al*. Beta fibrinogen gene polymorphisms are associated with plasma fibrinogen and coronary heart disease in patients with myocardial infarction. The ECTIM study. Etude Cas-Temoins sur l'Infarctus de Myocarde. *Circulation* 1996;**93**:440–9.

21 Humphries SE, Cook M, Dubowitz M, Stirling Y, Meade TW. Role of genetic variation at fibrinogen locus in determination of plasma fibrinogen concentrations. *Lancet* 1987;**i**:1452–5.

22 Haught WH, Mansour M, Rothlein R *et al*. Alterations in circulating intercellular adhesion molecule-1 and L-selectin: further evidence for chronic inflammation in ischaemic heart disease. *Am Heart J* 1996;**132**:1–8.

23 Munro JM, Cotran RS. The pathogenesis of atherosclerosis: atherogenesis and inflammation. *Lab Invest* 1988;**58**:249–61.

24 Heinrich J, Schulte H, Schonfeld R, Kohler E, Assmann G. Association of variables of coagulation, fibrinolysis and acute-phase with atherosclerosis in coronary and peripheral arteries and those arteries supplying the brain. *Thromb Haemostasis* 1995;**73**:374–9.

25 Miche E, Baller D, Gleichmann U, Mannebach H, Schmidt H, Prohaska W. Fibrinogen and leukocyte number in coronary heart disease. Correlation with angiography and clinical degree. *Z Kardiol* 1995;**84**:92–7.

26 Mori T, Sasaki J, Kawaguchi H *et al.* Serum glycoproteins and severity of coronary atherosclerosis. *Am Heart J* 1995;**129**:234–8.

27 Mendall MA, Carrington D, Strachan D. Chlamydia pneumoniae: risk factors for seropositivity and association with coronary heart disease. *J Infect* 1995;**30**:121–8.

28 Niemela S, Kartunen T, Korhonen T *et al.* Could Helicobacter pylori infection increase the risk of coronary heart disease by modifying serum lipid concentrations? *Heart* 1996;**75**:573–5.

29 Whincup PH, Mendall MA, Perry IJ, Strachan DP, Walker M. Prospective relations between *Helicobacter pylori* infection, coronary heart disease, and stroke in middle aged men. *Heart* 1996;**75**:568–72.

30 Mendall MA, Goggin PM, Molineaux N *et al.* Relation of *Helicobacter pylori* infection and coronary heart disease. *Br Heart J* 1994;**71**:437–9.

31 Patel P, Mendall MA, Carrington D *et al.* Association of *Helicobacter pylori* and *Chlamydia pneumoniae* infections with coronary heart disease and cardiovascular risk factors. *BMJ* 1995;**311**(7007):711–14.

32 Leinonen M. Pathogenic mechanisms and epidemiology of *Chlamydia pneumoniae*. *Eur Heart J* 1993;**14**(suppl. K):57–61.

33 Mendall MA, Patel P, Ballam L, Strachan D, Northfield TC. C reactive protein and its relation to cardiovascular risk factors: a population based cross sectional study. *BMJ* 1996;**312**(7038):1049–50.

34 Thom DH, Grayston JT, Siscovick DS, Wang SP, Weiss NS, Daling JR. Association of prior infection with *Chlamydia pneumoniae* and angiographically demonstrated coronary artery disease. *JAMA* 1992;**268**:68–72.

35 Linnanmaki E, Leinonen M, Mattila K, Nieminen MS, Valtonen V, Saikku P. *Chlamydia pneumoniae*-specific circulating immune complexes in patients with chronic coronary heart disease. *Circulation* 1993;**87**:1130–4.

36 Saikku P, Leinonen M, Tenkanen L *et al.* Chronic *Chlamydia pneumoniae* infection as a risk factor for coronary heart disease in the Helsinki Heart Study. *Ann Intern Med* 1992;**116**:273–8.

37 Beck J, Garcia R, Heiss G, Vokonas PS, Offenbacher S. Periodontal disease and cardiovascular risk. *J Periodontol* 1996;**67**(suppl. 10):1123–37.

38 Loesche WJ. Periodontal disease as a risk factor for heart disease. *Compendium* 1994;**15**:978–82.

39 Mattila KJ, Nieminen MS, Valtonen VV *et al.* Association between dental health and acute myocardial infarction. *BMJ* 1989;**298**(6676):779–81.

40 Mattila KJ. Dental infections as a risk factor for acute myocardial infarction. *Eur Heart J* 1993;**14**(suppl. K):51–3.

41 Mattila KJ, Valle MS, Nieminen MS, Valtonen VV, Hietaniemi KL. Dental infections and coronary atherosclerosis. *Atherosclerosis* 1993;**103**:205–11.

42 Kohchi K, Takebayashi S, Hiroki T, Nobuyoshi M. Significance of adventitial inflammation of the coronary artery in patients with unstable angina: results of autopsy. *Circulation* 1985;**71**:709–16.

43 Biasucci LM, Vitelli A, Liuzzo G. Elevated levels of IL-6 in unstable angina. *Circulation* 1996;**94**:874–7.

44 Berk BC, Weintraub WS, Alexander RW. Elevation of C-reactive protein in "active" coronary artery disease. *Am J Cardiol* 1990;**65**:168–72.

45 Liuzzo G, Biasucci LM, Rebuzzi AG *et al.* Plasma protein acute phase response in unstable angina is not induced by ischemic injury. *Circulation* 1996;**94**:2372–80.

46 Haverkate F, Thompson SG, Pyke SD, Gallimore JR, Pepys MB. Production of C-reactive protein and risk of coronary events in stable and unstable angina. European Concerted Action on Thrombosis and Disabilities Angina Pectoris Study Group. *Lancet* 1997;**349**(9050):462–6.

47 Montgomery HE, Clarkson P, Nwose OM *et al.* The acute rise in plasma fibrinogen concentration with exercise is influenced by the G-453-polymorphism of the beta-fibrinogen gene. *Arteriosclerosis Thromb Vasc Biol* 1996;**16**:386–91.

48 Saikku P, Leinonen M, Mattila K *et al.* Serological evidence of an association of a novel Chlamydia, TWAR, with chronic coronary heart disease and acute myocardial infarction. *Lancet* 1988;**ii**(8618):983–6.

49 Saikku P. *Chlamydia pneumoniae* infection as a risk factor in acute myocardial infarction. *Eur Heart J* 1993;**14**(suppl. K):62–5.

50 Dobson AJ, Alexander HM, Al-Roomi K *et al.* Coronary events in the Hunter region of New South Wales, Australia: 1984–1986. *Acta Med Scand* 1988;**728**(suppl. 1):84–9.

51 Stout RW, Crawford V. Seasonal variations in fibrinogen concentrations among elderly people. *Lancet* 1991;**338**:9–13.

52 Group E. Cold exposure and winter mortality from ischaemic heart disease, and all causes in warm and cold regions of Europe. The Eurowinter Group. *Lancet* 1997;**349**(9062):1341–6.

53 Mittleman MA, Maclure M, Tofler GH, Sherwood JB, Goldberg RJ, Mullers JE. Triggering of acute myocardial infarction by heavy physical exertion. Protection against triggering by regular exertion. *N Engl J Med* 1993;**329**:1678–83.

54 Willich SN, Lewis M, Lowel H, Arntz HR, Schubert F, Schroder R. Physical exertion as a trigger of acute myocardial infarction. *N Engl J Med* 1993;**329**:1684–90.

55 Heinrich PC, Castell JV, Andus T. Interleukin-6 and the acute phase response. *Biochem J* 1990;**265**:621–36.

56 Jansky L, Pospisilova D, Honova S. Immune system of cold-exposed and cold-adapted humans. *Eur J Appl Physiol* 1996;**72**:445–50.

57 Mohamed-Ali V, Bulmer K, Clarke D, Goodrick S, Coppack SW, Pinkey JH. Beta-Adrenergic regulation of proinflammatory cytokines in humans. *Int J Obes Relat Metab Disord* 2000;**24(Suppl 2)**:154–5.

58 Tracy RP, Lemaitre RN, Psaty BM *et al.* Relationship of C-reactive protein to risk of cardiovacular disease in the elderly. Results from the Cardiovascular Health Study and the Rural Health Promotion project. *Arteriosclerosis Thromb Vasc Biol* 1997;**17**:1121–7.

59 Nieman DC. Immune response to heavy exertion. *J Appl Physiol* 1997;**82**:1385–94.

60 Romano M, Sironi M, Toniatti C *et al.* Role of IL-6 and its soluble receptor in induction of chemokines and leukocyte recruitment. *Immunity* 1997;**6**:1–20.

61 Dalmon J, Laurent M, Courtois G. The human beta fibrinogen promotor contains a hepatocyte nuclear factor 1-dependent interleukin-6-responsive element. *Mol Cell Biol* 1993;**13**:1183–93.

62 Thomas AE, Green FR, Kelleher CH *et al.* Variation in the promotor region of the β fibrinogen gene is associated with plasma fibrinogen levels in smokers and non-smokers. *Thromb Haemostasis* 1991;**65**:487–90.

63 Omoto M, Furuichi S, Imai T, Nomura R, Hokama Y, Igarashi M. Changes in the FDP (fibrin and fibrinogen degradation products) value under mental and physical stress. II. Simultaneous observations of FDP and other indices of fatigue in persons under experimentally loaded stress. *Sangyo Igaku* 1982;**24**:616–27.

64 Maes M, Song C, Lin A *et al.* The effects of psychological stress on humans: increased production of pro-inflammatory cytokines and a Th1-like response in stress-induced anxiety. *Cytokine* 1998;**10**:313–18.

65 Nukina H, Sudo N, Komaki G, Yu X, Mine K, Kubo C. The restraint stress-induced elevation in plasma interleukin-6 negatively regulates the plasma TNF-alpha level. *Neuroimmunomodulation* 1998;**5**:323–7.

66 Shizuya K, Komori T, Fujiwara R, Miyahara S, Ohmori M, Nomura J. The expressions of mRNAs for interleukin-6 (IL-6) and the IL-6 receptor (IL-6R) in the rat hypothalamus and midbrain during restraint stress. *Life Sci* 1998;**62**:2315–20.

67 Glaser R, Kielcolt-Glaser JK, Malarkey WB, Sheridan JF. The influence of psychological stress on the immune response to vaccines. *Ann NY Acad Sci* 1998;**1**:649–55.

68 Marucha PT, Kielcolt-Glaser JK, Favagehi M. Mucosal wound healing is impaired by examination stress. *Psychosom Med* 1998;**60**:362–5.

69 Fishman D, Faulds G, Jeffery R *et al.* The effect of novel polymorphisms in the interleukin-6 gene (IL-6) on IL-6 transcription and plasma IL-6 levels, and an association with systemic-onset juvenile chronic arthritis. *J Clin Invest* 1998;**102**:1369–76.

70 Jones KG, Brull DJ, Brown LC, Sian M, Greenhalgh RM, Humphries SE, Powell JT. Interleukin-6, (IL-6) and the prognosis of abdominal aortic aneurysms. *Circulation* 2001;**103**:2260–65.

71 Koenig W. Haemostatic risk factors for cardiovascular diseases. *Eur Heart J* 1998;**19**(suppl. C):C39–43.

72 Sueishi K, Ichikawa K, Kato K, Nakagawa K, Chen YX. Atherosclerosis: coagulation and fibrinolysis. *Semin Thromb Hemostasis* 1998;**24**:255–60.

73 Haines AP, Howarth D, North WRS *et al.* Haemostatic variables and outcome of acute myocardial infarction. *Thromb Haemostasis* 1983;**50**:800–3.

74 Green F, Humphries S. Control of plasma fibrinogen levels. *Baillière's Clin Haematol* 1989;**2**:945–59.

75 Thompson SG, Kienast J, Pyke SDM, Haverkate F, Van de Loo JCW. Hemostatic factors and the risk of myocardial infarction or sudden death in patients with angina pectoris. *N Engl J Med* 1995;**332**:635–41.

76 Shah P, Chander R, Daly K. Plasma fibrinogen level and other risk factor profile; association with coronary artery disease. *Br Heart J* 1995;**71**:P25.

77 Meade TW, Mellows S, Brozovic M *et al.* Hemostatic function and ischaemic heart disease: principal results of the Northwick Park Heart Study. *Lancet* 1986;**ii**:533–7.

78 Yarnell JW, Baker IA, Sweetnam PM *et al.* Fibrinogen, viscosity, and white blood cell count are major risk factors for ischaemic heart disease. *Circulation* 1991;**83**: 836–44.

79 Stone MC, Thorp JM. Plasma fibrinogen—a major coronary risk factor. *J R Coll Gen Pract* 1985;**35**:565–9.

80 Di Minno G, Mancini M. Measuring plasma fibrinogen to predict stroke and myocardial infarction. *Arteriosclerosis* 1990;**10**:1–7.

81 Lassila R, Pltonen S, Lepantalo M, Saarinen O, Kauhanen P, Manninen V. Severity of peripheral atherosclerosis is associated with fibrinogen and degradation of cross-linked fibrin. *Arteriosclerosis Thromb* 1993;**13**:1738–42.

82 Lowe GDO, Drummond MM, Lorimar AR. Relation between extent of coronary artery disease and blood viscosity. *BMJ* 1980;**i**:673–4.

83 Grotta JC, Yatsu TM, Pettigrew LC *et al.* Prediction of carotid stenosis progression by lipid and hematological measurements. *Neurology* 1989;**39**:1325–31.

84 Resch K, Ernst E, Matrai A, Paulsen H. Fibrinogen and viscosity as risk factors for subsequent cardiovascular events in stroke survivors. *Ann Intern Med* 1992;**117**:371–5.

85 Martin JF, Bath PM, Burr ML. Influence of platelet size on outcome after myocardial infarction. *Lancet* 1992;**338**:1409–11.

86 Cristal N, Slonim A, Bar-Ilan I, Hart A. Plasma fibrinogen levels and the clinical course of acute myocardial infarction. *Angiology* 1983;**34**:693–8.

87 Ernst E, Resch KL. Fibrinogen as a cardiovascular risk factor: a meta-analysis and review of the literature. *Ann Intern Med* 1993;**118**:956–63.

88 Pyke SD, Thompson SG, Buchwalsky R, Kienast J. Variability over time of haemostatic and other cardiovascular risk factors in patients suffering from angina pectoris. ECAT Angina Pectoris Study Group. *Thromb Haemostasis* 1993;**70**:743–6.

89 Jern C, Manhem K, Eriksson E, Tengborn L, Risberg B, Jern S. Hemostatic responses to mental stress during the menstrual cycle. *Thromb Haemostasis* 1991;**66**:614–18.

90 Ishizaki M, Tsuritani I, Noborisaka Y, Yamada Y, Tabata M, Nakagawa H. Relationship between job stress and plasma fibrinolytic activity in male Japanese workers. *Int Arch Environ Health* 1996;**68**:315–20.

91 Kop WJ, Hamulyak K, Pernot C, Appels A. Relationship of blood coagulation and fibrinolysis to vital exhaustion. *Psychosom Med* 1998;**60**:352–8.

92 Frimerman A, Miller HI, Laniado S, Keren G. Changes in hemostatic function at times of cyclical variation in occupational stress. *Am J Cardiol* 1997;**79**:72–5.

93 Biondi G, Farrace S, Mameli G, Marongiu F. Is there a hypercoagulable state in military fighter pilots? *Aviat Space Environ Med* 1996;**67**:568–71.

94 Morimoto A, Watanabe T, Myogin T, Murakami N. Restraint induced stress elicits acute-phase response in rabbits. *Pflugers Arch* 1987;**410**:554–6.

95 Jern C, Eriksson E, Tengborn L, Risberg B, Wadenvik H, Jern S. Changes of plasma coagulation and fibrinolysis in response to mental stress. *Thromb Haemostasis* 1989;**62**:767–71.

96 Siegrist J, Pater R, Cremer P, Seidel D. Chronic work stress is associated with atherogenic lipids and elevated fibrinogen in middle-aged men. *J Intern Med* 1997;**242**:149–56.

97 Davis MC, Matthews KA. Are job characteristics related to fibrinogen levels in middle-aged women? *Health Psychol* 1995;**14**:310–18.

98 Kario K, Matsuo T, Kayaba K, Soukejima S, Kagamimori S, Shimada K. Earthquake-induced cardiovascular disease and related risk factors in focusing on the Great Hanshin-Awaji Earthquake. *J Epidemiol* 1998;**8**:131–9.

99 Matsuo T, Kobayashi H, Kario K, Suzuki S, Matsuo M. Role of biochemical and fibrinolytic parameters on cardiac events associated with Hanshin-Awaji earthquake-induced stress. *Rinsho Byori* 1998;**46**:593–8.

100 Baumann RE, Henschen AH. Linkage disequilibrium relationships among four polymorphisms within the human fibrinogen gene cluster. *Hum Genet* 1994;**94**:165–70.

101 Roy SN, Mukhopadhyay G, Redman CM. Regulation of fibrinogen assembly: transfection of hep G2 cells with Bbeta cDNA specifically enhances synthesis of the three component chains of fibrinogen. *J Biol Chem* 1990;**265**:6389–93.

102 Scarabin PY, Bara L, Ricard S *et al*. Genetic variation at the β-fibrinogen locus in relation to plasma fibrinogen concentrations and risk of myocardial infarction. The ECTIM study. *Arteriosclerosis Thromb* 1993;**13**:886–91.

103 Humphries SE, Ye S, Talmud P, Bara L, Wilhelmsen L, Tiret L. European Atherosclerosis Research Study: genotype at the fibrinogen locus (G455-A beta-gene) is associated with differences in plasma fibrinogen levels in young men and women from different regions in Europe. Evidence for gender–genotype–environment interaction. *Arteriosclerosis Thromb Vasc Biol* 1995;**15**:96–104.

104 Camus G, Poortmans J, Nys M *et al*. Mild endotoxaemia and the inflammatory response induced by a marathon race. *Clin Sci Colch* 1997;**92**:415–22.

105 Weinstock C, Konig D, Harnischmacher R, Keul J, Berg A, Northoff H. Effect of exhaustive exercise stress on the cytokine response. *Med Sci Sports Exerc* 1997;**29**:345–54.

106 Hallsten Y, Frandsen U, Orthenblad N, Sjodin B, Richter EA. Xanthine oxidase in human skeletal muscle following eccentric exercise: a role in inflammation. *J Physiol* 1997;**498**:239–48.

107 Ross R, Glomset JA. The pathogenesis of atherosclerosis. *N Engl J Med* 1976;**295**:369–77.

108 Ross R. The pathogenesis of atherosclerosis—an update. *N Engl J Med* 1986;**314**:488–500.

109 Tofler GH, Brinski D, Schafer AI *et al*. Concurrent morning increase in platelet aggregability and the risk of myocardial infarction and sudden cardiac death. *N Engl J Med* 1987;**316**:1514–21.

110 Fitgerald DJ, Roy L, Catella F, Fitzgerald GA. Platelet activation in unstable coronary disease. *N Engl J Med* 1986;**315**:983–7.

111 Elwood PC, Renaud S, Sharp DS, Beswick AD, O'Brien JR, Yarnell JW. Ischaemic heart disease and platelet aggregation. The Caerphilly Heart Disease Study. *Circulation* 1991; **83**:38–44.

112 Burnstein SA, Downs T, Friese P *et al*. Thrombocytopoiesis in normal and sublethally irradiated dogs: response to human interleukin-6. *Blood* 1992;**80**:420–4.

113 Peng J, Friese P, George JN, Dale GL, Burnstein SA. Alteration of platelet function in dogs mediated by interleukin-6. *Cytokine* 1994;**8**:717–21.

114 Kaushansky K. Thrombopoietin: the primary regulator of platelet production. *Blood* 1995;**86**:419–31.

115 Souyri M, Vigon I, Penciolelli JF, Heard JM, Tambourin P, Wendling F. A putative truncated cytokine receptor gene transduced by the myeloproliferative leukaemia virus immortalizes hemopoietic progenitors. *Cell* 1990;**63(6)**:1137.

116 Erusalimsky JD, Martin JF. The regulation of megakaryocyte polyploidization and its implications for coronary artery occlusion. *Eur J Clin Invest* 1993;**23**:1–9.

117 Kristensen SD, Martin JF. Megakaryocytes and atherosclerosis. *Clin Sci* 1992;**82**:353–5.

118 Brown AS, Hong Y, de Belder A *et al*. Megakaryocyte ploidy and platelet changes in human diabetes and atherosclerosis. *Arteriosclerosis Thromb Vasc Biol* 1997;**17**:802–7.

119 Bath PM, Missouris CG, Buckenham T, MacGregor GA. Increased platelet volume and platelet mass in patients with atherosclerotic renal artery stenosis. *Clin Sci Colch* 1994;**87**:253–7.

120 Pizzulli L, Yang A, Martin JF, Luderitz B. Changes in platelet size and count in unstable angina compared to stable angina or non cardiac chest pain. *Eur Heart J* 1998;**19**:80–4.

121 Hendra TJ, Oswald GA, Yudkin JS. Increased mean platelet volume after acute myocardial infarction related to diabetes and to cardiac failure. *Diabetes Res Clin Pract* 1988;**5**:63–7.

122 Martin JF, Bath PM, Burr ML. Influence of platelet size on outcome after myocardial infarction. *Lancet* 1991;**338**:1409–12.

123 Kishk YT, Trowbridge EA, Martin JF. Platelet volume subpopulations in acute myocardial infarction: an investigation of their homogeneity for smoking, infarct size and site. *Clin Sci* 1985;**68**:419–25.

124 Heptinstall S, Mulley GP, Taylor PM, Mitchell JRA. Platelet-release reaction in myocardial infarction. *BMJ* 1981;**i**:80–1.

125 Cameron HA, Philips R, Ibbotson RM, Carson PHM. Platelet size in myocardial infarction. *BMJ* 1983;**287**:449–51.

126 Arkel YS, Haft JI, Kreutner W, Sherwood J, Williams R. Alteration in second phase platelet aggregation associated with an emotionally stressful activity. *Thromb Haemostasis* 1977;**38**:552–61.

127 Naesh O, Haedersdal C, Hindberg I, Trap-Jensen J. Platelet activation in mental stress. *Clin Physiol* 1993;**13**:299–307.

128 Rostrup M, Mundal HH, Kjeldsen SE, Gjesdal K, Eide I. Awareness of high blood pressure stimulates platelet release reaction. *Thromb Haemostasis* 1990;**63**:367–70.

129 Levine SP, Towell BL, Suarez AM, Knieriem LK, Harris MM, George JN. Platelet activation and secretion associated with emotional stress. *Circulation* 1985;**71**:1129–34.

130 Grignani G, Pacchiarini L, Zucchella M *et al*. Effect of mental stress on platelet function in normal subjects with coronary artery disease. *Haemostasis* 1992;**22**:138–46.

131 Wallen NH, Held C, Rehnqvist N, Njemdahl P. Effects of mental and physical stress on platelet function in patients with stable angina pectoris and healthy controls. *Eur Heart J* 1997;**18**:807–15.

132 Fortunato JS, Pinheiro MJ, Monteiro MC, Rodrigues MA, Amaral I. Acute effects of adrenaline on platelet aggregation and kinetics in vivo. *J Nucl Biol Med* 1991; **35**:105–10.

133 Markovitz JH, Matthews KA. Platelets and coronary heart disease: potential psychophysiologic mechanisms. *Psychosom Med* 1991;**53**:643–68.

134 Murata M, Matsubara Y, Kawano K *et al*. Coronary artery disease and polymorphisms in a receptor mediating shear stress-dependent platelet activation. *Circulation* 1997; **96**:3281–6.

135 Gardemann A, Humme J, Stricker J *et al*. Association of the platelet glycoprotein IIIa *PLA1/A2* gene polymorphism to coronary artery disease but not to nonfatal myocardial infarction in low risk patients. *Thromb Haemostasis* 1998;**80**:214–17.

136 Anderson JL, King GJ, Bair TL *et al*. Associations between a polymorphism in the gene encoding glycoprotein IIIa and myocardial infarction or coronary artery disease. *J Am Coll Cardiol* 1999;**33**:727–33.

137 Kastrati A, Schomig A, Seyfarth M *et al*. PIA polymorphism of platelet glycoprotein IIIa and risk of restenosis after coronary stent placement. *Circulation* 1999;**99**:1005–10.

138 Senti M, Aubo C, Bosch M *et al*. Platelet glycoprotein IIb/IIIa genetic polymorphism is associated with plasma fibrinogen levels in myocardial infarction patients. The REGICOR Investigators. *Clin Biochem* 1998;**31**:647–51.

139 Senti M, Aubo C, Bosch M. The relationship between smoking and triglyceride-rich lipoproteins is modulated by genetic variation in the glycoprotein IIIa gene. *Metabolism* 1998;**47**:1040–1.

140 Gonzalez-Conejero R, Lozano ML, Rivera J *et al*. Polymorphisms of platelet membrane glycoprotein Ib associated with arterial thrombotic disease. *Blood* 1998; **92**:2771–6.

141 Spalding A, Vaitkevicius H, Dill S, MacKenzie S, Schmaier A, Lockette W. Mechanism of epinephrine-induced platelet aggregation. *Hypertension* 1998;**31**:603–7.

142 Greenberg BD, Tolliver TJ, Huang SJ, Li Q, Bengel D, Murphy DL. Genetic variation in the serotonin transporter promoter region affects serotonin uptake in human blood platelets. *Am J Med Genet* 1999;**88**:83–97.

143 Coleman CA, Friedman AG, Burright RG. The relationship of daily stress and health-related behaviours to adolescents' cholesterol levels. *Adolescence* 1998;**33**:447–60.

144 Muldoon MF, Herbert TB, Patterson SM, Kameneva M, Raible R, Manuck SB. Effects of acute psychological stress on serum lipid levels, hemoconcentration, and blood viscosity. *Arch Intern Med* 1995;**155**:615–20.

145 Shirom A, Westman M, Shamai O, Carel RS. Effects of work overload and burnout on cholesterol and triglyceride levels: the moderating effects of emotional reactivity among male and female employees. *J Occup Health Psychol* 1997;**2**:275–88.

146 Vogele C. Serum lipid concentrations, hostility and cardiovascular reactions to mental stress. *Int J Psychophysiol* 1998;**28**:167–79.

147 Schneider RH, Nidich SI, Salerno JW *et al*. Lower lipid peroxide levels in practitioners of the Transcendental Meditation program. *Psychosom Med* 1998;**60**:38–41.

148 Sapolsky RM, Mott GE. Social subordinance in wild baboons is associated with suppressed high density lipoprotein-cholesterol concentrations: the possible role of chronic social stress. *Endocrinology* 1987;**121**:1605–10.

149 Clark VR, Moore CL, Adams JH. Cholesterol concentrations and cardiovascular reactivity to stress in African American college volunteers. *J Behav Med* 1998;**21**: 505–15.

150 Brennan FX, Cobb CL, Silbert LH, Watkins LR, Maier SF. Peripheral beta-adrenoceptors and stress-induced hypercholesterolemia in rats. *Physiol Behav* 1996;**60**:1307–10.

151 Wahrenberg H, Lonnqvist F, Hellmer J, Arner P. Importance of beta-adrenoceptor function in fat cells for lipid mobilization. *Eur J Clin Invest* 1992;**22**:412–19.

152 Reynisdottir S, Wahrenberg H, Carlstrom K, Rossner S, Arner P. Catecholamine resistance in fat cells of women with upper-body obesity due to decreased expression of beta 2-adrenoceptors. *Diabetologia* 1994;**37**:428–35.

153 Lonnqvist F, Wahrenberg H, Hellstrom L, Reynisdottir S, Arner P. Lipolytic catecholamine resistance due to decreased beta 2-adrenoceptor expression in fat cells. *J Clin Invest* 1992;**90**:2175–86.

154 Marcus C, Bolme P, Karpe B, Bronnegard M, Sellden H, Arner P. Expression of beta 1- and beta 2-receptor genes and correlation to lipolysis in human adipose tissue during childhood. *J Clin Endocrinol Metab* 1993;**76**:879–84.

155 Timmermann B, Li GH, Luft FC, Lund-Johansen P, Skrabal F, Hoehe MR. Novel DNA sequence differences in the beta2-adrenergic receptor gene promoter region. *Hum Mutat* 1998;**11**:343–4.

156 Large V, Hellstrom L, Reynisdottir S *et al.* Human beta-2 adrenoceptor gene polymorphisms are highly frequent in obesity and associate with altered adipocyte beta-2 adrenoceptor function. *J Clin Invest* 1997;**199**:3005–13.

157 McGraw DW, Forbes SL, Kramer LA, Liggett SB. Polymorphisms of the 5′ leader cistron of the human beta 2-adrenergic receptor regulate receptor expression. *J Clin Invest* 1998;**102**:1927–32.

158 Koper JW, Stolk RP, de Lange P *et al.* Lack of association between five polymorphisms in the human glucocorticoid receptor gene and glucocorticoid resistance. *Hum Genet* 1997;**99**:663–8.

159 Huizenga NA, Koper JW, DeLange P *et al.* A polymorphism in the glucocorticoid receptor gene may be associated with an increased sensitivity to glucocorticoids in vivo. *J Clin Endocrinol Metab* 1998;**83**:144–51.

160 Panarelli M, Holloway CD, Fraser R *et al.* Glucocorticoid receptor polymorphism, skin vasoconstriction, and other metabolic intermediate phenotypes in normal human subjects. *J Clin Endocrinol Metab* 1998;**83**:1846–52.

161 Lehman CD, Rodin J, McEwan B, Brinton R. Impact of environmental stress on the expression of insulin-dependent diabetes mellitus. *Behav Neurosci* 1991;**105**:241–5.

162 Zhou D, Kusnecov AW, Shurin MR, DePaoli M, Rabin BS. Exposure to physical and psychological stressors elevates plasma interleukin-6: relationship to the activation of the hypothalamic–pituitary–adrenal axis. *Endocrinology* 1993;**133**:2523–30.

163 Mastorakos G, Chrousos GP, Weber JS. Recombinant interleukin-6 activates the hypothalamo–pituitary–adrenal axis in humans. *J Clin Endocrinol Metab* 1993;**77**:1690–4.

164 Brunner EJ, Marmot MG, Nanchahal K *et al.* Social inequality in coronary risk: central obesity and the metabolic syndrome: evidence from the Whitehall II Study. *Diabetologia* 1997;**40**:1341–9.

165 Montgomery H, Clarkson P, Barnard M *et al.* Angiotensin-converting-enzyme gene insertion/deletion polymorphism and response to physical training. *Lancet* 1999;**353**:541–5.

166 Proudler AJ, Crook D, Godsland IF, Collins P, Rosano GM, Stevenson JC. Serum angiotensin-I-converting enzyme activity in women with cardiological syndrome X: relation to blood pressure and lipid and carbohydrate metabolic risk markers for coronary heart disease. *J Clin Endocrinol Metab* 1995;**80**:696–9.

167 Hennes MM, O'Shaughnessy IM, Kelly TM, LaBelle P, Egan BM, Kissebah A. Insulin-resistant lipolysis in abdominally obese hypertensive individuals. Role of the renin–angiotensin system. *Hypertension* 1996;**28**:120–6.

168 Henriksen EJ, Jacob S, Augustin HJ, Dietze GJ. Glucose transport activity in insulin-resistant rat muscle. Effects of angiotensin-converting-enzyme inhibitors and bradykinin antagonism. *Diabetes* 1996;**45**(suppl. 1):S125–8.

169 Chiu KC, McCarthy JE. The insertion allele at the angiotensin I-converting enzyme gene locus is associated with insulin resistance. *Metabolism* 1997;**46**:395–9.

170 Katsuya T, Horiuchi M, Chen YD *et al*. Relations between deletion polymorphism of the angiotensin-converting enzyme gene and insulin resistance, glucose intolerance, hyperinsulinemia, and dyslipidemia. *Arteriosclerosis Thromb Vasc Biol* 1995;**15**:779–82.

171 Panahloo A, Andres C, Mohamed-Ali V *et al*. The insertion allele of the ACE gene I/D polymorphism. A candidate gene for insulin resistance? *Circulation* 1995;**92**:3390–3.

172 Katz AM. Cardiomyopathy of overload: a major determinant of prognosis in congestive cardiac failure. *N Engl J Med* 1990;**322**:100–10.

173 Massie BM, Tubau JF, Szlachcic J, O'Kelly BF. Hypertensive heart disease: the critical role of left ventricular hypertrophy. *J Cardiovasc Pharm* 1989;**13**(suppl. 1):s18–24.

174 Vogt M, Motz WH, Schwartzkopf B, Strauer BE. Pathophysiology and clinical aspects of hypertensive hypertrophy. *Eur Heart J* 1993;**14**(suppl. D):2–7.

175 Kamarck TW, Everson SA, Kaplan GA *et al*. Exaggerated blood pressure responses during mental stress are associated with enhanced carotid atherosclerosis in middle-aged Finnish men: findings from the Kuopio Ischemic Heart Disease Study. *Circulation* 1997;**96**:3842–8.

176 Manuck SB, Adams MR, McCaffrey JM, Kaplan JR. Behaviorally elicited heart rate reactivity and atherosclerosis in ovariectomized cynomolgus monkeys (*Macaca fascicularis*). *Arteriosclerosis Thromb Vasc Biol* 1997;**17**:1774–9.

177 Carmelli D, Chesney MA, Ward MM, Rosenman RH. Twin similarity in cardiovascular stress response. *Health Psychol* 1985;**4**:413–23.

178 Friedman R, Iwai J. Genetic predisposition and stress-induced hypertension. *Science* 1976;**193**(4248):161–2.

179 Horikoshi Y, Tajima I, Igarashi H, Inui M, Kasahara K, Noguchi T. The adreno-sympathetic system, the genetic predisposition to hypertension, and stress. *Am J Med Sci* 1985;**289**:186–1.

180 Danser AH, Schalekamp MA, Bax WA *et al*. Angiotensin converting enzyme in the human heart. Effect of the deletion/insertion polymorphism. *Circulation* 1995; **92**:1387–8.

181 Dzau VJ. Multiple pathways of angiotensin production in the blood vessel wall: evidence, possibilities, and hypotheses. *J Hypertens* 1989;**7**:933–6.

182 Berge KE, Berg K. No effect of insertion/deletion polymorphism at the ACE locus on normal blood pressure level or variability. *Clin Genet* 1994;**45**:169–74.

183 Friedl W, Krempler F, Sandhofer F, Paulweber B. Insertion/deletion polymorphism in the angiotensin-converting-enyme gene and blood pressure during ergometry in normal males. *Clin Genet* 1996;**50**:541–4.

184 Jian M, Cao X, Huang J *et al*. Polymorphism of angiotensin I converting enzyme gene in the older Chinese: linked to ambulatory blood presure levels and circadian rhythm. *Int J Cardiol* 1996; **55**:33–40.

185 Chrostowska M, Narkiewicz K, Bigda J *et al*. Ambulatory systolic blood pressure is related to the deletion allele of the angiotensin I converting enzyme gene in young normotensives with parental history of hypertension. *Clin Exp Hypertens* 1998;**20**:283–94.

186 Dominiak P. Modulation of sympathetic control by ACE inhibitors. *Eur Heart J* 1993;**14**(suppl. I):169–72.

187 Beinlich CJ, White GJ, Baker KM, Morgan HE. Angiotensin II and left ventricular growth in newborn pig heart. *J Mol Cell Cardiol* 1991;**23**:1031–8.

188 Montgomery HE, Clarkson P, Dollery CM *et al*. Association of angiotensin-converting enzyme gene I/D polymorphism with change in left ventricular mass in response to physical training. *Circulation* 1997;**96**:741–7.

189 Montgomery HE. Should the contribution of *ACE* gene polymorphism to left ventricular hypertrophy be reconsidered? *Heart* 1997;**77**:502–5.

16: Psychosocial interventions in coronary heart disease

MATTHEW BURG AND LISA BERKMAN

There has been a great deal of research on the identification of social and psychological factors that predict the onset and course of cardiovascular disease. However, far fewer studies have addressed psychosocial interventions and cardiovascular disease; of these, many have reported equivocal results, provide little or no detail regarding the precise nature of the intervention (such as intervention content, training of interventionists, and treatment adherence), are directed towards all patients rather than those at risk due to some psychosocial factor, and/or rely on self help interventions.[1,2] This chapter describes several large scale interventions in more detail than is generally provided, to encourage others to replicate and build on these efforts, and discusses the issues that we believe inhibit the development of research efforts on interventions for stress in CHD.

The Recurrent Coronary Prevention Project

The goals of the Recurrent Coronary Prevention Project (RCPP) were to use group therapy to reduce type A behaviour, and to demonstrate that this approach would effectively reduce type A and cardiac endpoints (for example, reinfarction and cardiac death).[3] Participants in the RCPP were randomly assigned to either a cardiac counselling condition ($n = 270$) or a type A counselling condition ($n = 592$). Those in the cardiac counselling group received counselling aimed at increasing knowledge and adherence to the treatment regimen prescribed by their physician, including efforts to reduce lifestyle risk factors such as diet and exercise; they were invited to attend a total of 33 monthly sessions of 90 minutes duration over the course of the study. Those in the type A counselling group received cardiac counselling and also a comprehensive package designed to address and alter the specific type A behaviours in the participants' behavioural repertoire[4]; they were invited to attend a total of 62 (initially weekly, fading to monthly after 1 year) sessions over the course of the study. Mean attendance for both conditions averaged 67% of sessions.[5]

278

Study findings

At study outset, the two groups were found to be equivalent with regard to a range of medical and sociodemographic factors, while approximately 98% were found to exhibit some significant degree of type A behaviour.[6] At the end of 3 years, the cardiac counselling group evidenced a combined coronary recurrence rate of 13%, while the type A counselling group evidenced a combined coronary recurrence rate of 7.2% ($p > 0.005$), a difference primarily accounted for by non-fatal events.[5] The latter group also showed a marked reduction in type A behaviour. In addition, those who showed a reduction of type A behaviour, regardless of group assignment, evidenced one fifth of the cardiac recurrence rate of those showing no significant reduction in type A behaviour. Lastly, reductions in type A behaviour after termination of treatment were found to persist after 1 year.[7] Hence, the RCPP demonstrated the viability of treatment efforts targeting a stress related cognitive and behavioural factor associated with cardiac endpoints, and the significant impact on hard endpoints of such an intervention.

Treatment description and overview

The intention of the RCPP treatment was to:

- educate participants regarding various aspects of type A behaviour
- increase their understanding of how type A behaviour contributed to their disease
- facilitate the development of the participants' awareness of their own type A behaviour
- teach them specific strategies for physical and psychological relaxation
- help them recognise and ultimately modify underlying type A attitudes, thoughts, and beliefs
- help them develop an alternative, healthier repertoire of non-type A behaviours
- reduce their insecurities while promoting healthier means for maintaining self-esteem.

Small groups (10–12 participants) took part in sessions lasting 90 minutes to 2 hours; methods relied on didactic, cognitive behavioural, and existential humanistic orientations.[8]

A group approach was selected because it provided regular opportunities for participants to learn by listening to others, thereby reducing experienced threat to self esteem; opportunities for feedback on behaviour from several peers (rather than from one "expert"), thereby making the feedback more effective and palatable; and opportunities for social support to develop within the group, thereby enhancing esteem and connectedness. An important part was played by the group leaders; these leaders required a working knowledge of type A and a thorough appreciation of their own type A behaviour. They needed to be actively involved in the alteration of this

279

behaviour, providing them with experience and insight into the process of such change, and able to present themselves as respected and accomplished professionals. They needed to communicate in a simple, straightforward, and sincere manner, and exercise a sense of humour when discussing the material of the group session, when working with participants around the issues presented, and when describing their personal experiences with their own type A behaviour.

Therapeutic techniques

A number of novel approaches were developed for the RCPP. For example, the use of metaphor was found to be helpful. One particularly powerful metaphor was that of a "bomb and fuse".[9] The "bomb" was the patient's acute coronary event or the progressive development of coronary disease. The "fuse" to this bomb was represented by such things as type A behaviour (particularly anger or impatience), or becoming emotionally or mentally aroused. The acronym AIAI—anger, irritation, aggravation, impatience—was also used to facilitate this process. Group members were encouraged to describe the potential fuse situations that preceded their coronary event, and to identify and describe the various fuse situations that they experienced between group sessions. These descriptions were then used to prompt discussions of ways in which such fuses could be avoided in future.

A second useful metaphor was that of the "self monitor". This assisted the patient in detaching from the distress that accompanied fuse situations and in focusing instead on the occurrence of distress itself. The patient thereby adopted a metacognitive perspective: a "third party" awareness and appreciation of the emotions, rationalisations, and behaviours that contribute to the fuse situation.[8] Videotapes and audiotapes of AIAI events proved useful in helping patients develop an awareness of fuse situations and responses, thereby improving their self monitoring skills. Group discussion and feedback in a trusting, accepting atmosphere was essential for patients to first accept their reactions to the fuse and then develop a stance for the self monitor that is respectful, curious, and interested in understanding.[10] The development and use of a self monitor was a critical component for reducing the anger and hostility components of type A behaviour in particular.

A third metaphor that also proved valuable for the reduction of anger and hostility was that of "bait" and "hooks".[11] Within this metaphor, the individual is viewed as a fish, swimming through the unpredictable waters of daily life. Provocative situations were then viewed as the "bait" encountered in daily living. The critical part of this metaphor set was the "hook"—the patient's own perception and interpretation of "bait" situations. For example, the "bait" of a coworker's careless mistake becomes a "hook" only when the type A attitude regarding the incompetence of others and the consequence of being slowed by others' errors comes into play. The ability to avoid such "hooks" by first slowing down and noticing one's emotional reactions (for example, through the work of the self monitor) and then developing an alternative point of view regarding the "bait", helped patients either avoid "hooks" or employ healthier responses to them.

In addition to examining and modifying underlying type A beliefs, patients were taught how to respond to "bait" and similar situations with assertiveness rather than aggressiveness. This required a guided examination of the consequences of aggressive responses, which illuminated not only the short-term compliance of others, but also the longer term maintenance of a hostile atmosphere, rejection from others, and feelings of guilt. Patients worked to reduce the intensity of the emotional experiences that gave rise to aggressive responses, while learning to consider the various aspects of the provocative situation and to take on the perspective of the other people with whom they were engaged in that situation. This was further used as a means to develop both respect for self and for others.

Relaxation training was used to reduce the excessive physiological and emotional arousal that was a regular part of the type A experience. Relaxation exercises were typically used at the start of the group sessions. The immediate positive consequences of this practice were then examined, focusing on the impact it had in modulating emotion and thoughtfulness. In this way, the use of relaxation in daily life (many techniques were taught) was gradually modelled, prompted, and shaped.

A final component of the RCPP intervention was the daily behavioural practice. A "drill book" helped to guide patients in the institution of new behavioural practices (for example, not wearing a watch, walking more slowly, verbalising affection to a family member, practising smiling while remembering three happy events of the past), with an entry for each day of the week listing the behaviour to practise. The group leader provided the rationale, modelling, and encouragement for patients to use the "drill book", while group discussion about the obstacles and resistances to practice of daily drills served to illuminate underlying type A attitudes. Over time, patients were encouraged to institute their own more personally relevant set of daily drills.

The ENRICHD study

The Enhancing Recovery in Coronary Heart Disease (ENRICHD) study is a multicenter, randomised, controlled clinical trial funded by the National Heart, Lung and Blood Institute, designed to determine the impact on subsequent morbidity and mortality in patients with acute myocardial infarction (MI) of treating depression and low perceived social support (LPSS). A total of 2481 patients were recruited for this trial, with near equal representation of women and men, and of whites and other races (minority groups). Primary endpoints were cardiovascular mortality and recurrent non-fatal MI; secondary endpoints included all cause mortality, incidence of revascularisation procedures, cardiovascular hospitalisations, and change in risk factor profile. Secondary psychosocial endpoints included severity of depression, degree of social support, and health related quality of life. Patients were eligible for randomisation to a usual care or intervention arm within 28 days of their index cardiac event if they met DSM–IV criteria for major depression, minor depression with a history of major depression, or dysthymia, or if they achieved a criterion score on the ENRICHD Social Support Instrument, a six-item, Likert scored scale composed of items found in other studies to be predictive of morbidity and mortality following MI.[12–15] A more comprehensive report of the eligibility and recruitment aspects of ENRICHD is provided elsewhere.[16]

Treatment description

A rapid and aggressive treatment approach (designed to have an immediate impact on behavioural targets) was necessitated for ENRICHD because the greatest risk for poor outcome is found in the months immediately after the index event.[17] In addition, with its focus on cardiac endpoints rather than treatment efficacy, the intervention needed to rely upon the most effective treatment approach described in the literature.[18] It also needed to be cost effective, while ensuring rapid intervention and accommodating the needs of patients with severe depression. Lastly, the intervention had to be standardised and uniformly administered across eight clinical centres, while also needing to be flexible enough to allow counsellors to address realistic situations and the regional, cultural, and ethnic diversity of the ENRICHD clinical sites, which ranged from large, densely populated inner city settings, to small, thinly populated rural settings. Hence, cognitive behaviour therapy (CBT)[19,20] and social learning approaches[20,21] were used. In addition, a combination of individual and group treatment was selected, while adjunctive pharmacotherapy was included for participants with more severe or unresponsive depression.

Clinical trials typically recruit patients by placing advertisements for free treatment of the conditions of interest to both the study and the patient. The ENRICHD participants, however, were often sanguine about their feelings of depression or LPSS and were mostly unaware of the risk this status incurred; they were therefore correspondingly reluctant to engage in therapy. Overcoming barriers to participation in treatment was therefore an important task during the recruitment and treatment process.

Structure

Treatment started with a reliance on individual therapy. This allowed treatment to begin immediately after randomisation and very soon after the index myocardial event. Shorter and/or more frequent sessions were used first when patients were easily fatigued or overwhelmed, thereby reducing the burden of participation for the recently discharged or slowly recuperating patient. Sessions longer than an hour were also used, especially for participants with both depression and LPSS. Treatment duration ranged from six sessions to a maximum of 6 months, depending on treatment progress. Success in treatment was criterion based, and largely determined by both a sufficient reduction in symptoms and a demonstrated capacity for self therapy.

A patient's course of treatment was completed, where possible, by open membership group therapy. While individual treatment was rapid and aggressive, the group component provided a cost effective way to reinforce and extend early progress. A participant could join a group at any point in a 12 session continuum, after completing three individual sessions, but no later than 6 months after enrolling in the trial; patients could attend both individual and group therapy concurrently. For some of the ENRICHD sites there were often too few patients to form a therapy group at any one time, but the curricular nature of the intervention allowed the group material to be presented within the context of individual therapy sessions.

Therapeutic techniques

A typical ENRICHD treatment session would begin with the setting of an agenda. Common points for discussion included the participant's reaction to the previous session, homework from the previous session, and problems and accomplishments since that session. The therapist used the participant's experiences to reinforce previously learnt concepts and introduce new ones. The session ended with an assignment of homework and feedback from the participant regarding the session.

The development of a supportive collaboration was essential. Counsellors presented themselves as a potentially useful resource for the patient undergoing postinfarction adjustment. The counsellor described how the ENRICHD programme could be useful in the patient's particular circumstances. Participants were encouraged to "tell their story", describing the circumstances that led up to their infarction, and the circumstances they currently face in their lives, leaving the participants with a sense of being understood and cared about.

Behavioural activation, a second feature of this approach, was targeted toward increasing pleasurable and socially supportive activities, and was associated with an increase in a sense of satisfaction, accomplishment, and support. Active problem solving was applied to the circumstances that were believed to contribute to depression or LPSS, while a focus on dysfunctional automatic thoughts that contributed to problematic affect and behaviour allowed a guided exploration of more accurate or flexible points of view. Stress reduction techniques (such as relaxation training), and behavioural skills training (such as communication and assertiveness skills) were also used.

The ENRICHD patients had many anxieties related to health (for example, overcoming unwarranted fears about, and avoidance of, returning to work, leisure activities, and sexual intercourse), and were prone to "catastrophising" in response to mild exertional fatigue, "fortune telling" in response to fears of abandonment, and "black and white thinking" in response to shifting from medically risky leisure activities to safer alternatives. Patients were taught to identify these negative or dysfunctional automatic thoughts, using such techniques as induced fantasy or role playing. They were then taught to see the relationship between these automatic thoughts and the emotions they subsequently experienced. Through guided discovery they came to see how these automatic thoughts represent distortions of reality and trigger symptoms of depression, or actions that are socially isolating. They also came to understand the underlying assumptions, beliefs, and attitudes that gave rise to automatic thoughts. Toward the end of treatment, participants were expected to be able to apply the skills learned in treatment to their life situations and daily events as needed.

In adapting conventional material to this patient population, it was important to recognise that, while MI could serve as the precipitant of depression and LPSS, many patients with MI have a premorbid history of these problems. Further, this premorbid history had in many cases left the ENRICHD patient particularly susceptible to a recurrent problem in the face of their newly or further compromised medical condition. Hence, the intervention provided for a focus on general life issues as well as more medically relevant issues. Nevertheless, the key features of cognitive behaviour therapy, and the relatively brief, goal oriented, collaborative and emotionally supportive features of this treatment were particularly relevant to the patients enrolled in the trial. Through the use of these processes and techniques, counsellors and (where relevant) other group members help patients develop an ability to identify the problem situations and associated cognitions that promote problematic feelings, apply the cognitive and behavioural skills learned during treatment as needed in their daily life, appraise their thoughts and beliefs about current problematic situations or issues, and apply skills learned during treatment to problematic situations in the future.

Special features

Adjunctive pharmacotherapy, managed by study psychiatrists, was also used for patients with severe depression and for those whose response to treatment was slow. Sertraline, a selective serotonin reuptake inhibitor (SSRI), was used as the initial agent (unless contraindicated), based on its efficacy and safety in patients with cardiovascular disease. Patients unable to tolerate sertraline, or judged to have an inadequate response to treatment after 4 weeks, were considered for alternative treatment with another SSRI or with nortriptyline. The therapeutic agent was given for 12 months; if treatment beyond 12 months was needed, the patient was referred to community resources.

The problem of low perceived social support provided a unique opportunity for ENRICHD. Although LPSS is a risk factor for poor medical outcome after acute MI, it is not psychopathological, and there are no standard treatments with tested efficacy. Cognitive behaviour therapy and social learning approaches provided a framework for the treatment of LPSS, however. Special features of treatment included an ongoing multimodal assessment that identified the patient's instrumental and emotional needs, and revealed the cognitions, attitudes, and beliefs that related to the patient's social ties and network. It also identified the degree of social integration, current satisfaction with specific sources of support, and the importance to the patient of—and preference for—specific types of support. It determined the sophistication of the patient's social planning, communication, and problem solving skills, and whether social anxiety or phobia was contributing to LPSS. Modular treatment components were developed to dovetail with this assessment. These addressed remediation of behavioural and social skill deficits, modification of cognitive factors contributing to a perception or maintenance of unsatisfying levels of social support, and social outreach and network development efforts.

Treatment progress

To monitor progress in treatment for depression, the Beck Depression Inventory was administered at every session. Individual treatment continued until the patient completed at least six sessions, was in at least partial remission, had developed self therapy skills, and scored below 7 on the inventory for two consecutive assessments. For patients who met these criteria but who relapsed within 6 months of enrolment, individual therapy was resumed.

To monitor progress in treatment for LPSS, a modified version of the Perceived Social Support Scale (PSSS) was administered at every session.[22] Individual treatment continued until the participant was engaged in at least one satisfying and supportive social relationship (other than with the counsellor), was capable of self therapy, and had achieved a criterion score on the modified PSSS for at least two consecutive sessions. As with the treatment for depression, participants who achieved success but relapsed within 6 months of randomisation resumed individual therapy.

In summary, ENRICHD provides an important opportunity to examine the impact of a psychosocial intervention on hard medical endpoints in a population with identified disease and risk. In addition, it offers an important model for the provision of such treatment within the context of the difficult conditions associated with modern medical care.

Other approaches

The Ischemic Heart Disease Life Stress Monitoring Program and the Montreal Heart Attack Readjustment Trial

Interventions to relieve distress associated with disease and its treatment offer an additional promising avenue for stress reduction in the cardiac population. These approaches typically rely upon a wide range of techniques, ranging from relaxation training and group psychoeducation, to more individually tailored approaches. One of the most important distress mitigation approaches demonstrated with cardiac patients has been the

Ischemic Heart Disease Life Stress Monitoring Program.[23–25] In this study, 461 male patients recovering from MI were randomised to a stress monitoring intervention or usual care. The hypothesis of this investigation was that targeting life stress through a coordinated programme of screening and multimodal intervention would reduce the risk of cardiac recurrence and death. Patients were contacted by telephone on a regular basis and screened for symptoms of stress and distress. Those in the intervention group who showed an increasing trend in symptoms of stress received home nursing interventions consisting of individually tailored combinations of education, support, collaborative problem solving, and referral. Nursing visits were continued until there was a significant reduction in symptoms of stress. After 1 year, follow up revealed that the programme had a significant impact on stress symptoms, and that control patients had twice the risk of death due to cardiac causes as their intervention counterparts.[23] After 7 years, the mortality differences between the two groups were found to persist, with the greatest impact being on sudden cardiac death.[24] The success of this trial led to the subsequent Montreal Heart Attack Readjustment Trial, designed to treat life stress in a larger cohort of 1376 men and women who had survived MI; this trial unfortunately showed no benefit for the intervention group. Indeed, a significant increase in cardiac and all cause mortality was observed among women in the intervention group.[25] Further analyses of the data, however, revealed that patients who responded to the support intervention within two home visits showed improved medical outcomes, while those who continued to display high levels of distress worsened.[18] This indicates the importance of interventions that have a significant effect on the presenting psychosocial problem, and of using staff who have the background and experience needed to address the complex stress related problems of patients with coronary heart disease. Indeed, interventions with equivocal results may share this problem of failing to intervene sufficiently on the target problem and of not using appropriately trained personnel.[1]

The Lifestyle Heart Trial

Stress reduction for cardiac patients has also been explored in the context of a comprehensive programme of risk factor reduction for patients with ischaemic heart disease. The Lifestyle Heart Trial was a randomised, controlled trial in which 28 men participated in a short-term, comprehensive lifestyle intervention.[26–28] The intervention consisted of a low fat vegetarian diet, smoking cessation (where appropriate), moderate exercise, stress management, and a support discussion group led by a psychologist; 20 other participants received standard cardiologic care. The effect of this intervention on progression of coronary lesions was compared for the two groups. After 1 year, coronary lesions were found to have significantly regressed in 82% of the experimental group. A further study has shown that the benefits of this intervention are detectable after 5 years.[29]

The daily stress reduction component of the intervention consisted of 20 minutes of stretching, 15 minutes of progressive relaxation, 5 minutes of diaphragmatic breathing, 15 minutes of meditation, and 5 minutes of directed imagery. In addition, the programme included communication skills training and other techniques for increasing intimacy with family, friends, and the other participants in the trial. Participants met twice weekly with the study psychologist to discuss the progress they were making with the programme, and any problems they had encountered that they wanted to raise with the other members of the group.

Ornish describes how group support meetings became a powerful avenue for the achievement of intimacy among participants, enabling group members to let down their guards and express their feelings.[30] This had a profound effect in reinforcing the efforts of participants to make necessary lifestyle changes. More importantly as regards the focus of this chapter, this aspect of the programme led Ornish to realise the essential connection between stress, support, and intimacy, and their combined role in heart disease. As he points out, intimacy is associated with safety—the safety necessary to show one's self as one really is, "warts and all". If people do not have a place where they feel safe enough to show how they really are, or anyone with whom they can really be themselves, the result is essential isolation and chronic stress. The ability to be oneself leads to self acceptance, which allows one to be at peace with one's failures and shortcomings. This state has a profound impact on what may be described as the essential underpinnings of the occurrence and experience of stress.[30] Hence, while the Lifestyle Heart Trial has been described as focusing on comprehensive lifestyle change, Ornish places the stress reduction component in a larger context: the opening of the heart to feelings, to inner peace, and most importantly, to others, through altruism, compassion, and forgiveness, thereby providing a way to "heal the isolation that leads to stress, suffering, and illness" (p. 215).[30]

Transient ischaemia in CAD

Transient myocardial ischaemia is common in patients with coronary artery disease (CAD). Up to 75% of occurrences are without symptom, and most often in the absence of physical exertion. The presence of this phenomenon may be a significant predictor of both fatal and non-fatal cardiac events.[31-36] Studies have shown that mental stress can trigger ischaemic episodes in susceptible individuals,[37-42] and that ischaemia induced by mental stress under controlled conditions in the laboratory is associated with an increased likelihood of ischaemia in naturalistic settings, during routine daily experience.[41-44]

Blumenthal et al. evaluated the impact of a stress management intervention (v exercise training and usual care) on clinical outcomes and myocardial ischaemia in 136 men and women with CAD.[45] Patients underwent baseline and follow up evaluations at the conclusion of a 4 month intervention, including an assessment of changes in myocardial

287

ischaemia during exercise and mental stress testing, and during ambulatory electrocardiographic monitoring. Follow up of adverse events, including non-fatal MI, death, and revascularisation secondary to progressive angina, was conducted yearly. Compared with the control group, the stress management group had a lower relative risk of an event (0.26; 95% confidence interval 0.07–0.93, $p = 0.04$), even after adjusting for baseline ejection fraction, history of MI, and age. Patients in the stress management group showed a reduction in wall motion abnormalities during post-treatment mental stress testing ($p < 0.004$), and significantly fewer ischaemic episodes ($p = 0.05$) and angina than those in usual care. In addition, those receiving stress management who had more severe pretreatment wall motion abnormalities during mental and exercise testing showed the greatest improvement ($p < 0.001$). Patients in the stress management condition also showed the greatest effect for measures of distress ($p < 0.001$).

Stress management

For this study, the stress management programme was based on a cognitive–social learning model of behaviour. Within this model, stress is seen as a function of an interaction between the social environment and aspects of an individual's personality traits that predispose to responding to situations in potentially cardiotoxic ways. This approach further assumes that emotion and behaviour are largely determined by an individual's perceptions of—and automatic thoughts about—routine events experienced throughout the day. The programme consisted of 16 sessions of 90 minutes each, conducted in a group of eight patients. Elements from the Recurrent Coronary Prevention Project and the Ischemic Heart Disease Life Stress Monitoring Program described above were incorporated, as well as cognitive behavioural therapy.[19–21] The initial sessions were largely psychoeducational and provided information about coronary disease, the structure and function of the heart, risk factors, and stress. Subsequent sessions involved instruction in specific skills to reduce the affective, behavioural, cognitive, and physiologic components of stress. Participants performed graded task assignments; monitored stress levels during routine daily events; concurrently monitored the irrational and stress provoking automatic thoughts that occurred in response to these routine daily events; and received instruction and practice in the generation of alternative interpretations of these events or stress provoking thought patterns. Patients were additionally taught progressive muscle relaxation techniques and the incorporation of progressive muscle relaxation into their daily routine. Each patient also received at least two individual sessions of electromyographic biofeedback training in addition to the 16 group sessions.

While a number of similarities exist between this work and that of the RCPP and the Montreal experience, the work of Blumenthal also highlights a number of important aspects of the treatment of stress in cardiac populations. This study demonstrates the potential importance of such an approach on intermediate endpoints such as transient ischaemic events and wall motion abnormalities, in addition to mortality based endpoints. Of perhaps greatest interest was the finding of a positive impact during mental stress testing. In this condition, patients are exposed to provocative and demanding laboratory tasks (for example, time pressured mental arithmetic, or recall of an anger provoking incident). The positive findings related to the stress management intervention hint at a chronic and generalised effect. The implications are not just that the patient learns ways to reduce stress when it is occurring, but rather that the patient learns to approach life circumstances in new ways so that previously provocative (routine daily) events are no longer so. The ability to achieve this with a relatively quick and inexpensive intervention further highlights the importance of such an approach, and the potential role that stress reduction and management interventions can play in the treatment of coronary heart disease.

The future

As we reflected upon what might account for the dearth of interventions or randomised clinical trials in this area, we identified three issues that might inhibit the development of interventions.

- Investigators who are responsible for developing interventions do not believe the observational evidence. They view it as inconsistent, poorly specified, or not causally linked to CHD.
- Investigators believe the evidence, but do not know how to change the psychosocial conditions, or they believe it is too difficult to change these conditions in an efficacious way.
- Investigators believe the evidence, know how to change the conditions, but believe it is not within their purview to do so, owing to professional, political, ethical, or legal obligations.

We suspect that the primary reasons behind the reluctance to launch major interventions are related more to issues of implementation than to strength of evidence. In the USA, National Institutes of Health recommendations and commentaries have made the case that behavioural and social scientists, for a number of reasons, rarely make use of all phases of clinical trial research in the development of interventions. As a result of funding incentives, investigators often jump to the final phases of clinical trial research (such as testing effectiveness) before developing interventions they know will alter risk; this is akin to testing whether a putative cholesterol lowering drug decreases the risk of MI before knowing whether it effectively lowers cholesterol level. We also suspect that intervention research has not blossomed in the area of psychosocial conditions because of the discomfort that medically trained clinicians experience in integrating psychological and social interventions with medical practice. A similar issue is the reluctance of social scientists concerned with the social environment to integrate their work with medicine and public health. Lastly, we have been surprised by the lack of transparency of many psychosocial interventions. Such transparency would make these interventions more readily reproducible.

In an effort to stimulate intervention work across a number of levels (structural, community, and individual) as well as across phases of work, we present a taxonomy of intervention approaches that we hope will promote more novel interventions to improve cardiovascular health by improving social and psychological conditions. Our proposed taxonomy cuts across four dimensions and is illustrated in Figure 16.1.

In this taxonomy, the first axis is related to the definition of the psychosocial risk under investigation. We might think of such conditions along a continuum from clearly psychological (such as depression, hostility, or vital exhaustion) through those that are psychosocial (such as social support or work strain) to those that are more purely structural (such as socioeconomic position, structure of network ties, and social capital). The second axis is related to the level at which we intervene. Again, this ranges from interventions aimed at the individual, to those aimed at some collective or system (such as small groups, family, or worksite), to larger ones aimed at community and societal levels. The third axis relates to the point along the spectrum of disease at which we intervene: we might, for instance, intervene at the level of secondary prevention, at the subclinical level of disease development, or at the level of primary prevention, before any evidence of

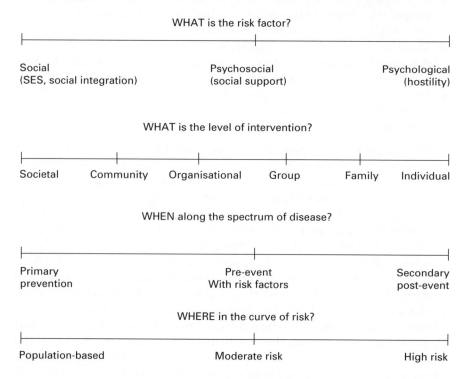

Figure 16.1   Taxonomy of psychosocial interventions.

disease is present. Finally, we come to the question posed by Rose, of whether we should pursue a high risk strategy, intervening in cases at highest psychosocial risk, or whether we should pursue a population based strategy.[46]

Perhaps what is so remarkable about our review of interventions is that these interventions "line up" along the left side of each of these domains. Thus, even when investigators have chosen to intervene on a risk factor that is social in nature, they have chosen an individually oriented intervention approach or a high risk intervention strategy. We therefore believe that research on interventions to reduce risk for coronary heart disease associated generically with "stress" would benefit substantially from greater innovation. Such innovation could apply the taxonomy provided as a structure to rethink the nature of the standard approach, and thereby expand the potential for risk reduction.

References

1 Jones DA, West RR. Psychological rehabilitation after myocardial infarction: multicentre randomized controlled trial. *BMJ* 1996;**313**:1517–21.

2 Lewin B, Robertson IH, Cay EL, Irving JB, Campbell M. Effects of self-help post-myocardial infarction rehabilitation on psychological adjustment and use of health services. *Lancet* 1992;**339**(8800):1036–40.

3 Friedman M, Thoresen CE, Gill JJ *et al.* Feasibility of altering Type A behavior pattern after myocardial infarction. Recurrent coronary prevention project study: Methods, baseline results and preliminary findings. *Circulation* 1982;**66**:83–92.

4 Friedman M, Rosenman RH. *Type A behavior and your heart.* New York: Knopf, 1974.

5 Friedman M, Thoresen CE, Gill J *et al.* Alteration of Type A behavior and its effects on cardiac recurrences in post-myocardial infarction patients: Summary results of the Recurrent Coronary Prevention Project. *Am Heart J* 1986;**112**:653–65.

6 Friedman M, Thoresen CE, Gill J *et al.* Alteration of Type A behavior and reduction in cardiac recurrences in postmyocardial infarction patients. *Am Heart J* 1984;**108**:237–48.

7 Friedman M, Powell LH, Thoresen CE *et al.* Effect of discontinuance of type A behavioral counseling on type A behavior and cardiac recurrence rate in post myocardial infarction patients. *Am Heart J* 1987;**114**:483–90.

8 Powell LH, Thoresen CE. Small group treatment of Type A behavior. In Blumenthal JA, McKee DC, eds. *Applications in behavioral medicine and health psychology: A clinician's sourcebook.* Sarasota: Professional Resource Exchange, 1987.

9 Friedman M, Ulmer DK. *Treating type A behavior and your heart.* New York: Knopf, 1984.

10 Thoresen CE, Bracke P. Reducing coronary recurrences and coronary-prone behavior: A structured group treatment approach. In Spira JL, ed. *Group therapy for medically ill patients.* New York: Guilford, 1997.

11 Powell LH. The hook: A metaphor for gaining control of emotional reactivity. In Allen R, Scheidt S, eds. *Heart and mind: The practice of cardiac psychology.* Washington, DC: American Psychological Association, 1996.

12 Berkman LF, Leo-Summer L, Horwitz RI. Emotional support and survival after myocardial infarction. *Ann Intern Med* 1992;**117**:1003–9.

13 Williams RB, Barefoot JC, Califf RM *et al.* Prognostic importance of social and economic resources among medically treated patients with angiographically documented coronary artery disease. *JAMA* 1992;**267**:520–4.

14 Ruberman W, Weinblatt E, Goldberg JD, Chaudhary BS. Psychosocial influences on mortality after myocardial infarction. *N Engl J Med* 1984;**311**:552–9.

15 Gorkin L, Schron EB, Brooks MM *et al.* for the CAST Investigators. Psychosocial predictors of mortality in the Cardiac Arrhythmia Suppression Trial-1 (CAST-1). *Am J Cardiol* 1993;**71**:263–7.

16 The ENRICHD Investigators. Enhancing recovery in coronary heart disease patients (ENRICHD): Study design and methods. *Am Heart J* 2000;**139**:1–9.

17 Carney RM, Rich MW, Freedland KE. Psychiatric depression, anxiety, and coronary heart disease: Implications for treatment. *Compr Ther* 1989;**15**:8–13.

291

18 Cossette S, Fraser-Smith N, Lesperance F. Impact of improving psychological distress in post-MI patients. *Psychosom Med* 1999;**61**:93[abstr.].

19 Beck JS. *Cognitive Therapy: Basics and Beyond*. New York: Guilford, 1995.

20 Bandura A. *Social foundations of thought and action: A social cognitive theory*. Englewood Cliffs: Prentice-Hall, 1986.

21 Tobin DL, Reynolds RVC, Holroyd KA, Creer TL. Self-management and Social Learning Theory. In Holroyd KA, Creer TL, eds. *Self-management of chronic disease: Handbook of clinical interventions and research*. Orlando: Academic, 1986.

22 Blumenthal JA, Burg MM, Barefoot J, Williams RB, Haney T, Zimet G. Social support, type A behavior, and coronary artery disease. *Psychosom Med* 1987;**44**:331–40.

23 Fraser-Smith N, Prince R. The Ischemic Heart Disease Life Stress Monitoring Program: Impact on mortality. *Psychosom Med* 1985;**47**:431–45.

24 Fraser-Smith N, Prince R. Long-term follow-up of the Ischemic Heart Disease Stress Monitoring Program. *Psychosom Med* 1989;**51**:485–513.

25 Fraser-Smith N, Lesperance F, Prince R *et al*. Randomized trial of home based psychosocial nursing intervention for patients recovering from myocardial infarction. *Lancet* 1997;**350**:473–9.

26 Ornish D, Scherwitz LW, Billings JH *et al*. Intensive lifestyle changes for reversal of coronary heart disease. *JAMA* 1998;**280**:2001–7.

27 Ornish D, Scherwitz LW, Doody RS *et al*. Effects of stress management training and dietary changes in treating ischemic heart disease. *JAMA* 1983;**249**:54–9.

28 Ornish D, Brown SB, Scherwitz LW *et al*. Can lifestyle change reverse coronary heart disease? *Lancet* 1990;**336**:129–33.

29 Gould KL, Ornish D, Scherwitz L *et al*. Changes in myocardial perfusion abnormalities by positron emission tomography after long-term, intense risk factor modification. *JAMA* 1995;**274**:894–901.

30 Ornish DM. *Dr. Dean Ornish's program for reversing heart disease*. New York: Random House, 1990.

31 Rocco MB, Nabel EG, Campbell S *et al*. Prognostic importance of myocardial ischemia detected by ambulatory monitoring in patients with stable coronary artery disease. *Circulation* 1988;**78**:877–84.

32 Yeung AC, Barry J, Orav J *et al*. Effects of asymptomatic ischemia on long-term prognosis in chronic stable coronary disease. *Circulation* 1991;**83**:1598–604.

33 Deedwania PC, Carbajal EV. Silent ischemia during daily life is an independent predictor of mortality in stable angina. *Circulation* 1990;**81**:748–56.

34 Gottlieb SO, Weisfeldt ML, Ouyang P *et al*. Silent ischemia as a marker for early unfavorable outcomes in patients with unstable angina. *N Engl J Med* 1986;**314**:1214–19.

35 Gill JB, Cairns JA, Roberts RS *et al*. Prognostic importance of myocardial ischemia detected by ambulatory monitoring early after acute myocardial infarction. *N Engl J Med* 1996;**334**:65–70.

36 Trauner MA, Jiang W, Blumenthal JA. Prognostic significance of silent myocardial ischemia. *Ann Behav Med* 1994;**16**:24–34.

37 Gullette ECD, Blumenthal JA, Babyak M *et al*. Mental stress triggers myocardial ischemia during daily life. *JAMA* 1997;**277**:1521–6.

38 Rozanski A, Bairey CN, Krantz DS *et al*. Mental stress and the induction of myocardial ischemia in patients with coronary artery disease. *N Engl J Med* 1988;**318**:1005–11.

39 Deanfield JE, Shea M, Kensett M. Silent ischemia due to mental stress. *Lancet* 1984;**ii**:1001–5.

40 Krantz DS, Helmers KF, Bairey CN, Nebel LE, Hedges SM, Rozanski A. Cardiovascular reactivity and mental stress-induced myocardial ischemia in patients with coronary artery disease. *Psychosom Med* 1991;**53**:1–12.

41 Blumenthal JA, Jiang W, Waugh RA *et al*. Mental stress-induced ischemia in the laboratory and ambulatory ischemia during daily life: association and hemodynamic features. *Circulation* 1995;**92**:2102–8.

42 Gabbay FH, Krantz DS, Kop WJ *et al*. Triggers of myocardial ischemia during daily life in patients with coronary artery disease: physical and mental activities, anger, and smoking. *J Am Coll Cardiol* 1996;**27**:585–92.

43 Gottdiener JS, Krantz DS, Howell RH *et al*. Induction of silent myocardial ischemia with mental stress testing: relation to the triggers of ischemia during daily life activities and to ischemic functional severity. *J Am Coll Cardiol* 1994;**24**:1645–51.

44 Legault SE, Langer A, Armstrong PW, Freeman MR. Usefulness of ischemic response to mental stress in predicting silent myocardial ischemia during ambulatory monitoring. *Am J Cardiol* 1995;**75**:1007–11.

45 Blumenthal JA, Jiang W, Babyak M *et al.* Stress management and exercise training in cardiac patients with myocardial ischemia: Effects on prognosis and evaluation of mechanisms. *Arch Intern Med* 1997;**157**:2213–23.

46 Rose G. *The strategy of preventive medicine.* Oxford: Oxford University Press, 1992.

Index

Page numbers in **bold** type refer to figures; those in *italics* refer to tables or boxed material.